UCLA Symposia on Molecular and Cellular Biology, New Series

Series Editor, C. Fred Fox

Please contact the publisher for information about previous titles in this series.

Cellular and Molecular Biology of Tumors and Potential Clinical Applications

Cellular and Molecular Biology of Tumors and Potential Clinical Applications

Proceedings of an Abbott-UCLA Symposium
Held in Steamboat Springs, Colorado, January 20–25, 1986

Editors

John Minna
W. Michael Kuehl
NCI-Navy Medical Oncology
National Navy Hospital
Bethesda, Maryland

Alan R. Liss, Inc. • New York

Library of Congress Cataloging-in-Publication Data

Abbott-UCLA Symposium (1986 : Steamboat Springs, Colo.)
   Cellular and molecular biology of tumors and potential
clinical applications.

   (UCLA symposia on molecular and cellular biology ;
new ser., v. 56)
   Includes bibliographies and index.
   1. Carcinogenesis—Congresses. 2. Cancer cells—
Congresses. 3. Oncogenes—Congresses. 4. Pathology,
Molecular—Congresses. I. Minna, John D., 1905–
II. Kuehl, W. Michael. III. Abbott Laboratories.
IV. University of California, Los Angeles. V. Title.
VI. Series. [DNLM: 1. Cell Transformation, Nepolastic—
congresses. 2. Growth Substances—physiology—
congresses. 3. Neoplasms—physiopathology—congresses.
4. Oncogenes—congresses. W3 U17N new ser. v.56   /
QZ   202   A1325c   1986]
   RC268.5.A23   1986   616.99'2071   87-17061
   ISBN 0-8451-2655-5

Pages 1–158 of this volume are reprinted from the Journal of Cellular Biochemistry, Volumes 31, 32, 33, and 34. The Journal is the only appropriate literature citation for the articles printed on these pages. The page numbers in the table of contents, contributors list, and index of this volume correspond to the page numbers at the foot of these pages.

The table of contents does not necessarily follow the pattern of the plenary sessions. Instead, it reflects the thrust of the meeting as it evolved from the combination of plenary sessions, poster sessions, and workshops, culminating in the final collection of invited papers, submitted papers, and workshop summaries. The order in which articles appear in this volume does not follow the order of citation in the table of contents. Many of the articles in this volume were published in the Journal of Cellular Biochemistry, and they are reprinted here. These articles appear in the order in which they were accepted for publication and then published in the Journal. They are followed by papers which were submitted solely for publication in the proceedings.

Contents

I. ONCOGENE ACTIVATION AND AMPLIFICATION

Contributors

Frederick Alt, Department of Biochemistry and Biophysics, Columbia Presbyterian Medical Center, Columbia University, New York, NY 10032 **[97]**

Steven Anderson, Merck Sharp and Dohme Research Laboratories, West Point, PA 19486 **[269]**

Ralph B. Arlinghaus, Johnson and Johnson Biotechnology Center, La Jolla, CA 92037 **[25]**

Robert C. Ash, Medical College of Wisconsin, Milwaukee, WI 53226 **[47]**

Herman Autrup, Laboratory of Environmental Carcinogenesis, The Fibiger Institute, DK-2100 Copenhagen Ø, Denmark **[137]**

Rebecca S. Bahn, Mayo Clinic and Foundation, Rochester, MN 55905 **[47]**

Timothy P. Bender, National Cancer Institute, NCI-Navy Medical Oncology Branch, Naval Hospital, Bethesda, MD 20814-2015 **[239]**

Avri Ben-Zeev, Department of Genetics, The Weizmann Institute of Science, Rehovot 76100, Israel **[247]**

Jonas Bergh, Departments of Pathology and Oncology, University of Uppsala, University Hospital, S-751 85 Uppsala, Sweden **[9]**

Virginia Bertness, NCI-Navy Medical Oncology Branch, National Cancer Institute, National Institutes of Health, National Naval Medical Center, Bethesda, MD 20814 **[35]**

N.M. Bleehen, MRC Clinical Oncology and Radiotherapeutics Unit, MRC Center, Cambridge, CB2 2QH England **[107]**

Mark Blick, Department of Clinical Immunology and Biological Therapy, The University of Texas, M.D. Anderson Hospital and Tumor Institute, Houston, TX 77030 **[17]**

P. Borst, Division of Molecular Biology, The Netherlands Cancer Institute, 1066 CX Amsterdam, The Netherlands **[147]**

Karim Braham, Groupe d'Immunobiologie des Tumeurs, CNRS UA 1156, Institute Gustave Roussy, 94805 Villejuif Cedex, France **[1]**

Garrett Brodeur, Washington University School of Medicine, St. Louis, MO 63110 **[167]**

Gail Bruns, Department of Pediatrics, Harvard Medical School, Boston, MA 02114 **[167]**

W.P. Carney, Biomedical Products Department, E.I. du Pont de Nemours and Company, Inc., North Billerica, MA 01862 **[59]**

J.E. Chin, Center for Genetics, University of Illinois College of Medicine at Chicago, Chicago, IL 60612 **[287]**

K. Choi, Center for Genetics, University of Illinois College of Medicine at Chicago, Chicago, IL 60612 **[287]**

Britta Christensen, Laboratory of Environmental Carcinogenesis, The Fibiger Institute, DK-2100 Copenhagen Ø, Denmark **[137]**

Robert Collum, Department of Biochemistry and Biophysics, Columbia Presbyterian Medical Center, Columbia University, New York, NY 10032 **[97]**

The number in brackets is the opening page number of the contributor's article.

G. Cooper, Department of Pathology, Dana Farber Cancer Institute, Boston, MA 02115 **[59]**

Carlo M. Croce, The Wistar Institute, Philadelphia, PA 19104 **[159]**

Mark M. Davis, Department of Medical Microbiology, Stanford University School of Medicine, Stanford, CA 94305-5402 **[261]**

John R. Dedman, Departments of Physiology and Cell Biology, University of Texas Medical School, Houston, TX 77225 **[75]**

Koussay Dellagi, Département d'Immunopathologie et d'Hématologie, INSERM U108, Hopitâl Saint Louis, 75475 Paris Cédex 10, France **[1]**

Ronald DePinho, Department of Biochemistry and Biophysics, Columbia Presbyterian Medical Center, Columbia University, New York, NY 10032 **[97]**

Gordon W. Dewald, Mayo Clinic and Foundation, Rochester, MN 55905 **[47]**

Tim Donlon, Department of Pediatrics, Harvard Medical School, Boston, MA 02114 **[167]**

Jon P. Durkin, Cell Physiology Group, Division of Biological Sciences, National Research Council of Canada, Ottawa, Ontario, Canada K1A 0R6 **[89]**

Sean E. Egan, The Manitoba Institute of Cell Biology, University of Manitoba, Winnipeg, Manitoba, Canada R3E 0V9 **[279]**

Daniel Eliyahu, Department of Chemical Immunology, The Weizmann Institute of Science, Rehovot 76100, Israel **[247]**

Pierre Ferrier, Department of Biochemistry and Biophysics, Columbia Presbyterian Medical Center, Columbia University, New York, NY 10032 **[97]**

Lawrence R. Finger, The Wistar Institute, Philadelphia, PA 19104 **[159]**

A. Fojo, Laboratory of Molecular Biology, National Cancer Institute, Bethesda, MD 20892 **[287]**

Douglas J. Franks, Cell Physiology Group, Division of Biological Sciences, National Research Council of Canada, Ottawa, Ontario, Canada K1A 0R6; and Department of Pathology, Faculty of Health Sciences, University of Ottawa, Ottawa, Ontario, Canada K1H 8M5 **[89]**

Marsha L. Frazier, Department of Medical Oncology, The University of Texas, M.D. Anderson Hospital and Tumor Institute, Houston, TX 77030 **[17]**

Charlotte M. Fryling, Frederick Cancer Research Facility, National Cancer Institute, Frederick, MD 21701-1013; present address: Meloy Laboratories, Inc., Springfield, VA 22151 **[75]**

Gary E. Gallick, Departments of Neuro-Oncology, Tumor Biology, and Clinical Immunology, The University of Texas, M.D. Anderson Hospital and Tumor Institute at Houston, Houston, TX 77030 **[25]**

Brenda L. Gallie, Departments of Ophthalmology, Hematology, and Genetics, Hospital for Sick Children, University of Toronto, Toronto, Canada M5G 1X8 **[67]**

Ellen A. Garber, The Rockefeller University, New York, NY 10021 **[191]**

Adi F. Gazdar, NCI-Navy Medical Oncology Branch, National Cancer Institute and Naval Hospital, Bethesda, MD 20814 **[297]**

David Givol, Department of Chemical Immunology, The Weizmann Institute, Rehovot 76100, Israel **[275]**

Christo Goridis, Centre d'Immunologie de Marseille-Luminy, 13288 Marseille Cedex 9, France **[1]**

M.M. Gottesman, Laboratory of Molecular Biology, National Cancer Institute, Bethesda, MD 20892 **[287]**

Arnold H. Greenberg, The Manitoba Institute of Cell Biology, University of Manitoba, Winnipeg, Manitoba, Canada R3E 0V9 **[279]**

Philip R. Greipp, Mayo Clinic and Foundation, Rochester, MN 55905 **[47]**

P. Gros, Center for Cancer Research and Department of Biology, Massachusetts Institute of Technology, Cambridge, MA 02139 **[287]**

Jordan U. Gutterman, Departments of Neuro-Oncology, Tumor Biology, and Clinical Immunology, The University of Texas, M.D. Anderson Hospital and Tumor Institute at Houston, Houston, TX 77030 **[25]**

Gordon Hager, Laboratory of Tumor Virus Genetics, National Cancer Institute, Bethesda, MD 20205 **[279]**

Frank G. Haluska, The Wistar Institute, Philadelphia, PA 19104 **[159]**

P. Hamer, Biomedical Products Department, E.I. du Pont de Nemours and Company, Inc., North Billerica, MA 01862 **[59]**

Hidesaburo Hanafusa, The Rockefeller University, New York, NY 10021 **[191]**

Teruko Hanafusa, The Rockefeller University, New York, NY 10021 **[191]**

William R. Hargreaves, Frederick Cancer Research Facility, National Cancer Institute, Frederick, MD 21701-1013 **[75]**

Peter Harris, Department of Pediatrics, Harvard Medical School, Boston, MA 02114; Howard Hughes Medical Institute, Washington University School of Medicine, St. Louis, MO 63110 **[167]**

Kimi Hatton, Department of Biochemistry and Biophysics, Columbia Presbyterian Medical Center, Columbia University, New York, NY 10032 **[97]**

Parul Hazarika, Departments of Physiology and Cell Biology, University of Texas Medical School, Houston, TX 77225 **[75]**

Michael Heartlein, Department of Pediatrics, Harvard Medical School, Boston, MA 02114 **[167]**

Lee Helman, Molecular Genetics Section, Pediatric Branch COP, National Cancer Institute, National Institutes of Health, Bethesda, MD 20892 **[301]**

E. Hes, Division of Molecular Biology, The Netherlands Cancer Institute, 1066 CX Amsterdam, The Netherlands **[147]**

Gregory F. Hollis, NCI-Navy Medical Oncology Branch, National Cancer Institute, National Institutes of Health, National Naval Medical Center, Bethesda, MD 20814 **[35]**

D.E. Housman, Center for Cancer Research and Department of Biology, Massachusetts Institute of Technology, Cambridge, MA 02139 **[287]**

W. Robert Hudgins, Frederick Cancer Research Facility, National Cancer Institute, Frederick, MD 21701-1013 **[75]**

J.M. Ibson, Ludwig Institute for Cancer Research, Cambridge, CB2 2QH England **[107]**

Tatsuro Irimura, Department of Tumor Biology, The University of Texas, M.D. Anderson Hospital and Tumor Institute, Houston, TX 77030 **[17]**

Mark A. Israel, Molecular Genetics Section, Pediatric Branch COP, National Cancer Institute, National Institutes of Health, Bethesda, MD 20892 **[301]**

Lenka Jarolim, The Manitoba Institute of Cell Biology, University of Manitoba, Winnipeg, Manitoba, Canada R3E 0V9 **[279]**

Jan Jongstra, Department of Medical Microbiology, Stanford University School of Medicine, Stanford, CA 94305-5402; present address: Toronto Western Hospital, McLaughlin Pavilion, Toronto, Ontario M5T 2S5, Canada **[261]**

Richard Jove, The Rockefeller University, New York, NY 10021 **[191]**

Naotoshi Kanda, Department of Pediatrics, Harvard Medical School, Boston, MA 02114 **[167]**

John Kang, Department of Pediatrics, Harvard Medical School, Boston, MA 02114 **[167]**

Ilan R. Kirsch, NCI-Navy Medical Oncology Branch, National Cancer Institute, National Institutes of Health, National Naval Medical Center, Bethesda, MD 20814 **[35]**

William S. Kloetzer, Johnson and Johnson Biotechnology Center, La Jolla, CA 92037 **[25]**

Murray Korc, Department of Internal Medicine, University of Arizona, Tucson, AZ 85724 **[179]**

Bruce Korf, Department of Pediatrics, Harvard Medical School, Boston, MA 02114 **[167]**

Ronald Kriz, Genetics Institute, Cambridge, MA 02138 [97]

Wiebe Kruijer, The Salk Institute, San Diego, CA 92138; present address: Hubrecht Laboratorium, Uppsalalaan, Utrecht, The Netherlands [225]

W. Michael Kuehl, National Cancer Institute, NCI-Navy Medical Oncology Branch, Naval Hospital, Bethesda, MD 20814-2015 [xxi, 239]

Robert A. Kyle, Mayo Clinic and Foundation, Rochester, MN 55905 [47]

Ronald A. LaBiche, Department of Tumor Biology, The University of Texas, M.D. Anderson Hospital and Tumor Institute, Houston, TX 77030 [17]

Samuel Latt, Department of Pediatrics, Harvard Medical School, Boston, MA 02114; Howard Hughes Medical Institute, Washington University School of Medicine, St. Louis, MD 63110 [167]

M. Lefebvre, Department of Pathology, Dana Farber Cancer Institute, Boston, MA 02115 [59]

Edith Legouy, Department of Biochemistry and Biophysics, Columbia Presbyterian Medical Center, Columbia University, New York, NY 10032 [97]

Gilbert M. Lenoir, International Agency for Research on Cancer, 69372 Lyon Cédex 2, France [1]

K.B. Leslie, The Walter and Eliza Hall Institute of Medical Research, P.O. Royal Melbourne Hospital, Victoria 3050, Australia; present address: The Biomedical Research Centre, The University of British Columbia, Vancouver, British Columbia, Canada V6T 1W5 [129]

Marc Lipinski, Groupe d'Immunobiologie des Tumeurs, CNRS UA 1156, Institute Gustave Roussy, 94805 Villejuif Cédex, France [1]

Douglas R. Lowy, Laboratory of Cellular Oncology, National Cancer Institute, Bethesda, MD 20892 [203]

C. MacLeod, University of California at San Diego Cancer Center, La Jolla, CA 92093 [307]

H. Masui, Memorial Sloan Kettering Cancer Center, New York, NY 10021 [307]

Steve A. Maxwell, Departments of Neuro-Oncology, Tumor Biology, and Clinical Immunology, The University of Texas, M.D. Anderson Hospital and Tumor Institute at Houston, Houston, TX 77030 [25]

Bruce J. Mayer, The Rockefeller University, New York, NY 10021 [191]

Grant A. McClarty, The Manitoba Institute of Cell Biology, University of Manitoba, Winnipeg, Manitoba, Canada R3E 0V9 [279]

Catherine McKeon, Molecular Genetics Section, Pediatric Branch COP, National Cancer Institute, National Institutes of Health, Bethesda, MD 20892 [301]

Paul S. Meltzer, Department of Pediatrics, University of Arizona, Tucson, AZ 85724 [179]

John Mendelsohn, Memorial Sloan Kettering Cancer Center, and Cornell University Medical College, New York, NY 10021 [307,313]

Dan Michalovitz, Department of Chemical Immunology, The Weizmann Institute of Science, Rehovot 76100, Israel [247]

John Minna, NCI-Navy Medical Oncology, National Navy Hospital, Bethesda, MD 20814-2015 [xxi]

Richard L. Mitchell, The Salk Institute, San Diego, CA 92138 [225]

Lisa Mitsock, Genetics Institute, Cambridge, MA 02138 [97]

Richard P. Moser, Departments of Neuro-Oncology, Tumor Biology, and Clinical Immunology, The University of Texas, M.D. Anderson Hospital and Tumor Institute at Houston, Houston, TX 77030 [25]

Garth L. Nicolson, Department of Tumor Biology, The University of Texas, M.D. Anderson Hospital and Tumor Institute, Houston, TX 77030 [17]

Kenneth Nilsson, Department of Pathology, University of Uppsala, University Hospital, S-751 85 Uppsala, Sweden [9]

Perry Nisen, Department of Pediatrics, Schneider Children's Hospital of LI Jewish Medical Center, New Hyde Park, NY 11042 [97]

Allen Oliff, Merck Sharp and Dohme Research Laboratories, West Point, PA 19486 **[269]**

Moshe Oren, Department of Chemical Immunology, The Weizmann Institute of Science, Rehovot 76100, Israel **[247]**

David N. Orth, Division of Endocrinology, Vanderbilt University, Nashville, TN 37232 **[75]**

Alex G. Papageorge, Laboratory of Cellular Oncology, National Cancer Institute, Bethesda, MD 20892 **[203]**

Robert L. Pardue, Departments of Physiology and Cell Biology, University of Texas Medical School, Houston, TX 77225 **[75]**

I. Pastan, Laboratory of Molecular Biology, National Cancer Institute, Bethesda, MD 20892 **[287]**

D. Petit, Biomedical Products Department, E.I. du Pont de Nemours and Company, Inc., North Billerica, MA 01862 **[59]**

Irène Philip, Centre Léon Bérard, 69373 Lyon Cedex, France **[1]**

Thierry Philip, Centre Léon Bérard, 69373 Lyon Cedex, France **[1]**

Orit Pinhasi-Kimhi, Department of Chemical Immunology, The Weizmann Institute of Science, Rehovot 76100, Israel **[247]**

P.H. Rabbitts, Ludwig Institute for Cancer Research, Cambridge, CB2 2QH England **[107]**

H. Rabin, Biomedical Products Department, E.I. du Pont de Nemours and Company, Inc., North Billerica, MA 01862 **[59]**

Christopher L. Reading, Department of Tumor Biology, The University of Texas, M.D. Anderson Hospital and Tumor Institute, Houston, TX 77030 **[17]**

N. Richert, Laboratory of Molecular Biology, National Cancer Institute, Bethesda, MD 20892 **[287]**

I.B. Roninson, Center for Genetics, University of Illinois College of Medicine at Chicago, Chicago, IL 60612 **[287]**

Elise Rose, Department of Pediatrics, Harvard Medical School, Boston, MA 02114 **[167]**

Varda Rotter, Department of Cell Biology, The Weizmann Institute of Science, Rehovot, Israel **[17]**

Kazuo Sakai, Department of Pediatrics, Harvard Medical School, Boston, MA 02114 **[167]**

Kalle Saksela, Department of Virology, University of Helsinki, 00290 Helsinki, Finland **[9]**

J.W. Schrader, The Walter and Eliza Hall Institute of Medical Research, P.O. Royal Melbourne Hospital, Victoria 3050, Australia; present address: The Biomedical Research Centre, The University of British Columbia, Vancouver, British Columbia, Canada V6T 1W5 **[129]**

S. Schrader, The Walter and Eliza Hall Institute of Medical Research, P.O. Royal Melbourne Hospital, Victoria 3050, Australia; present address: The Biomedical Research Centre, The University of British Columbia, Vancouver, British Columbia, Canada V6T 1W5 **[129]**

David Schubert, The Salk Institute, San Diego, CA 92138 **[225]**

Robert Seeger, Department of Pediatrics, UCLA School of Medicine and the Children's, Cancer Study Group, Los Angeles, CA 90024 **[167]**

D.-W. Shen, Laboratory of Molecular Biology, National Cancer Institute, Bethesda, MD 20892 **[287]**

Yosef Shiloh, Department of Pediatrics, Harvard Medical School, Boston, MA 02114 **[167]**

Jonathan Silver, Laboratory of Viral Diseases, National Institute of Allergy and Infectious Diseases, National Institutes of Health, Bethesda, MD 20205 **[35]**

Jan Skouv, Laboratory of Environmental Carcinogenesis, The Fibiger Institute, DK-2100 Copenhagen Ø, Denmark **[137]**

R. Soffir, Center for Genetics, University of Illinois College of Medicine at Chicago, Chicago, IL 60612 **[287]**

Ira Spiro, Division of Radiation Oncology, George Washington University, Washington, DC 20037 **[279]**

Dennis W. Stacey, Roche Institute of Molecular Biology, Roche Research Center, Nutley, NJ 07110 **[213]**

Peter A. Steck, Departments of Neuro-Oncology, Tumor Biology, and Clinical Immunology, The University of Texas, M.D. Anderson Hospital and Tumor Institute at Houston, Houston, TX 77030 **[25]**

Helene Stroh, Department of Pediatrics, Harvard Medical School, Boston, MA 02114; Howard Hughes Medical Institute, Washington University School of Medicine, St. Louis, MO 63110 **[167]**

Kurt Stromberg, Frederick Cancer Research Facility, National Cancer Institute, Frederick, MD 21701-1013 **[75]**

H. Sunada, Memorial Sloan Kettering Cancer Center, New York, NY 10021 **[307]**

Abeba Tesfaye, Department of Biochemistry and Biophysics, Columbia Presbyterian Medical Center, Columbia University, New York, NY 10032 **[97]**

Carol J. Thiele, Molecular Genetics Section, Pediatric Branch COP, National Cancer Institute, National Institutes of Health, Bethesda, MD 20892 **[301]**

Jeffrey M. Trent, Department of Radiation Oncology and Internal Medicine, University of Arizona College of Medicine, Cancer Center Division, Tucson, AZ 85724 **[179,185]**

Robert J. Tressler, Department of Tumor Biology, The University of Texas, M.D. Anderson Hospital and Tumor Institute, Houston, TX 77030 **[17]**

Yoshihide Tsujimoto, The Wistar Institute, Philadelphia, PA 19104 **[159]**

Thomas Tursz, Groupe d'Immunobiologie des Tumeurs, CNRS UA 1156, Institute Gustave Roussy, 94805 Villejuif Cedex, France **[1]**

P.R. Twentyman, MRC Clinical Oncology and Radiotherapeutics Unit, MRC Center, Cambridge, CB2 2QH England **[107]**

Charles Van Beveren, The Salk Institute, San Diego, CA 92138 **[225]**

A.M. Van Der Bliek, Division of Molecular Biology, The Netherlands Cancer Institute, 1066 CX Amsterdam, The Netherlands **[147]**

T. Van Der Velde-Koerts, Division of Molecular Biology, The Netherlands Cancer Institute, 1066 CX Amsterdam, The Netherlands **[147]**

William C. Vass, Laboratory of Cellular Oncology, National Cancer Institute, Bethesda, MD 20892 **[203]**

Inder M. Verma, The Salk Institute, San Diego, CA 92138 **[225]**

J.J. Waters, Department of Cytogenetics, Addenbrooke's Hospital, Cambridge, CB2 2QH England **[107]**

James F. Whitfield, Cell Physiology Group, Division of Biological Sciences, National Research Council of Canada, Ottawa, Ontario, Canada K1A 0R6 **[89]**

Joëlle Wiels, Biochemical Oncology and Membrane Research, Fred Hutchinson Cancer Research Center, Seattle, WA 98104 **[1]**

Berthe M. Willumsen, University Microbiology Institute, 1353 Copenhagen, Denmark **[203]**

H. Wolfe, Department of Pathology, Tufts University Medical School, Boston, MA 02115 **[59]**

Gayle E. Woloschak, Mayo Clinic and Foundation, Rochester, MN 55905 **[47]**

Ronald G. Worton, Departments of Ophthalmology, Hematology, and Genetics, Hospital for Sick Children, University of Toronto, Toronto, Canada M5G 1X8 **[67]**

Jim A. Wright, The Manitoba Institute of Cell Biology, University of Manitoba, Winnipeg, Manitoba, Canada R3E 0V9 **[279]**

George Yancopoulos, Department of Biochemistry and Biophysics, Columbia Presbyterian Medical Center, Columbia University, New York, NY 10032 **[97]**

W.K. Alfred Yung, Departments of Neuro-Oncology, Tumor Biology, and Clinical Immunology, The University of Texas, M.D. Anderson Hospital and Tumor Institute at Houston, Houston, TX 77030 **[25]**

H.J. Ziltener, The Walter and Eliza Hall Institute of Medical Research, P.O. Royal Melbourne Hospital, Victoria 3050, Australia; present address: The Biomedical Research Centre, The University of British Columbia, Vancouver, British Columbia, Canada V6T 1W5 **[129]**

Kathy Zimmerman, Department of Biochemistry and Biophysics, Columbia Presbyterian Medical Center, Columbia University, New York, NY 10032 **[97]**

Preface

During the past ten years, clinical research on cancer treatment has resulted in some spectacular successes. For example, it is now possible to cure many childhood leukemias, Hodgkin's disease, aggressive histology lymphomas, and testicular tumors. Unfortunately, however, the vast majority of human malignancies remain recalcitrant to our best clinical efforts directed toward prevention or treatment. During this same period there has been a virtual explosion of information regarding the cellular and molecular biology of tumors. We are now able to identify and isolate genes which are aberrant in structure or expression, thereby determining fundamental properties of tumor cells such as malignant transformation, tumor progression, enhanced metastatic potential, and resistance to various therapeutic modalities. The fact that cancer can now be viewed as a molecular disease resulting from multiple genetic abnormalities suggests new strategies for prevention, diagnosis, and treatment based on our ability to identify the relevant genetic abnormalities.

The purpose of this Abbott-UCLA symposium was to achieve a useful dialogue among diverse scientists who perform basic research on cancer and clinicians who are responsible for prevention, diagnosis, and treatment of human malignancies. The major emphasis of the meeting was on recent results in cellular and molecular biology which begin to define fundamental and objective biological properties of cancer cells. These results include oncogene identification, activation, products, and functions; growth factors and receptors; chromosomal abnormalities; relationships of tumors and differentiation; phenotypic, karyotypic, and genetic heterogeneity of tumors; and tumor progression, metastasis, and resistance to drug therapy. In addition, there were presentations and discussions regarding antibodies and other biological response modifiers as preventive, diagnostic, and therapeutic agents, and analysis of human tumor lines in vitro to permit rational selection of potentially effective therapeutic agents.

Overall, the symposium was extremely successful in achieving a useful dialogue among diverse scientists and clinicians. At the outset, it was clear that the basic scientists would succeed in presenting state of the art cellular and molecular biological approaches to cancers, unifying hypotheses and mechanisms which provide the present and future basis for understanding the biology of tumor cells, and a catalog of genes that are likely to be deranged in cancer cells. However, it was a pleasant surprise to find that some of the best fundamental work in cancer biology is actually occurring in a clinical setting for a variety of human tumor systems. Several examples from the symposium are cited below, even though not all of them are included as manuscripts in this volume. A first example is the work of B. Gallie and co-workers, who have described how genetic events unmask recessive alleles to cause malignancy. A second example is the work of J. Minna and co-workers, who describe the potential importance of a neuroendocrine peptide (gastrin-releasing peptide) as an autocrine growth factor in small cell lung cancer. A third example is the work of M. Israel and co-workers, who describe how patterns of oncogene expression permit classification of histopathologically similar tumors. A fourth example is the work of R. Levy and co-workers, who describe the use of monoclonal antibodies directed against the clonal surface immunoglobulin on adult B-cell lymphomas as a potentially specific therapy. Despite the apparent clinical failure of this therapeutic approach, a careful analysis indicates frequent successes in elimination of the target cells, despite ultimate clinical failure due to selection of variants resulting from somatic mutation in the tumor immunoglobulin gene. Finally, the last session in the meeting described major progress in understanding the biology of lung, breast, and neuroectodermal human solid tumors. This is particularly gratifying since lung and breast cancer represent tumors which are the major causes of cancer mortality for men and women, respectively.

In planning and implementing the program of this symposium, we would like to thank all of our colleagues in the NCI-Navy Medical Oncology Branch, especially James Battey, Gregory Hollis, and Lanny Kirsch. In addition, we appreciate the contributions of our workshop chairpersons (Adi Gazdar, David Givol, John Mendelsohn, and Jeffery Trent). Finally, we received invaluable assistance from the UCLA symposium staff, in particular, Robin Yeaton, Betty Handy, and Hank Harwood.

John Minna, M.D.
W. Michael Kuehl, M.D.

Acknowledgments

We thank Abbott Laboratories for their generous sponsorship of this meeting. We also wish to acknowledge additional financial support from Meloy Laboratories, Merck Sharp & Dohme Research Laboratories, Bristol-Myers Company, Pharmaceutical Research and Development Division, Genetics Institute, Pfizer Central Research, Pfizer, Inc., Damon Biotech, Inc., and Smith Kline & French Laboratories.

Journal of Cellular Biochemistry 31:289–296 (1986)
Cellular and Molecular Biology of Tumors and
Potential Clinical Applications   1–8

Phenotypic Characterization of Ewing Sarcoma Cell Lines With Monoclonal Antibodies

Marc Lipinski, Karim Braham, Irène Philip, Joëlle Wiels, Thierry Philip,
Koussay Dellagi, Christo Goridis, Gilbert M. Lenoir, and Thomas Tursz

Groupe d'Immunobiologie des Tumeurs, CNRS UA 1156, Institute Gustave Roussy, 94805
Villejuif Cedex (M.L., K.B., T.T.), Centre Léon Bérard, 69373 Lyon Cedex (I.P., T.P.),
Département d'Immunopathologie et d'Hématologie, INSERM U108, Hôpital Saint Louis,
75475 Paris Cedex 10 (K.D.), Centre d'Immunologie de Marseille-Luminy, 13288 Marseille
Cedex 9 (C.G.), International Agency for Research on Cancer, 69372 Lyon Cedex 2
(G.M.L.), France, and Biochemical Oncology and Membrane Research, Fred Hutchinson
Cancer Research Center, Seattle, Washington 98104 (J.W.)

The histogenesis of Ewing sarcoma, the second most frequent bone tumor in humans, remains controversial. Four Ewing cell lines were analyzed by immunological methods. A panel of antibodies directed to T, B, and myelomonocytic markers gave negative results. Surface antigens recognized on Ewing cells were found to be related to the neuroectoderm lineage. Ganglioside GD_2, a marker of neuroectodermal tissues and tumors, was present on all lines. These were also stained by the mouse monoclonal antibody HNK-1, which detects a carbohydrate epitope present on several glycoconjugates of the nervous system, including two glycoproteins, the myelin-associated glycoprotein and the neural cell-adhesion molecule (N-CAM), and an acidic glycolipid of the peripheral nervous system. The P61 monoclonal antibody, which reacts with a peptide moiety of N-CAM, and a rabbit antiserum, raised to purified mouse N-CAM and not recognizing the HNK-1-defined epitope, were also reactive. By contrast, all antibodies specific for hematopoietic cell surface antigens were totally negative. Besides these antigenic features, Ewing sarcoma cells are characterized by a specific t(11;22)(q24;q12) translocation also observed in neuroepithelioma, a neuroectodermal tumor, suggesting a possible evolutionary related origin. The recent finding that the human N-CAM gene is located at the vicinity of the breakpoint on chromosome 11 indicates that it might be involved in genetic rearrangements occurring in this region.

Key words: histogenesis, antigenic phenotype, flow cytometry, N-CAM, HNK-1 monoclonal antibody

Received February 12, 1986; revised and accepted April 22, 1986.

Ewing sarcoma, a childhood tumor, was first described in 1921 [1]. It is the second most frequent bone tumor in humans, but also occurs in extraskeletal localizations. Because of its morphological aspect, it belongs to the group of small round cell tumors that, because of absence of unequivocal features of differentiation, poses many problems to the pathologists [2]. For the same reason, the histogenesis of Ewing sarcoma is still debated: The postulated endothelial origin proposed by Ewing has not received confirmation, and most authors consider it to derive from a mesenchymal cell [3,4].

We have used cell lines with the characteristic translocation t(11;22)(q24;q12) [5] also described in fresh Ewing sarcoma [6] to investigate the immunological phenotype of Ewing cells. In the large panel of antibodies used, all those found positive detected antigens whose expression is related to the neuroectoderm lineage, thus supporting our previous hypothesis [7,8] of a developmental relationship between Ewing sarcoma and the neuroectoderm.

MATERIALS AND METHODS

Cell Lines

Four continuous Ewing tumor-derived cell lines were established at the International Agency for Research on Cancer (IARC-EW1, IARC-EW3, and IARC-EW7) and at the Centre Léon Bérard (IARC-EW11), from metastatic cells of different sites of origin in four different patients. The karyotypic analysis of these lines has been performed by Turc-Carel et al and has led to the original description of the t(11;22)(q24;q12) translocation [5].

The HNK-1 hybridoma was purchased from the American Type Culture Collection (Rockville, MD).

All lines were grown as monolayers or in suspension and were carried in RPMI 1640 medium supplemented with 10% heat-inactivated fetal calf or horse serum. Adherent cells were usually resuspended using trypsin (1:250, 0.05%)/EDTA (ethylenediamine tetraacetic acid, 0.02%) (Flow Laboratories, UK) with no effect on surface antigen expression, as assessed by comparative staining on cells resuspended with EDTA alone.

Staining Antibodies

Monoclonal antibodies used in this study originated from hybridoma grown in our laboratory or were kindly made available to us. Mouse antibody HNK-1 was initially shown to detect a blood cell population with NK activity [9] but later shown by us and others to identify a neuroectoderm-associated antigen [10–12]. Rat antibody P61 has been raised to purified mouse neural cell-adhesion molecule (N-CAM) [13] and shown to detect a peptide determined epitope of this molecule [14]. This antibody also reacts with N-CAM proteins from all major species tested including man. Mouse antibodies 126 and MB3.6 were donated by David Cheresh (Scripps Clinic, La Jolla, CA). They are directed to gangliosides GD_2^* and GD_3, respectively, both highly enriched in neuroectodermal tumors [16]. Antibodies UJ127:11, UJ13A, UJ181, and

*According to the nomenclature of Svennerholm [15].

UJ167, obtained after immunization with human fetal brain and used in a panel of anti-neuroblastoma reagents [17], were provided by John Kemshead (ICRF, London). Human monoclonal IgM antibodies with reactivity to purified myelin-associated glycoprotein (MAG) originated from patients with peripheral neuropathy [18].

A rabbit antiserum was obtained as described [19] after immunization with purified mouse N-CAM. This antiserum does not contain antibodies recognizing the HNK-1-determined epitope [20] and reacts with typical N-CAM proteins in immunoblot from human brain.

Indirect Immunofluorescence Assay

Indirect immunofluorescence assays were performed as described [10] by incubating cells with hybridoma supernatant, ascites fluid, purified antibody, or antiserum at the appropriate dilutions. Reactions were revealed with fluoresceinated goat antisera to mouse Ig or IgM, rat Ig, rabbit Ig, or human IgM, as necessary. Fluorescence of live cells was quantitatively analyzed by flow cytometry (Epics C, Coulter, Margency, France) as described [21], or examined under a fluorescence microscope. Negative controls were included in every experiment and consisted of cells incubated with irrelevant antibodies or in the absence of first antibody.

Neuraminidase Treatment

EW3 cells (10^6) were incubated for 30 min in 50 mM sodium acetate, pH 5.5, 37°C, in the presence or absence of 5 μU of neuraminidase (Calbiochem, Behring Diagnostics, La Jolla, CA), and washed three times in RPMI 1640 supplemented with 2% fetal calf serum prior to immunofluorescence staining.

RESULTS

Immunofluorescence studies using a panel of monoclonal and polyclonal antibodies were carried on cell suspensions from Ewing cell lines EW1, EW3, EW7, and EW11, and analyzed by flow cytometry. All Ewing lines expressed human lymphocyte antigen (HLA) class I but not class II antigens. None was stained by monoclonal antibody 9.4 to the common leukocyte antigen T200. A series of antibodies from the panels of the Second International Workshop on Leukocyte Antigens that are directed to antigens associated with the B, T, and myelomonocytic cell lineages and define clusters of differentiation CD2, CD3, CD4, CD5, CD6, CD8, CD10, CD11, and CDw14 were tested and remained constantly negative (data not shown). By contrast, several molecules associated with the neuroectoderm lineage were demonstrated at the surface of the cells.

Antibody 126, directed to the ganglioside GD_2, stained all Ewing lines (Fig. 1). That the antigenic site resided upon the sialic acid residues of the conjugate was demonstrated by the abrogation of the reactivity with antibody 126 after treatment of the cells with neuraminidase (Fig. 2). Interestingly, antibody MB3.6, directed to GD_3, the metabolic precursor of GD_2, was totally unreactive on these same lines.

Antibody HNK-1 also stained the four Ewing lines to a varying degree (Fig. 3). Two distinct glycoproteins, MAG and N-CAM, both expressed in neuroectodermal tissues, have been reported to carry the HNK-1-defined carbohydrate epitope [20]. Human monoclonal antibodies whose reactivity to purified MAG had been verified by immunoblotting were also tested on Ewing cell lines. They produced similar,

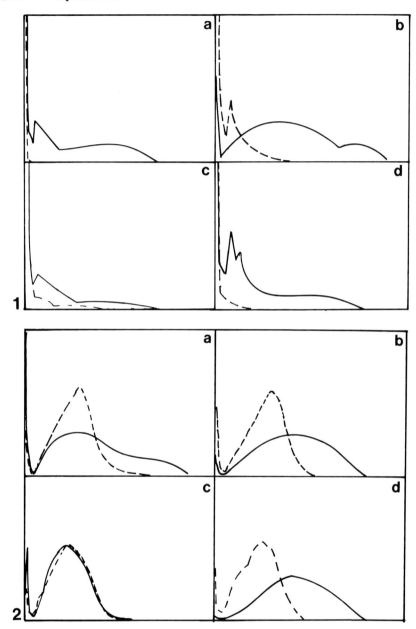

Fig. 1.   Immunofluorescence staining of Ewing sarcoma lines EW1 (a), EW3 (b), EW7 (c), and EW11 (d). Cells were incubated for 30 min with 50 μl of hybridoma supernatant containing antibody 126 to GD_2. The reaction was revealed by a fluoresceinated goat antimouse IgM antiserum, analyzed by flow cytometry (——) and compared to controls (- - - - -) obtained with first antibody omitted or replaced by antibody MB3.6 to GD_3. Histograms appear with fluorescence plotted on a logarithmic scale on the x-axis.

Fig. 2.   Immunofluorescence staining of neuraminidase and mock-treated cells from Ewing sarcoma line EW3. Cells were incubated for 30 min at pH 5.5, 37°C in the absence (a,b) or presence (c,d) of neuraminidase, then stained with antibody 126 (a,c) or HNK-1 (b,d). Revelation, analysis, and display as in Figure 1.

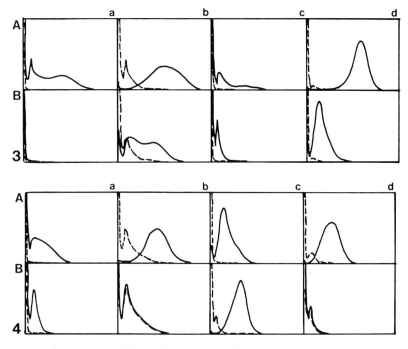

Fig. 3.   Immunofluorescence staining of Ewing sarcoma lines EW1 (a), EW3 (b), EW7 (c), and EW11 (d) with mouse monoclonal antibody HNK-1 (A) and with a human monoclonal antibody with MAG reactivity (B). The reaction was as in Figure 1 except that a fluoresceinated antiserum to human IgM was used in B as a developing reagent. Analysis and display as in Figure 1.

Fig. 4.   Immunofluorescence staining of Ewing sarcoma lines EW1 (a), EW3 (b), EW7 (c), and EW11 (d) with a rabbit anti-N-CAM antiserum (A) and with the rat monoclonal antibody P61 (B). The reaction was as in Figure 1 except that the reaction was revealed with fluoresceinated antisera to rabbit or rat Ig, respectively. Analysis and display as in Figure 1.

although less intense, stainings. Profiles obtained with one such antibody are shown in Figure 3.

We investigated the reactivity of Ewing lines with two reagents raised to purified mouse N-CAM, a rabbit antiserum and a rat monoclonal antibody that both cross-react with human N-CAM. The rabbit serum bound all Ewing lines (Fig. 4). With this reagent, lines EW3 and EW11 proved more reactive than EW1 and EW7. By contrast, antibody P61 that detects a peptide epitope carried by the 140- and 180-kd species of the N-CAM molecule produced totally different staining profiles, as line EW7 was the most brightly stained, even more so than neuroblastoma cell lines used as controls (data not shown). Line EW1 was more weakly stained while lines EW3 and EW11 seemed to entirely lack the P61 determinant at their cell surface (Fig. 4).

A third glycoconjugate, an acidic glycolipid present in the ganglioside fraction of the peripheral nervous system, also binds HNK-1 antibody [22]. Preliminary results indicate that HNK-1 does detect such a molecule purifying in the trisialo ganglioside fraction extracted from Ewing cell lines EW1 and EW3 (data not shown). That sialic acid residues do not carry the epitope is shown by the persistence of the staining after treatment with neuraminidase in condition that totally abrogated the detection of surface ganglioside GD_2 (Fig. 2).

Finally, we assayed the reactivity of four antibodies to neuroblastoma cells [17]. As shown in Table I, all antibodies but one reacted with one or two Ewing lines.

DISCUSSION

We have used an immunological approach to attempt to clarify the question of the histogenesis of Ewing sarcoma. A preliminary study of Ewing lines had led us to postulate a neuroectodermal origin for Ewing cells [7,8]. We have now obtained additional evidence that the antigens expressed at the surface of Ewing cell lines are indeed related to this lineage.

Ganglioside GD_2 was detected on all Ewing lines. Its expression has previously been analyzed in detail and shown to be restricted to normal tissues and tumors of neuroectodermal origin [23]. The epitope recognized probably contains the sialic acid residues of GD_2 since the reactivity was lost after neuraminidase treatment.

Antibody HNK-1 was also found to bind all four Ewing lines. Staining of a large panel of human solid tumors with this reagent has indicated that its reactivity was restricted to neuroectoderm-derived tumors [12]. HNK-1 has been shown to react with a ganglioside of peripheral nerves [22], but its binding to Ewing cells was not affected by neuraminidase treatment. However, when gangliosides were purified from Ewing cells, HNK-1 was found to detect a moiety present in the trisialoganglioside-containing fraction. This reactivity is likely to be identical with that already described in peripheral nerves [22].

The same carbohydrate epitope seems to be carried by several glycoproteins of the nervous system, including MAG and N-CAM. These two structures are highly glycosylated molecules suspected to play an important role in the nervous system, MAG as a minor constituent of myelin sheaths [24], and N-CAM as a major ligand implicated in the phenomenon of neural-neural cell binding [25]. Also, the antigenic epitope detected by HNK-1 is extremely well conserved during evolution, suggesting that it might exert a major function in the nervous tissues [26]. In this respect, its presence on Ewing cells provides a further indication of the expression on this tumor of neuroectoderm associated structures.

Finally, all Ewing lines tested reacted with an anti-N-CAM antiserum, and furthermore lines EW1 and EW7 were stained by antibody P61 that detects a peptide epitope restricted to the 140- and 180-kd species of the N-CAM molecule [14]. The importance of the finding of neuroectodermal antigens on Ewing cells is strengthened

TABLE I. Binding on Ewing Cell Lines of Monoclonal Antibodies Reacting With Neuroblastoma*

Staining antibody	Ewing cell lines			
	EW1	EW3	EW7	EW11
UJ127:11	+	−	−	+
UJ13A	−	+	−	+
UJ181	−	−	−	+
UJ167	−	−	−	−

*Target cells were incubated for 30 min with staining antibody. The reaction was revealed with a fluoresceinated goat anti-mouse Ig antiserum. Cells were smeared on a slide, and live cells were examined for fluorescence under a fluorescence microscope. Results were scored as positive (+) or negative (−) by comparison with control fluorescence obtained with target cells incubated with second step only.

by the absence of reactivity of these cells with a panel of antibodies directed to differentiation antigens of the B, T, and myelomonocytic lineages. By contrast, monoclonal antibodies raised to human fetal brain that all bind neuroblastoma cells [17] displayed some degree of reactivity with one or two Ewing lines.

To the pathologist, Ewing sarcoma is often difficult to differentiate from other small round cell tumors of neuroectodermal origin [2]. Most often, investigations of specific enzymatic activities and electron microscopic features will nevertheless allow discrimination of a bone metastasis of neuroblastoma from a Ewing sarcoma. Also, neuroblastoma cells usually express very low levels of HLA class I molecules [27], in contrast with Ewing cells. Even more strikingly, the expression of the N-*myc* oncogene is specifically amplified in neuroblastoma [28]. We did not observe such an amplification in DNA from two Ewing lines analyzed here with a specific N-*myc* probe (provided by Frederick Alt, NY) (data not shown). Thus, a variety of biological criteria clearly delineate Ewing sarcoma from neuroblastoma.

The comparison of Ewing sarcoma with peripheral neuroepithelioma raises more problems, as recently underlined [29]. In 1983, the description of a specific translocation t(11;22)(q24;q12) in Ewing sarcoma cells [5,6] provided the first means of positive diagnostic for this malignancy until the same translocation was reported as well in peripheral neuroepithelioma [30] and in another rare neuroectodermal tumor of the thoracopulmonary region [31] described by Askin et al [32], raising questions about the possible implications of this repetitive chromosomal accident.

During normal differentiation of the B cell lineage, genetic rearrangements take place on chromosomes 14, 2, and 22 in the genes coding for heavy and light Ig chains, respectively [33]. Burkitt lymphoma, a B cell malignancy, is characterized by a translocation between chromosome 8 where the c-*myc* oncogene is normally located and one of the Ig gene carrying chromosomes [34]. New DNA configurations are thus obtained that can affect the structure of c-*myc* or the regulation of its expression [35].

Two proto-oncogenes have been localized in the vicinity of the breakpoints observed in Ewing cells: c-*ets* on chromosome 11q23–24, and c-*sis* on chromosome 22 distal to q11. Neither one seems to be involved in the oncogenetic process since, despite being translocated, c-*sis* is neither rearranged nor amplified [36], and c-*ets* has not been found rearranged in five different Ewing tumors [37].

It is nevertheless tempting to imagine that the t(11;22) translocation of Ewing sarcoma and neuroepithelioma could also point to chromosomal breakpoints involved in normal genetic rearrangements occurring during neuroectodermal differentiation. With this hypothesis in mind, it becomes striking that the human N-CAM gene has recently been localized to chromosome 11q23 [38]. Whether this gene is actually translocated in Ewing cells resulting in the transcription of new RNA messengers and expression of abnormal cell surface molecules is presently under investigation at the molecular level.

ACKNOWLEDGMENTS

We thank David Cheresh and John Kemshead for providing monoclonal antibodies and Cécile Tétaud and Gilbert Hue for excellent technical assitance. This work was supported, in part, by grants 83D7 from the Institut Gustave Roussy and 2098 from the Association pour la Recherche sur le Cancer.

REFERENCES

1. Ewing J: Proc NY Pathol Soc 21:17, 1921.
2. Reynolds CP, Smith RG, Frenkel EP: Cancer 48:2088, 1981.
3. Miettinen M, Lehto VP, Virtainen I: Virchows Arch 41:277, 1982.
4. Navas-Palacios JJ, Aparicio-Duque R, Valdes MD: Cancer 53:1882, 1984.
5. Turc-Carel C, Philip I, Berger MP, Philip T, Lenoir GM: N Engl J Med 309:497, 1983.
6. Aurias A, Rimbaut C, Buffe D, Dubousset J, Mazabraut A: N Engl J Med 309:496, 1983.
7. Lipinski M, Braham K, Tursz T: (Abstract) Fed Proc 43:1510, 1984.
8. Lipinski M, Braham K, Caillaud JM, Philip I, Philip T, Lenoir GM, Tursz T: In Peeters H (ed): "Protides of the Biological Fluids, Proceedings of the Thirty-Second Colloquium." Oxford: Pergamon Press, 1984, pp 491–494.
9. Abo T, Balch CM: J Immunol 127:1024, 1981.
10. Lipinski M, Braham K, Caillaud JM, Carlu C, Tursz T: J Exp Med 158:1775, 1983.
11. Schuller-Petrovic S, Gebhart W, Lassmann H, Rumpold H, Kraft D: Nature 306:179, 1983.
12. Caillaud JM, Benjelloun S, Bosq J, Braham K, Lipinski M: Cancer Res 44:4432, 1984.
13. Gennarini G, Rougon G, Deagostini-Bazin H, Hirn M, Goridis C: Eur J Biochem 142:57, 1984.
14. Gennarini G, Hirn M, Deagostini-Bazin H, Goridis C: Eur J Biochem 142:65, 1984.
15. Svennerholm L: J Neurochem 10:613, 1963.
16. Cheresh DA, Harper JR, Schulz G, Reisfeld RA: Proc Natl Acad Sci USA 81:5767, 1984.
17. Kemshead JT, Goldman A, Fritschy J, Malpas JS, Pritchard J: Lancet i:12, 1983.
18. Dellagi K, Dupouey P, Brouet JC, Billecocq A, Gomez D, Clauvel JP, Seligmann M: Blood 62:280, 1983.
19. Sadoul H, Hirn M, Deagostini-Bazin H, Goridis C: Nature 304:347, 1983.
20. Kruse J, Mailhammer R, Wernecke H, Faissner A, Sommer I, Goridis C, Schachner M: Nature 311:153, 1984.
21. Herzenberg LA, Herzenberg LA: In Weir DM (ed): "Handbook of Experimental Immunology, 3rd Ed. Oxford: Blackwell, 1978, pp 22.1–22.21.
22. Ilyas AA, Quarles RH, Brady RO: Biochem Biophys Res Commun 122:1206, 1984.
23. Schulz G, Cheresh DA, Varki NM, Yu A, Staffileno LK, Reisfeld RA: Cancer Res 44:5914, 1984.
24. Trapp BD, Quarles RH, Suzuki K: J Cell Biol 99:594, 1984.
25. Rutishauser U, Hoffman S, Edelman GM: Proc Natl Acad Sci USA 79:685, 1982.
26. Tucker GC, Aoyama H, Lipinski M, Tursz T, Thiery JP: Cell Differ 14:223, 1984.
27. Lampson LA, Fisher CA, Wheelan JP: J Immunol 130:2471, 1983.
28. Brodeur GM, Seeger RC, Schwab M, Varmus HE, Bishop JM: Science 224:1121, 1984.
29. Jaffe R, Santamaria M, Yunis EJ, Hrinia Tannery N, Agostini RM, Medina J, Goodman M: Am J Surg Pathol 8:885, 1984.
30. Whang-Peng J, Triche TJ, Knutsen T, Miser J, Douglass EC, Israel MA: N Engl J Med 311:584, 1984.
31. De Chadarevian JP, Vekemans M, Seemayer TA: N Engl J Med 311:1702, 1984.
32. Askin FB, Rosai J, Sibley RK, Dehner LP, McAlister WH: Cancer 43:2438, 1979.
33. Tonegawa S: Nature 302:575, 1983.
34. Lenoir GM, Preud'homme JL, Bernheim A, Berger R: Nature 298:474, 1982.
35. Taub R, Moulding C, Battey G, Murphy W, Vasicek T, Lenoir GM, Leder P: Cell 36:339, 1984.
36. Bechet JM, Bornkamm GW, Freese UK, Lenoir GM: N Engl J Med 310:393, 1983.
37. De Taisne C, Gegonne A, Stehelin D, Berger A: Nature 310:581, 1984.
38. N'Guyen C, Mattei M-G, Mattei J-F, Santori M-J, Goridis C, Jordan BR: J Cell Biol 102:711, 1986.

Journal of Cellular Biochemistry 31:297–304 (1986)
Cellular and Molecular Biology of Tumors and
Potential Clinical Applications   9–16

Amplification of the N-*myc* Oncogene in an Adenocarcinoma of the Lung

Kalle Saksela, Jonas Bergh, and Kenneth Nilsson

Department of Virology, University of Helsinki, 00290 Helsinki, Finland (K.S.) and Departments of Pathology (J.B., K.N.) and Oncology (J.B.), University of Uppsala, University Hospital, S-751 85 Uppsala, Sweden

c-*myc* oncogene is the most extensively studied member of the *myc* gene family, which now consists of three characterized members, namely the c-*myc*, N-*myc*, and L-*myc* genes. Deregulation owing to amplification and/or rearrangements of the c-*myc* gene have been described in a variety of human malignancies. Several neuroblastomas have amplifications of the N-*myc* genes. The c-*myc*, N-*myc*, or L-*myc* oncogenes are also found amplified in different cell lines from small cell carcinomas of the lung. In this study, we have examined the c-*myc*, N-*myc*, and c-*erb*B oncogenes in 34 clinical and autopsy tumor specimens representing various histopathological types of human lung cancer, including nine small cell lung cancers. A 30-fold amplification of the N-*myc* gene was found in a tumor histopathologically and histochemically verified as a typical adenocarcinoma. No amplifications of the c-*myc* or c-*erb*B oncogenes were seen in any of the tumors. In the DNA of one small cell carcinoma, an extra c-*myc* and N-*myc* cross-hybridizing restriction fragment was observed, possibly owing to an amplification of a yet uncharacterized *myc*-related gene.

Key words: small cell lung cancer, c-*erb*B oncogene, EGF receptor, c-*myc* oncogene, *myc* gene family, squamous cell carcinoma, gene amplification, neuroblastoma, glioblastoma, neuron-specific enolase, cytokeratin, neuroendochine markers, variant form of small cell lung cancer

Amplifications of the c-*myc* oncogene have been described in many types of tumor cell lines, but they appear to be especially common in the cell lines of the variant form of small cell lung cancer [1–3]. In comparison with the classic small cell lung cancer (SCLC) cell lines, the cell lines of the variant form of SCLC have a faster doubling time and a higher cloning efficiency in culture [2,4]. The SCLC tumors with variant features have also been reported to behave more aggressively in vivo [5]. Since oncogene amplifications are typically found in tumors from patients with an advanced disease, a role for chemotherapy in the generation of c-*myc* amplifications has been discussed.

Received March 5, 1986; accepted April 22, 1986.

There may exist a sizable family of c-*myc* related genes. N-*myc* [6] and L-*myc* [7] are two other members of this gene family. Both of these genes have also been found amplified in different SCLC cell lines [7]. In neuroblastomas, N-*myc* amplification seems to correlate with an advanced clinical stage and a poor prognosis of the disease [8].

In all cases studied, the amplification of the c-*myc* gene has been accompanied by elevation of the levels of c-*myc* RNA and protein. However, very little is known of the cellular functions of the *myc* gene products. Homologies of the deduced amino acid sequences and functional similarities in transformation assays suggest that the protein products of c-*myc* and N-*myc* genes might have similar functions [9–11]. No c-*myc* protein or RNA has been found in cells having an amplified N-*myc* gene, nor have amplifications of more than one *myc*-related gene been observed in the same cells.

Induction of the c-*myc* protein is associated with the G0/G1 transition occurring after growth factor stimulation, but subsequent expression appears to be stable throughout the cell cycle [12]. The level of c-*myc* expression of normal cells has been correlated with mitogenic activity of the corresponding tissues [13], and elevated levels of c-*myc* transcripts have been found also in many tumor cells lacking chromosomal abnormalities that typically deregulate c-*myc* expression [14,15]. In culture, primary embryonic cells transfected with a constitutively highly expressed c-*myc* gene become susceptible to transformation by a complementing oncogene such as c-*ras* [16].

Besides SCLC, no amplifications of c-*myc* or related genes have been described in other types of human lung cancer tumors. We analyzed a series of lung tumors representing various histopathological types. Cloned DNA fragments of c-*myc* and N-*myc* oncogenes were used as probes in low- and high-stringency hybridization conditions. Because elevated levels of the EGF receptor have been described in several human squamous cell carcinoma cell lines and tumors [19], we found it also of interest to look for c-*erb*B amplifications in these tumor DNAs using cloned c-*erb*B cDNA as a probe. The c-*erb*B oncogene has been shown to code for the EGF receptor [17] and has been found amplified in human glioblastomas [18].

MATERIALS AND METHODS

Tumor Material

Fresh material was received from the Departments of Thorax Surgery and Otolaryngology, University of Uppsala, consisting of lung lobes (23 cases) or biopsies (6 cases) from 29 randomly selected and untreated patients with lung tumors. Parts of the tumors were removed and immediately frozen at $-70°C$. Material was also taken for routine histopathological examination. All tumor material was examined by two pathologists. The lung tumor that contained an amplified N-*myc* gene was also investigated with monoclonal antibodies against cytokeratin [20] and a sheep antiserum against neuron-specific enolase (NSE) [21], and part of the tumor was homogenized for radioimmunological determination of the NSE content [22]. The protein content was determined according to Lowry et al [23].

In addition, we received autopsy tumor material from five histopathologically verified SCLC patients from the Department of Pathology, University of Helsinki. In three out of these five cases metastatic material was also included in the study.

Isolation of DNA

High molecular weight DNA was isolated from the tumors. The tumors were first powdered with a microdismembranator (B-Braun, Melsungen AB, West Germany) at $-70°C$ and then dissolved in 0.5% sodium dodecyl sulfate (SDS), 0.1 M NaCl, 20 mM ethylamediamine tetracetic acid (EDTA), 50 mM Tris-HCl, pH 8.1. The cellular proteins were hydrolysed by incubating the lysates with 200 μg/ml proteinase K (Merck) for 1 hr at 37°C. The solution was extracted twice with phenol, and twice with an equal volume of butanol-propanol (7:3). Nucleic acids were precipitated with 3 volumes of ethanol, washed in absolute ethanol, and dried in a vacuum. The nucleic acids were then redissolved in 1 mM EDTA, 10 mM Tris-HCl, pH 8 (TE), and RNA was hydrolysed with 100 μg/ml pancreatic ribonuclease A at 37°C for 1 hr. Treatment with proteinase K, extraction with phenol and with butanol-propanol, and ethanol precipitation were performed as above. The DNA was dissolved and stored at 4°C in TE. The DNA concentrations of the preparations were estimated by their light absorbances at 260 nm.

Electrophoresis, Blotting, and Hybridizations

Aliquots of DNA were digested with restriction endonucleases, fractionated by electrophoresis through a 1% agarose gel, and transferred to nitrocellulose paper in 6 × SSC (1 × SSC is 0.15 M NaCl, 0.015 sodium citrate). Fragment sizes were calculated using lambda phage DNA cleaved with restriction endonuclease Hind III as a standard. Hybridization analyses were performed as described earlier [3].

RESULTS

DNA was extracted from the tumors of 34 lung cancer patients. Twenty-nine of the samples were clinical material, five of the samples were autopsy specimens, and all represented SCLC. Table I shows the histologic types and the origin of the tumors analyzed with radiolabeled probes detailed in the figure legends. In all but one of the tumor DNAs, the analysis revealed only the normal restriction fragments of the germ line proto-oncogenes. In one tumor (patient 18), an increased signal intensity was obtained from the 2-kbp Eco RI fragment of the N-*myc* oncogene (Fig. 1A, lanes Ad). This suggested that N-*myc* was amplified in the tumor DNA. DNA from normal lymphocytes of the patient and other tumors had a single-copy N-*myc* hybridization signal (Fig. 1A, lane C). The degree of amplification of N-*myc* was estimated from diluted DNA and found to be about 30-fold. The copy number of the gene for ornithine decarboxylase (ODC) was chosen for comparison, because it maps to the same chromosomal region (2p23-25) as N-*myc* [24]. The structure of amplified N-*myc* appeared normal in restriction endonuclease analysis of 13 kbp of DNA from the gene and its flanking sequences (Fig. 1B).

The morphology of tumor with the amplified N-*myc* gene was typical for an adenocarcinoma (Fig. 2) with prominent tubular structures, some of them containing mucin. Furthermore, the tumor cells contained cytokeratin in immunohistochemical staining. Scattered tumor cells were also strongly stained with the NSE antiserum (data not shown). The NSE value determined by radioimmunoassay (RIA) was found to be 0.31 μg/mg protein, a value in agreement with the histopathological classification of the tumor as an adenocarcinoma [22].

TABLE I. Lung Cancer Tumors Analyzed for *myc* Oncogenes*

Patient no.	Origin	Histopathologic diagnosis
1	B	SCLC
2	B	SCLC
3	L	SCLC
4	L	SCLC
5	L	SQC (poorly differentiated), SCLC?
6	L	SQC (minor SCLC component?)
7	B	SQC
8	L	SQC
9	L	SQC
10	L	SQC
11	L	SQC
12	L	SQC
13	L	SQC
14	L	LCC (poorly differentiated), SQC?
15	B	LCC
16	L	LCC (clear cell type)
17	L	ADC
18	L	ADC
19	B	ADC
20	L	ADC
21	L	ADC
22	L	ADC
23	L	ADC
24	L	BC (atypical)
25	L	BC
26	L	BC
27	L	BC
28	L	Neurilemmoma
29	B	Poorly differentiated lung cancer
30	A	SCLC
31	A	SCLC
32	A[†]	SCLC
33	A[†]	SCLC
34	A[†]	SCLC

*B, biopsy; L, lobectomy sample, A, autopsy sample; A†, metastatic material also analysed; SCLC, small cell lung cancer; SQC, squamous cell carcinoma; LCC, large cell carcinoma; ADC, adenocarcinoma; BC, bronchial carcinoid.

In one tumor DNA from an autopsy SCLC specimen (patient 33) we found extra restriction fragments cross-hybridizing with both the c-*myc* and N-*myc* probes (Fig. 3, and data not shown). The sizes of these restriction fragments were different from those described for the L-*myc* gene [7]. The same bands could be seen also in the DNA from the liver metastasis of the same patient, but more faintly. An extensive restriction enzyme study of the c-*myc* or N-*myc* genes of this DNA did not reveal any rearrangements. Different cross-hybridizing fragments were seen with both c-*myc* I exon and III exon-specific probes. No cross-hybridization was observed using plasmid DNA as a probe (data not shown). We are at the present studying the possibility that these abnormal bands emerged owing to the amplification of a still unknown *myc*-related gene.

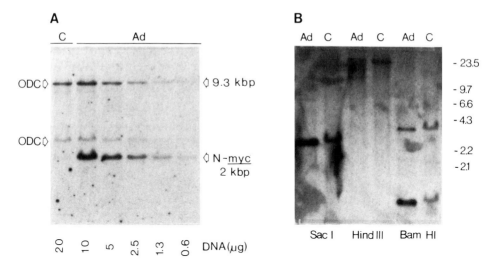

Fig. 1.   A) Analysis of the copy number of N-*myc* and ODC genes in tumor DNA. DNA was isolated from the adenocarcinoma tumor of patient 18 (lanes Ad) and from the SCLC tumor of paitent 5 (lane C), digested with Eco RI, electrophoresed, blotted, and hybridized with radioactively labeled DNA of the pNb-1 plasmid containing a 1-kbp Eco RI-Bam HI fragment from the second exon of N-*myc* [6] and with a radioactive insert of the human ornithine decarboxylase cDNA (plasmic pODC 10/2H [24], a kind gift from Dr. Olli Jänne). The blot was washed in high-stringency conditions and autoradiographed. It can be seen from the radioactive signal obtained from different amounts of adenocarcinoma DNA that the N-*myc* oncogene is amplified about 30-fold, whereas the signal from the ODC gene is of similar intensity in 10–20 μg of DNA from both adenocarcinoma and control DNA. B) Mapping of N-*myc* loci by restriction endonuclease analysis. DNA from the adenocarcinoma (Ad) was diluted 20-fold, and analyzed together with undiluted control DNA from the tumor of patient 5 (C). Three different endonuclease digestions are shown for comparison. The fragment lengths obtained with endonucleases Sac I, Hind III, and Bam HI were similar, except for the differences in mobility owing to loading of different amounts of DNA in the sample wells.

DISCUSSION

The c-*myc* oncogene has been found amplified in a subpopulation of in vitro grown cell lines of small cell carcinoma of the lung [1,3]. The cell lines with amplified c-*myc* in general have faster doubling times and fewer neuroendocrine markers [4]. A morphology typical for the SCLC cell lines with a c-*myc* amplification has been reported. These cell lines also seem to originate from SCLC tumors with variant morphological features [2]. Here we report oncogene DNA analysis in a series of lung cancer tumors, including nine SCLSs. None of the investigated tumors, except for one adenocarcinoma sample, disclosed amplifications of the c-*myc* or N-*myc* oncogenes.

The fact that no amplifications of the c-*myc* genes were seen in any of the SCLC tumors suggests that these amplifications are more common in established SCLC cell lines than in the clinical tumor material. The reason for the discrepancy between the in vitro situation and the in vivo situation is as yet unexplained. One alternative could be in vitro growth selection of clones with the amplified c-*myc* gene, already present but not detected in the tumor biopsy. Altered growth properties of the cells with c-*myc* amplifications may adapt them particularly well to culture conditions. On the other hand, no *myc* amplifications have been described to occur during the in vitro

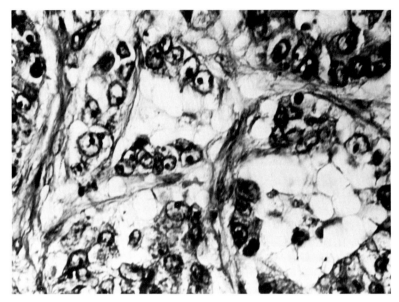

Fig. 2.   Histology of the adenocarcinoma tumor with the N-*myc* amplification. The picture shows cells with a large cytoplasm and prominent nucleolae, arranged in tubular structures typical for an adenocarcinoma (van Gieson stain, magnification about ×250).

cultivation of cells. Another explanation could be that six out of the nine examined SCLC tumor samples were from untreated patients, while the majority of established cell lines used in previous studies were obtained from drug-treated patients. This may have resulted in clonal selection of cells with altered geno- and phenotypes. A third alternative is that the number of examined SCLC tumors (nine) was too small to include variant subtypes. The present tumors could all represent "classic" SCLC, which should be expected to lack amplified c-*myc* oncogenes.

In this paper, we, for the first time, describe the presence of N-*myc* amplification in a primary lung adenocarcinoma. The adenocarcinoma diagnosis was based on a typical morphology with production of mucin, an epithelial phenotype reflected by the positive cytokeratin staining, and relatively low levels of NSE. However a value of 0.31 μg NSE/mg protein may even occur in some SCLC cell lines [25]. It should also be mentioned that NSE cannot be regarded as an ultimate marker for neuroendocrine differentiation, because unrelated human tumors such as lymphoblastoid cell lines, myeloma cell lines, and an Epstein-Barr virus-transformed chronic lymphocytic leukemia cell line have disclosed even higher NSE values [25].

The elevated level of *myc* expression owing to the amplifications of the *myc* genes give cells a growth advantage of as yet uncharacterized nature. This is often acquired by the SCLC cells, but amplification can occur in other tumors as well, as shown by the present results. Also, it may be that adenocarcinomas of the lung are a more heterogenous group of tumors than has been recognized. In part, then, our findings may merely reflect the difficulty in predicting the molecular and cellular biology of tumors on the basis of histopathologic diagnosis. After all, the major types of lung cancer are all histogenetically related [26].

The nature of the novel amplified 5.5 kbp *myc* cross-reacting fragment will be examined by molecular cloning. It may represent an additional gene of the *myc* family

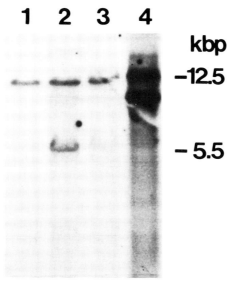

Fig. 3. Analysis of c-*myc*-related DNA sequences in lung cancer and colon carcinoma DNA. DNA from the SCLC tumor of patient 32 (lane 1), from the SCLC tumor of the patient 33 (lane 2), and from the liver metastasis of patient 33 (lane 3) were extracted and subjected to Southern blotting and hybridization analysis with a radioactive Cla I-Alu I-fragment from the III exon of c-*myc*. DNA from the colon carcinoma COLO 320 cells (lane 4) is analyzed as a positive control for c-*myc* amplification and rearrangement. As can be seen from the figure, the normal genomic 12.5 kbp Eco RI fragment of the c-*myc* oncogene is of similar size and intensity in all lung carcinoma DNAs, but there is an extra band hybridizing weakly in the DNA from liver metastasis and more strongly in the lung tumor. The size of the fragment is about 5.5 kbp, as can be interpolated from the mobilities of the Hind III fragments of bacteriophage lambda, indicated on the right.

similar to N-*myc* and L-*myc*, both of which were discovered by cross-hybridization of amplified, homologous DNA [6,7].

ACKNOWLEDGMENTS

We thank Dr. Lena Steinholtz from the Central Hospital in Västerås for providing us with clinical material, the staff of the Departments of Thorax Surgery and Otolaryngology for providing us with the fresh operation specimens, and Sven Påhlman and Ingegärd Hjertson for the RIA analyses. We also wish to thank Kirsi Pylkkänen for excellent technical assistance, Mervi Laukkanen for typing the manuscript, and Dr. Kari Alitalo for critical comments on the manuscript.

This study was supported by the Finnish Medical Foundation, the Finnish Cancer Research Organization, Svenska Nationalföreningen mot hjärt- och lungsjukdomar and The Swedish Cancer Society. Part of the work was carried out under contract with the Finnish Life and Pension Insurance Companies.

REFERENCES

1. Little CD, Nau MM, Carney DN, Gazdar AF, Minna JD: Nature 306:194, 1983.
2. Gazdar AF, Carney DN, Nau MM, Minna JD: Cancer Res 45:2924, 1985.
3. Saksela K, Bergh J, Lehto V-P, Nilsson K, Alitalo K: Cancer Res 45:1823, 1985.

4. Carney DN, Gazdar AF, Bepler G, Guccion JG, Marangos PJ, Moody TW, Zweig MH, Minna JD: Cancer Res 45:2913, 1985.

5. Radice PA, Matthews MJ, Ihde DC, Gazdar AF, Carney DN, Bunn PA, Cohen MH, Fossieck BE, Makuch RW, Minna JD: Cancer 50:2894, 1982.

6. Schwab M, Alitalo K, Klempnauer K-H, Varmus HE, Bishop JM, Gilbert F, Brodeur G, Goldstein M, Trent J: Nature 305:245, 1983.

7. Nau MM, Brooks BJ, Battey J, Sausville E, Gazdar AF, Kirsch IR, McBride OW, Bertness V, Hollis GF, Minna JD: Nature 318:69, 1985.

8. Seeger RC, Brodeur GM, Sather H, Dalton A, Siegel SE, Wong KY, Hammond D: N. Engl J Med 313:1111, 1985.

9. Schwab M, Varmus HE, Bishop JM: Nature 316:160, 1985.

10. Kohl NE, Legouy E, DePinho RA, Nisen PD, Smith RK, Gee CE, Alt FW: Nature 319:73, 1986.

11. Stanton LW, Schwab M, Bishop JM: Proc Natl Acad Sci USA 83:1772, 1986.

12. Hann SR, Thompson CB, Eisenman RN: Nature 314:366, 1985.

13. Stewart TA, Bellve AR, Leder P: Science 226:707, 1984.

14. Rothberg PG, Erisman MD, Diehl RE, Rovigatti UG, Astrin SM: Mol Cell Biol 4:1096, 1984.

15. Slamon D, de Kernion JB, Verma IM, Cline MJ: Science 224:256, 1984.

16. Land H, Parada LF, Weinberg RA: Nature 304:596, 1983.

17. Downward J, Yarden Y, Mayes E, Scrace G, Totty N, Stockwell P, Ullrich A, Schlessinger J, Waterfield MD: Nature 307:521, 1984.

18. Libermann TA, Nusbaum HR, Razon N, Kris R, Lax I, Soreq H, Whittle N, Waterfield MD, Ullrich A, Schlessinger J: Nature 313:114, 1985.

19. Ozanne B, Shum A, Richards CS, Cassells D, Grossman D, Trent J, Gusterson B, Hendler F: In: Feramisco J, Ozanne B, Stiles C, (eds): "Growth Factors and Transformation." Cold Spring Harbor, NY: Cold Spring Harbor Laboratory, 1985, pp 41–49.

20. Holthöfer H, Miettinen A, Lehto V-P, Lehtonen E, Virtanen I: Lab Invest 50:552, 1984.

21. Bergh, J, Esscher T, Steinholtz L, Nilsson K, Påhlman S: Am J Clin Pathol 84:1, 1985.

22. Påhlman S, Esscher T, Bergvall P, Odelstad L: Tumor Biol 5:127, 1984.

23. Lowry OH, Rosebrough NJ, Farr AL, Randell RJ: J Biol Chem 193:265, 1951.

24. Winqvist R, Mäkelä TP, Seppänen P, Jänne OA, Alhonen-Hongisto L, Jänne J, Grzeschik K-H, Alitalo K: Cytogenet Cell Genet (in press), 1986.

25. Påhlman S, Esscher T, Nilsson K: Lab Invest (in press), 1986.

26. Bergh J, Nilsson K, Dahl D, Andersson L, Virtanen I, Lehto V-P: Lab Invest 51:307, 1984.

Journal of Cellular Biochemistry 31:305–312 (1986)
Cellular and Molecular Biology of Tumors and
Potential Clinical Applications   17–24

Differential Expression of Metastasis-Associated Cell Surface Glycoproteins and mRNA in a Murine Large Cell Lymphoma

Garth L. Nicolson, Ronald A. LaBiche, Marsha L. Frazier, Mark Blick, Robert J. Tressler, Christopher L. Reading, Tatsuro Irimura, and Varda Rotter

Departments of Tumor Biology (G.L.N., R.A.L., C.L.R., R.J.T., T.I.), Medical Oncology (M.L.F.), and Clinical Immunology and Biological Therapy (M.B.), The University of Texas M.D. Anderson Hospital and Tumor Institute, Houston, Texas, and Department of Cell Biology, The Weizmann Institute of Science, Rehovot, Israel (V.R.)

A metastatic variant cell subline of the Abelson virus-transformed murine large lymphoma/lymphosarcoma RAW117 has been selected in vivo ten times for liver colonization. Highly metastatic subline RAW117-H10 forms greater than 200 times as many gross surface liver tumor nodules as the parental line RAW117-P. Analysis of cellular proteins and glycoproteins indicates reduced expression of murine Moloney leukemia virus-associated p15, p30, and gp70, and increased expression of a sialoglycoprotein, gp150, in the highly metastatic H10 cells. Northern analyses of oncogene expression suggested that mRNA of various oncogenes was expressed equally or not expressed in the RAW117 cells of differing metastatic potential. Differential gene expression was examined using a cDNA library of 17,600 clones established from poly A+ mRNA isolated from H10 cells. The cDNA library was screened by the colony hybridization technique using probes made from both RAW117-P and -H10 cells. Approximately 99.5% of these cDNA clones were expressed identically in P and H10 cells. Of the few differentially expressed cDNA clones (approx. 150/17,600), one-half of these were identified as Moloney leukemia virus sequences in a separate probing with a radiolabeled Moloney leukemia virus probe. The remainder of the differentially expressed mRNA detected by colony hybridization of the cDNA library were expressed at higher levels (approx. 1/6) or lower levels (approx. 1/3) in the highly metastatic H10 cells.

Key words: tumor metastasis, gene expression, oncogenes, virus antigens, glycoproteins

Highly malignant cells express unique properties that in combination with host environment are important in metastasis formation [1–6]. Some of these unique

Received February 13, 1986; revised and accepted May 5, 1986.

properties have been identified by comparing animal tumor cells of differing meta-static behaviors [1,2,4–6]. One such tumor cell model for large cell lymphoma metastasis has been established from the Abelson murine leukemia virus (AbMLV)-transformed cell line RAW117 [7]. The parental cell line (RAW117-P) of recent origin has a very low potential to metastasize to organs such as lung, liver, spleen, and lymph nodes in BALB/c mice; however, after ten sequential in vivo selections for liver colonization, a variant subline (RAW117-H10) was established that is highly metastatic to liver and rapidly kills its host [8]. This H10 subline forms more than 200 times as many gross surface liver tumor nodules after intravenous or subcuta-neous injection than does the parental line [8–10].

Comparison of the biochemical and immunological properties of RAW117-P and -H10 cells indicates that there are specific changes in the highly metastatic cells. For example, differences in the exposures of cell surface proteins [11] and glycopro-teins [10,12], amounts of viral antigens [10] and lectin-binding sites [12,13], partition-ing behavior in two-phase aqueous solutions [14], sensitivity to host effector systems [15,16], and presence of liver adhesion molecules [17] have been documented in the RAW117 system. We have examined whether these changes are related to the expres-sion of oncogenes or oncogene products [18], and whether the differential expression of RAW117 genes can be used to identify the genes responsible for the malignant behavior of RAW117-H10 cells.

MATERIALS AND METHODS
Cells and Metastasis Assays

RAW117 parental (RAW117-P) cells and a subline selected ten times for liver colonization (RAW117-H10) were established and grown in Dulbecco-modified Eagle's medium (DME) containing 10% fetal bovine serum (FBS) as described previously [8–10]. Cell cultures were used within ten passages from frozen stocks of low-passage cells to eliminate possible drift in metastatic and other properties [9]. Cultures were tested for the presence of *Mycoplasmas* using Hoechst 33258 staining [19] and were found to be negative. RAW117 sublines were assayed for organ colonization by intravenous injection of 5×10^3 viable tumor cells in 0.1 ml phosphate buffered saline (PBS) [5–10]. Mice were killed at specific times after injection, and visible surface tumor nodules were counted in all major organs and were confirmed by histologic examination [12].

Cellular Glycoproteins

Chemical pretreatment of separated RAW117 glycoproteins in polyacrylamide gels and reaction of the glycoproteins with ^{125}I-labeled lectins were performed as described by Irimura and Nicolson [20,21]. The lectins used were wheat germ agglutinin (WGA), *Lens culinaris* hemagglutinin (LCH), and concanavalin A (Con A). All lectins were purified by affinity chromatography and radiolabeled as described previously [20,21]. Standard glycoproteins with known carbohydrate chain structures were separated in adjacent lanes and stained simultaneously with the same ^{125}I-labeled lectins. Binding of ^{125}I-labeled lectins to the RAW117 cellular glycoproteins and to standard glycoproteins was assessed by autoradiography [10–13].

Analysis of mRNA

Total RNA was prepared [22,23] and polyadenylated (poly A+) mRNA was selected by oligo(dT)-cellulose chromatography [24]. Aliquots were heated at 60°C for 10 min and were electrophoresed in a 1.1% agarose gel containing 6.5% formaldehyde as described [18,25]. The RNA was transferred onto nitrocellulose paper [26], and hybridized to nick-translated plasmid inserts containing specific sequences [18,25,27].

cDNA Library

Double-stranded complementary DNA (ds-cDNA) made from RAW117-H10 poly A$^+$ RNA was cloned into pBR322 according to the method of Gubler and Hoffman [28] except that the *Pst* I site was used, and annealing was by homopolymeric tailing (C-tailed insert, G-tailed vector). Colonies were established and replicated by direct contact [29]. Probes were made from RAW117-P and -H10 poly A$^+$ RNA by preparing ds-cDNA [28], except that ^{32}P-dCTP was added to the second strand synthesis reaction. The filters were hybridized and washed prior to autoradiography [30].

RESULTS

Intravenous (IV) injection of $1-5 \times 10^3$ RAW117-P cells into groups of BALB/c mice produced few visible lung (median = 0) or liver (median = 0) surface tumor nodules within 2 wk, whereas injection IV of similar members of RAW117-H10 cells produced large numbers of liver tumor nodules (>200 in all animals) but few lung tumor nodules (median = 1). Differences in liver tumor colonies were also found when RAW117-P and -H10 cells were injected subcutaneously (SC) into BALB/c mice [10].

The cell surface glycoproteins of RAW117 cells have been identified by sodium dodecyl sulfate (SDS)-polyacrylamide slab gel electrophoresis and labeling of the gels with ^{125}I-lectins [10,12]. Labeling the separated glycoproteins from RAW117-P and -H10 cells with ^{125}I-Con A revealed a relative decrease in a $M_r \sim 70,000$ band and a relative increase in a $M_r \sim 150,000$ band in the RAW117-H10 cells (Table I) [10]. When ^{125}I-WGA or ^{125}I-LCH was used to label the separated glycoproteins after electrophoresis, similar increases were found in the amounts of a WGA-binding sialoglycoprotein component of $M_r \sim 130,000-200,000$ and a LCH-binding component of $M_r \sim 150,000$ (Table I) [13].

The $M_r \sim 70,000$ component that is dramatically reduced in expression on RAW117-H10 cells has been identified as gp70, the major Moloney leukemia virus

TABLE I. Expression of Some Viral and Cell Surface Proteins and Glycoproteins in RAW117 Cells

RAW117 subline	Relative amounts of RAW117 component expressed in parallel experiments				
	p15	p30	gp70	gp150	sialo-gp
P	1.00[a]	1.00[a]	1.00[a], 1.00[b]	1.00[b], 1.00[c]	1.00[d]
H5	0.57[a]	0.24[a]	0.26[a], 0.3[b]	1.8[b], ND[e]	ND[e]
H10	0.03[a]	0.03[a]	0.12[a], 0.1[b]	2.5[b], 2.2[c]	2.2[d]

[a]Determined by competition radioimmune assay [10].
[b]Estimated by binding of ^{125}I-Con A to SDS gels [10].
[c]Estimated by binding of ^{125}I-LCH to SDS gels [13].
[d]Estimated by binding of ^{125}I-WGA to SDS gels [13].
[e]ND, not determined

(MoMuLV)-encoded envelope glycoprotein. Competition radioimmune assays on other MoMuLV-encoded components, such as the internal proteins p15 and p30, also revealed lower amounts in the highly metastatic H10 cells (Table I) [10]. Examination of a variety of in vivo and in vitro selected sublines and clones indicated that the loss of gp70 directly correlated (r = 0.93) with increased malignancy [9].

RAW117 cells express a variety of transformation-related products. For example, the oncogene p53 was found to be expressed in RAW117 cells [25]. When the expression of p53 was compared in RAW117-P and -H10 cells, however, there was no detectable difference in the expression of the p53 message (Table II) or its encoded product [25]. Examination of the AbMuLV oncogene v-abl also revealed its equivalent expression of RAW117 cells of low or high metastatic potential (Table II) [18]. In addition, immunoprecipitation of abl-encoded p160 revealed similar amounts of this protein in RAW117-P and -H10 cells [18]. Other oncogenes, such as fos, myc, and myb were either not expressed or equivalently expressed in RAW117 cells of low or high metastatic potential (Table II) [18].

Since several MoMuLV-encoded and other proteins but not oncogenes were found to be expressed differentially in RAW117 cells of low and high malignant potential, we examined differences in gene expression by gene cloning and colony hybridization techniques. A pBR322 cDNA library of 17,600 clones was established from poly A$^+$ RNA of RAW117-H10 cells [30]. The H10 gene library was screened using the colony hybridization procedure by replicate exposure of the cDNA clones to ^{32}P-cDNA prepared from the poly A$^+$ RNA of RAW117-P (Fig. 1) and -H10 cells (Fig. 2). Several differences in gene expression were noted in the RAW117 system (Table III) [30]. Most of these differences were attributed to MoMuLV genes, as determined in a separate probing with a ^{32}P-labeled MoMuLV probe (Fig. 3). However, some non-MoMuLV mRNAs were expressed at higher levels in RAW117-P cells, and a few were expressed at higher levels in RAW117-H10 cells (Table III).

DISCUSSION

The numbers and locations of RAW117 metastases in BALB/c mice are determined by a number of tumor cell properties. In our studies, we have found that highly metastatic RAW117 cells progressively lose expression of MoMuLV antigens and glycoproteins [9,10,13] without loss of expression of the AbMuLV oncogene abl. These results suggest that host antitumor responses might be involved in selecting RAW117 cells that lose viral antigens and are less sensitive to host effector mechanisms. In an examination of various host antitumor response mechanisms active against RAW117 cells, we found that these cells were equally insensitive to T-cell, NK-cell, or NC-cell-mediated responses [15]. However, when we assayed RAW117

TABLE II. Expression of Oncogenes in RAW117 Cells by Northern Analysis

RAW117 subline	Relative amounts of oncogene mRNA expressed in parallel experiments[a]				
	abl	fos	myc	myb	p53
P	+++	−	+	+	++
H10	+++	−	+	+	++

[a]−, not detectable; +, detectable; ++, expressed in moderate amounts; +++, expressed in high amounts by Northern analysis [18, 25].

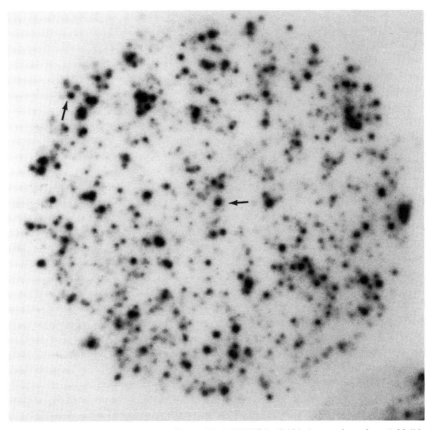

Fig. 1. Colony hybridization of library filter with RAW117-P cDNA (approximately ×1.32 life size). [^{32}P]dCTP-labeled probe derived from RAW117-P poly A$^+$ RNA was incubated with cloned RAW117-H10 cDNA fixed to nylon filters to detect homologous sequences. After subsequent autoradiography, the probe was stripped off to allow reprobing. Arrows indicate differentially hybridizing colonies.

cells for their sensitivities to macrophage-mediated cytolysis and cytostasis, we found that the highly metastatic RAW117-H10 cells were significantly less sensitive to macrophage-mediated responses [16]. Indeed, impairment of macrophage–mediated antitumor responses by administration of chlorine, silica, trypan blue, carrageenan, cyclosphosphamide, or pristane to animals before injection of RAW117 cells increased the malignancies of the low metastatic RAW117-P line [15]. In contrast to our findings, Thorgeirsson et al [31] found that NIH/3T3 cells transfected with T24 c-H-*ras* genes were metastatic in nude mice and were more sensitive to NK- and macrophage-mediated cytotoxicity than control NIH/3T3 cells.

Host antitumor responses may be important in determining the degree of metastasis in some tumor systems, but they are probably not very important in determining the locations of metastases [9,15]. The liver-selected RAW117-H series probably colonies liver, in part, because of an increased expression of liver-binding cell surface receptor(s) [9,17]. Blocking these surface receptors with F(ab′)$_2$ antibodies abolishes the ability of RAW117-H10 cells to colonize liver, but not lung [17]. In addition to cell surface receptors involved in organ homing, RAW117 cells selected for liver colonization also show differential growth characteristics in liver-conditioned me-

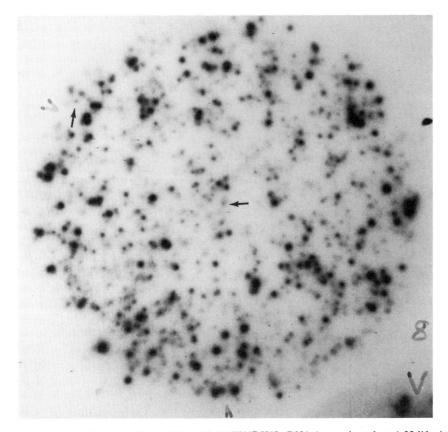

Fig. 2. Colony hybridization of library filter with RAW117-H10 cDNA (approximately ×1.32 life size). Procedure was the same as in Figure 1 except that the probe was derived from RAW117-H10 poly A⁺ RNA. Arrows indicate differentially hybridizing colonies.

TABLE III. Differential Gene Expression in RAW117 Cells by Colony Hybridization Analysis

Type	No. colonies	Percentage of abundance
Total library	17,600	100.00
Estimated differentially expressed	~160	~0.9
Estimated total MoMuLV	~75	~0.43
Estimated non-MoMuLV higher in P	~65	~0.36
Estimated non-MoMuLV higher in H10	~20	~0.12

dium, suggesting that the growth of metastatic cells is also regulated, in part, by organ microenvironment [32–34].

We have found that the increased abilities of RAW117 cells to metastasize to liver is not related to oncogene (*abl*, *fos*, *myc*, p53) expression [18,25]. Although examination of advanced neuroblastomas [35] and lung cancers [36] suggested that oncogene expression might be related to malignant properties, we have not found any evidence in the RAW117 system to support this possibility. In other metastatic tumor systems that have been examined for expression of oncogenes, differences were also not found [37], suggesting that overexpression of oncogenes is not a requirement for expression of the highly metastatic phenotype. Once cells are transformed, additional

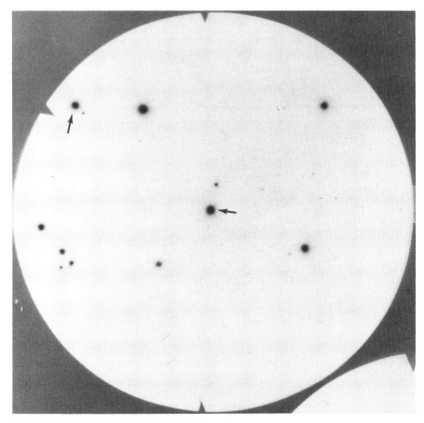

Fig. 3. Colony hybridization of library filter with MoMuLV cDNA (approximately ×1.32 life size). [32P]-labeled probe derived from cloned Moloney leukemia virus cDNA was incubated with cloned RAW117-H10 cDNA fixed to nylon filters to detect homologous sequences. Arrows indicate colonies that exhibited differential hybridization between RAW117-P and RAW117-H10 probes.

expression of oncogenes may not be required to achieve the metastatic phenotype [38,39].

We have identified several non-MoMuLV mRNAs that are differentially expressed in RAW117-P and -H10 cells. Presumably, some of these mRNAs code for proteins and glycoproteins whose expression is required to maintain the highly metastatic phenotype. Determining the identity of the encoded products of these differentially expressed genes could yield additional insights into the components and properties required for a cell to achieve the metastatic state.

REFERENCES

1. Nicolson GL: Biochim Biophys Acta 695:113, 1982.
2. Nicolson GL: Exp Cell Res 150:3, 1984.
3. Nicolson GL: Clin Exp Metastasis 2:85, 1984.
4. Nicolson GL, Poste G: Curr Prob Cancer 7(6):1, 1982.
5. Nicolson GL, Poste G: Curr Prob Cancer 7(7):1, 1983.
6. Nicolson GL, Poste G: Int Rev Exp Pathol 25:77, 1983.
7. Raschke WC, Ralph P, Watson J, Sklar M, Coon H: J Natl Cancer Inst 54:1249, 1975.
8. Brunson KW, Nicolson GL: J Natl Cancer Inst 61:1499, 1978.

9. Nicolson GL, Mascali JJ, McGuire EJ: Oncodev Biol Med 4:149, 1982.
10. Reading CL, Brunson KW, Torriani M, Nicolson GL: Proc Natl Acad Sci USA 77:5943, 1980.
11. Nicolson GL, Reading CL, Brunson KW: In Crispen RG (ed): "Tumor Progression." Amsterdam: Elsevier North Holland, 1980, pp 31–48.
12. Reading CL, Belloni PN, Nicolson GL: J Natl Cancer Inst 64:1241, 1980.
13. Irimura T, Tressler RJ, Nicolson GL: Exp Cell Res (in press), 1986.
14. Miner KM, Walter H, Nicolson GL: Biochemistry 20:6244, 1981.
15. Reading CL, Kraemer PM, Miner KM, Nicolson GL: Clin Exp Metastasis 1:135, 1983.
16. Miner KM, Nicolson GL: Cancer Res 43:2063, 1983.
17. McGuire EJ, Mascali JJ, Grady SR, Nicolson GL: Clin Exp Metastasis 2:213, 1984.
18. Rotter V, Wolf D, Blick M, Nicolson GL: Clin Exp Metastasis 3:77, 1985.
19. Chen TR: Exp Cell Res 104:255, 1977.
20. Irimura T, Nicolson GL: Carbohydr Res 115:209, 1983.
21. Irimura T, Nicolson GL: Cancer Res 44:791, 1984.
22. Auffray D, Rougeon F: Eur J Biochem 107:303, 1980.
23. Glisin W, Crkvenjakov R, Byus C: Biochemistry 13:2633, 1974.
24. Aviv H, Leder P: Proc Natl Acad Sci USA 69:1408, 1972.
25. Rotter V, Wolf D, Nicolson GL: Clin Exp Metastasis 2:199, 1984.
26. Thomas PS: Proc Natl Acad Sci USA 77:5201, 1970.
27. Rigby PW, Dieckmann M, Rhodes C, Berg P: J Mol Biol 113:237, 1977.
28. Gubler U, Hoffman BJ: Gene 25:263, 1983.
29. Hanahan D, Meselson M: Gene 10:63, 1980.
30. La Biche RA, Frazier ML, Brock WA, Nicolson GL: (in preparation), 1986.
31. Thorgeirsson UP, Turpeenniemi-Hujanen T, Williams JE, Westin EH, Heilman CA, Talmadge TE, Liotta LA: Mol Cell Biol 5:259, 1985.
32. Hart IR: Cancer Metastasis Rev 1:5, 1982.
33. Nicolson GL: In Welch DR, Bhuyan BK, Liotta LA (eds): "Cancer Metastasis: Experimental and Clinical Strategies." New York: Alan R. Liss, Inc., 1986, pp 25–43.
34. Nicolson GL, Dulski K: Int J Cancer (in press), 1986.
35. Brodeur GM, Seeger RC, Schwab M, Varmus H, Bishop J: Science 224:1121, 1984.
36. Little CD, Nau MM, Carney DN, Gazdar AF, Minna JD: Nature 306:194, 1983.
37. Kris RM, Avivi A, Bar-Eli M, Alon Y, Carmi P, Schlessinger J, Raz A: Int J Cancer 35:227, 1985.
38. Nicolson GL: Cancer Metastasis Rev 3:25, 1984.
39. Nicolson GL: Clin Exp Metastasis 2:85, 1984.

Journal of Cellular Biochemistry 32:1–10 (1986)
Cellular and Molecular Biology of Tumors and
Potential Clinical Applications 25–34

Expression of Epidermal Growth Factor Receptor and Associated Glycoprotein on Cultured Human Brain Tumor Cells

Peter A. Steck, Gary E. Gallick, Steve A. Maxwell, William S. Kloetzer, Ralph B. Arlinghaus, Richard P. Moser, Jordan U. Gutterman, and W.K. Alfred Yung

Departments of Neuro-Oncology, Tumor Biology, and Clinical Immunology, The University of Texas, M.D. Anderson Hospital and Tumor Institute at Houston, Texas 77030 (P.A.S., G.E.G., S.A.M., R.P.M., J.U.G., W.K.A.Y.) and Johnson and Johnson Biotechnology Center, La Jolla, California 92037 (W.S.K., R.B.A.)

The expression of epidermal growth factor (EGF-R) in normal glial and glioma cells grown in culture was examined by using several independent assays. Immunoprecipitation with the monoclonal antibody R1 of extracts from metabolically labeled glial and glioma cells revealed a protein of $M_r \sim 170,000$, with a migration in sodium dodecyl sulfate-polyacrylamide gels identical to the EGR-R of A431 epidermal carcinoma cells. Furthermore, in the majority of glioma extracts, a protein of $M_r \sim 190,000$ was specifically immunoprecipitated by this antibody. Similar results were obtained by immunoblotting with a second antibody directed against a synthetic peptide in the sequence of the v-erb-B oncogene. In cell lines expressing both proteins, each was specifically phosphorylated on tyrosine in immune complex kinase assays. The majority of glioma cells bound between 40,000 to 80,000 ^{125}I-labeled epidermal growth factor molecules per cell. These results suggest that the expression of EGF-R is common in cultured human glioma cells. In addition, a structurally related protein, is expressed in some of these cells.

Key words: epidermal growth factor, brain tumors, cell surface glycoproteins

Epidermal growth factor (EGF) is a mitogenic polypeptide for a variety of cells in vitro and in vivo and has been extensively studied in terms of its biochemistry and

Abbreviations used: EGF-R, epidermal growth factor receptor(s); EGF, epidermal growth factor; DME/F12, Dulbecco's modified minimal essential medium/Ham's F12 medium; PBS, phosphate-buffered saline; DPBS, Dulbecco's phosphate-buffered saline; EDTA, ethylenediaminetetraacetic acid; SDS, sodium dodecyl sulfate; PAGE; polyacrylamide gel electrophoresis; FBS, fetal bovine serum; Hepes, N-Z-hydroxyethylpiperazine-N'-Z-ethanesulfanic acid; BSA, bovine serum albumin. The single-letter amino acid nomenclature follows the rules as stated in J Biol Chem 250:14–42, 1985.

Received February 12, 1986; accepted June 9, 1986.

mode of action [1–4]. The binding of EGF to its target cells involves a specific membrane glycoprotein, epidermal growth factor receptor (EGF-R), and initiates a cascade of events resulting in cellular proliferation. An early response to the binding of EGF is the phosphorylation of a number of endogenous proteins [5,6]. The protein kinase activity has been shown to be associated with the EGF-R glycoprotein itself and to be a cyclic nucleotide-independent tyrosine protein kinase [7–9]. A major substrate of the in vitro phosphorylation appears to be EGF-R as identified by biochemical and immunological procedures. Furthermore, Downward et al [10] have shown sequence homology between EGF-R and the oncogene product v-erb B.

The overexpression of EGF-R has been reported for most squamous cell carcinomas [11], the A431 carcinoma cell line [5], and recently for some primary brain tumors [12]. Libermann et al [12] showed that the expression of EGF-R kinase activity was increased significantly in a number of non-neural brain tumor tissues over that in normal brain specimen without EGF stimulation. Furthermore, a few human malignant glioblastomas were observed to have an amplified and possibly rearranged EGF-R gene [13]. However, previous reports have demonstrated the similar binding of EGF to both human glioma and normal glial cells in culture [14]. To examine the difference in the binding of EGF to cells and the enzymatic activities of EGF-R, we investigated the expression of EGF-R on a number of human glial and glioma cells in culture with several independent assays. We observed the expression of the EGF-R ($M_r \sim 170,000$) on cells of glial origin. Furthermore, another protein of $M_r \sim 190,000$ cross-reacted with both antibody preparations. The possible relationship between EGF-R and the M_r 190,000 protein is discussed.

MATERIALS AND METHODS
Cells and Culture Conditions

Cell lines were derived from surgical specimens of primary brain tumors or from brain tissue specimens from patients with unrelated trauma. The glial origin of the cells was assessed by the presence of glial acidic fibrillary protein, DNA content, and morphologic histologic criteria as described [15]. The glioma cell lines (EFC-2, KE, LG, AO$_2$, MB, CT-3, CT-1, and PL-1) and normal glial cell lines (GB and CDG) were initiated from surgical specimens of human gliomas of different histological grades and of non-neoplastic brain tissues as previously described [15]. Human epidermoid carcinoma A431$_8$ cells were obtained from T. Hunter (Salk Institute, La Jolla, CA). Cells were routinely grown in a mixture of DME/F12 medium (Grand Island Biological Co., Grand Island, NY) containing 10% FBS (Hyclone Lab., Logan, UT) and no antibiotics. Cells were metabolically radiolabeled by incubating the cultures at 37° for 30 min with 1 mCi/ml of [^{3}H]leucine or 100 μCi/ml [^{35}S]methionine in DME/F12 medium, devoid of either leucine or methionine, respectively. Alternatively, the cells were labeled 24 hr with the radioactive precursors at 100 μCi/ml in DME/F12 medium at one tenth the usual concentration of the appropriate amino acid plus 10% FBS.

Immunoprecipitation of EGF-R

The metabolically radiolabeled cells were washed twice with cold PBS, lysed, and homogenized in a detergent-containing buffer (1% Triton X-100, 150 mM NaCl, 1 mM EDTA, 100 KIU /ml aprotinin in 20 mM sodium phosphte, pH 7.5). The lysates were cleared by centrifugation for 10 min at 8,000g, and 5 μl (1 mg/ml) of purified R1 monoclonal antibody R1 [16] was added. After 3 hr 60 μl of formalin-inactivated *Staphylococcus aureus* (Cowan strain) was added, and then precipitates were washed as described by Kessler [17]. The immunoprecipitates were then subjected to SDS-polyacrylamide gel electrophoresis according to the method of Laemmli [18] by using a 5–15% linear acrylamide gradient running gel. For gels containing ^{3}H-labeled or ^{35}S-labeled samples, the gels were processed by fluorography by treatment with Enhance (New England Nuclear, Boston, MA) and then were dried and exposed to x-ray film.

Autophosphorylation of Immunoprecipitated EGF-R Complexes

The cell extracts were prepared as previously described, except that the lysates were clarified by centrifugation in a Beckman Ti 50 rotor (Beckman Instruments, Fullerton, CA) at 100,000g for 60 min at 4°C. R1 antibody (5 μl) was added to the lysate and the mixture was incubated for 1 hr at 4°C, followed by another 15-min incubation after addition of 10 μl of pansorbin. The immune complex was washed twice with 3 ml of a mixture of 0.1% Triton X-100 and 150 mM NaCl in 10 mM sodium phosphate, pH 7.5, and was collected by centrifugation (8,000g, 10 min). The phosphorylation reaction was initiated by addition of 50 μl of 0.1% Triton X-100, 5 μCi of γ-[^{32}P]ATP (adenosine triphosphate, New England Nuclear, 2,000–3,000 Ci/mmol) and 6 mM MnCl$_2$ in 20 mM Hepes, pH 7.0, to the immunoprecipitated pellet. After 10 min on ice, the reaction was terminated by the addition of 3 ml of lysis buffer. The precipitates were washed again and then subjected to SDS-PAGE analysis as already described.

Western Blotting

Immunoblotting of the proteins was performed by a modification of the procedure as described by Towbin et al [19]. Briefly, equal aliquots (100 μg) of cell extracts were subjected to SDS-PAGE on a 5–15% polyacrylamide gradient gel, after which the proteins were electroblotted from the gel onto 0.1 μm nitrocellulose paper for 12–18 hr at 40 V in 20% ethyl alcohol, 5 mM sodium acetate, and 2 mM Hepes pH 8.2. The nitrocellulose paper was then incubated for 3 hr at 37°C in TNE/NP-40 (0.1% NP-40, 150 mM NaCl, 2 mM EDTA, in 50 mM Tris HCl, pH 7.5) containing 3% BSA. The blocking solution was removed and replaced with new buffer that contained antiserum (1:100 dilution) directed against a synthetic v-erb-B polypeptide (described below). Incubation proceeded for 3 hr at room temperature, followed by five washes with TNE/NP-40. Control immunoblots contained 100 μg synthetic polypeptide along with the antiserum. The filters were then incubated for 3 hr with 0.01 μCi/ml of ^{125}I-goat antirabbit IgG (40 μCi/μg; Amersham, Chicago, IL) in TNE/NP-40 plus 3% BSA. After the incubation, the filters were washed five times with TNE/NP-40 and then dried and exposed to x-ray film with intensifying screens. Densitometric scans of the exposed x-ray film were performed by using a Beckman DU-8 spectrophotometer with gel scan accessory.

The antiserum against a synthetic polypeptide of v-erb-B sequence was generated in a manner similar to the method previously described [20]. A hydrophobic domain of the v-erb-B gene product sequence with sequence homology of EGF-R [10] was chosen by using a computer program (Intelligenetics, Inc.) The amino acid sequence of v-erb B 421-437 (LMEEEDMEDIVDADEYL) was synthesized in a Vega solid-phase amino acid synthesizer (Vega Biotechnologies, Inc., Tucson, AZ) using standard procedures. An additional cysteine was added to the C-terminus of the peptide and was used to crosslink it to keyhole-limpet hemocyanin [21]. Antiserum was generated in rabbits by using an initial subcutaneous injection of 200 μg of the conjugate in Freund's complete adjuvant given at multiple sites. Two additional injections followed at 3-wk intervals—200 μg of conjugate in Freund's incomplete adjuvant.

Binding of ^{125}I-Labeled EGF to Glioma Cells

Receptor-grade EGF was purchased from Collaborative Research (Boston, MA) and was radiolabeled with ^{125}I (carrier free; ICN, Irvine, CA) as previously described [3]. Specific activity was determined to be 4.92×10^4 cpm/μg.

Binding assays followed the procedures previously described [3]. Briefly, cells were plated into multiwell plates ($0.5-1 \times 10^5$ cells/well) and cultured for 2 days. The medium was then aspirated, and the cells were washed once with DME/F12 followed by incubation an additional 24 hr in DME/F12 and no serum. The dishes were then washed twice in cold DPBS containing 0.2% BSA. To each well was added 1 ml of ^{125}I-labeled EGF at various concentrations in the DPBS/BSA solution, and then the plates were incubated for 1 hr at 4°C. The cultures were then washed five times with DPBS/BSA, the cells were lysed with 1% SDS in 100 mM NaOH, and radioactivity was determined with a Beckman 8000 gamma counter. Nonspecific binding was determined by using a 100-fold excess of unlabeled EGF.

RESULTS

Detection of EGF-R in Cultured Glioma Cells

Initially, to determine whether glioma cells expressed EGF-R, the ability of a monoclonal antibody, R1, to immunoprecipitated this protein was examined. Cells were metabolically radiolabeled with [^{3}H]leucine or [^{35}S]methionine for 30 min to minimize degradation; then EGF-R was immunoprecipitated as described in Materials and Methods. Figure 1 displays the SDS-PAGE profile from several cultured glioma cells. In most of the glial and glioma cells, a protein of M_r 170,000 was observed (Fig. 1, lowest arrow). These bands migrated in the same position as did an immunoprecipitated protein from A431 cells, which had been demonstrated previously to be EGF-R. In addition to the 170,000 protein (p170), a band with a slower migration M_r 190,000 (p190; Fig. 1, top arrow) was observed in most cells of glial origin. The p190 was not observed to be immunoprecipitated in cultured human fibroblasts, colon, breast, or head and neck carcinoma cells (unpublished observation). A more slowly migrating band (M_r 220,000), observed in CT-3 cells was identified in other experiments as fibronectin, which had been previously observed to bind nonspecifically to *S aureus* protein A. In two cell lines, AO$_2$ and NG-1, no bands were observed at either the 170,000 or the 190,000-dalton molecular weight range. To determine whether this result was due to a slow metabolism rate in these cells, the metabolic labeling period was increased to 24 hr. Under these conditions, a p170 and p190 were observed in AO$_2$ cells. However, these proteins were not observed in NG-1 cells. Two immunoprecipitated bands were consistently seen in the NG-1 cells (with relative molecular weights of 150,000 and 95,000); these bands migrated with the same relative mobility as did immunoprecipitated bands from A431 cells. Preliminary

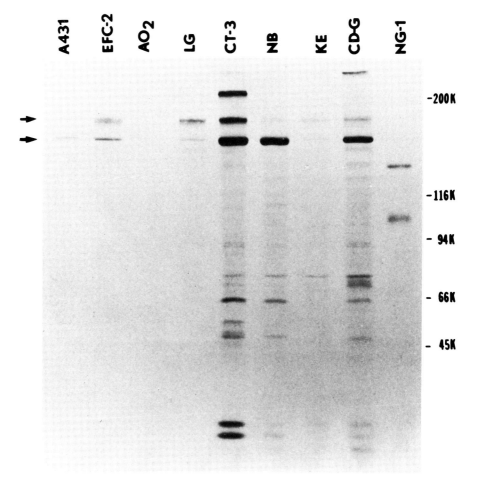

Fig 1.   Immunoprecipitations of glioma, glial, and A431 cell extracts of established cultured cells with a monoclonal antibody directed against EGF-R, followed by SDS-PAGE. Immunoprecipitation was performed as described in Materials and Methods. The top arrow is for an observed band at M_r 190,000, and the bottom arrow is directed toward a band at 170,000 (EGF-R). The protein standards include myosin, galactosidase, phosphorylase b, bovine serum albumin, and ovalbumin, with M_rs ($\times 10^3$) of 200, 116, 94, 66, and 45, respectively.

Southern analysis has suggested that NG-1 cells may contain a rearranged EGF-receptor gene, which may account for this result (unpublished observation).

Immunoblotting

Several explanations might account for the presence of the p190 in R1 monoclonal antibody immunoprecipitates of glial and glioma cell extracts. To determine whether the p190 was a coprecipitating band or whether it shared other similar antigenic determinants with EGF-R, proteins from glial and glioma cell extracts were separated by SDS-PAGE and then were electroblotted onto nitrocellulose paper. Proteins were reacted with an antiserum generated against a synthetic peptide with sequence homology to v-erb B and then with ^{125}I-labeled *S aureus* protein A as described in Materials and Methods. An example of the reactivity with KE cell extracts is shown in Figure 2. Both a p170 and p190 are observed. In contrast, when the specific reactivity of the antiserum is blocked by prior addition of excess free peptide, little or no reactivity is observed in the M_r 170,000–190,000 region (Fig. 2b, blocked). A densitometric scan of the difference in intensities in this region is shown in Figure 2a and indicates that both the p170 and p190 react specifically with this serum. Thus, the ability of a v-erb-B antiserum to react independently with the p170 and p190 suggests that these proteins share antigenic determinants.

Phosphorylation of p170 and p190 in Immune Complex Kinase Assays

To further characterize the p170 and p190 peptides, their ability to undergo posttranslational modifications was examined. In metabolic labeling experiments followed by immunoprecipitation with the R1 monclonal antibody, both p170 and p190 were found to incorporate $[^{32}P]O_4$ and $[^3H]$mannose. Incorporation of mannose

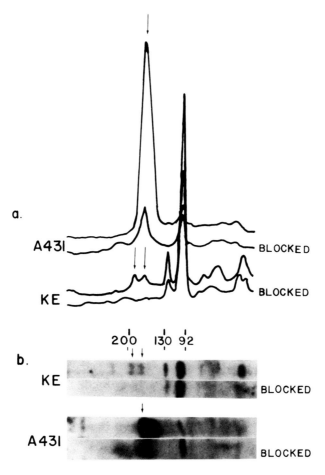

Fig. 2. Immunoblots of A431 and glioma cell KE cell extracts with an antisera generated against a synthetic polypeptide with homology to v-erb-B (see Materials and Methods) after SDS-PAGE. a) The densitometric tracings of the immunoblots shown in (b). The arrows (left to right) show p190 and p170, respectively in (a) and (b). The blocked lanes show that the immunoblot performed in the presence of the synthetic polypeptide. The molecular weight standards are myosin, β-galactosidase, and phosphory-lase b.

into p170 was increased approximately fourfold over that of p190 by similar metabolic labeling (data not shown). Because p170 has been demonstrated to be a tyrosine protein kinase, it was of considerable interest to determine whether the immunoprecipitate proteins had associated kinase activity. Immunoprecipitates containing these proteins were incubated with [^{32}P]ATP as described in Materials and Methods for immunocomplex-kinase assay. The results of the proteins after SDS-PAGE analysis are shown in Figure 3. In each of the glial and glioma cells in which a p170 and p190 were present in immunoprecipitation, these proteins were also found phosphorylated in immune complex kinase assays. Whether p190 is itself also a kinase or is phosphorylated by the kinase associated with EGF-R remains to be determined. Furthermore, both proteins were found to be phosphorylated on tyrosine residues.

Quantitation of Cell-Surface EGF-R

Although direct immunoblotting techniques are not a good quantitative measured of an antigen, both immunoblotting and immunoprecipitation experiments suggested that EGF-R was not significantly overexpressed in normal glial and glioma cells compared with EGF-R expression on A431 cells. To directly measure the number of EGF-R on the cell surface, the binding of ^{125}I-labeled EGF to cells in culture was performed at 4°C. Scatchard plots of the binding data were performed for each of the cell lines, and the calculated number of EGF-R is shown in Table I. For A431 cells, 1.5×10^6 molecules of EGF per cell were bound, in agreement with the published number of receptor sites for these cells [7]. Furthermore, two affinity

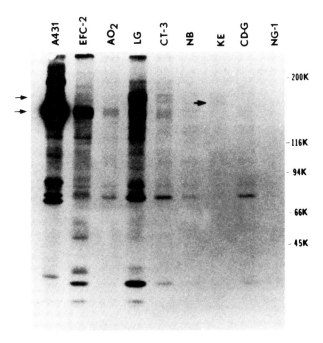

Fig. 3.   Gel electrophoresis of autophosphorylated EGF-R immunoprecipitated with R1 monoclonal antibody from the various cultured glial/glioma cells. Immunoprecipitation of EGF-R-complex kinases were performed as described in Materials and Methods. The top arrow shows phosphorylation of a band of M_r 190,000, and the bottom arrow shows the EGF-R, also demonstrated by A431 cells. The protein standards are the same as those described in Figure 1.

TABLE I. Epidermal Growth Factor Receptor Expression on Cultured Human Glioma Cells

Cell line	Immuno-precipitation[a]	Immunocomplex kinase[a]	Immuno-blot[a]	Binding sites/cell[b]	K_d[b] $(\times 10^{-10})$
A431	170K	170K	170K	1.3×10^6	900
				2.4×10^5	2
EFC-2	170K	170K	170K	4.5×10^4	17
	190K	190K	190K		
KE	170K	170K	170K	7.2×10^4	44
	190K	190K	190K		
LG	170K	170K	170K	14.1×10^4	10
	190K	190K	190K		
AO$_2$	170K	170K	170K	5.4×10^4	6
	190K	190K	190K		
NG-1	120K	—	ND[c]	0	—
	80K				
MB	190K	170K	—	2×10^4	500
	170K				
PL-1	190K	190K	170K	12.2×10^4	6
	170K	170K	150K		
CT-3	170K	170K	—	3×10^4	700
	190K	190K			
CDG	190K	170K	170	5×10^4	2

[a]The immunoprecipitation, immunocomplex kinase and immunoblot was performed as described in Materials and Methods and Figures 1–3. The 170K or 190K refers to the presence of either a p170 or a p190 band.

[b]The binding sites per cell and apparent dissociation constants (K_d) were determined by Scatchard analysis of the binding of ^{125}I-labeled EGF to the various cells as described in Materials and Methods. The analysis was performed by using linear regression by computer.

[c]Not detectable. Due to the high background of nonspecific bands at less than $M_r \sim 130$, specific binding could not be determined.

classes of binding sites were observed for the A431 cells as represented by a biphasic Scatchard plot. The majority of glial and glioma cells were calculated to express between 40,000 and 80,000 EGF-R. Scatchard analysis suggested only one class of binding site (linear relationship), in cells which expressed mainly p170, as well as in cells which expressed both p170 and p190. Whether the single observed class of EGF binding sites is due to experimental limitations or to the interaction of EGF-R with a specific component, particularly p190, cannot be ascertained presently. Studies are underway to examine these possibilities. However, no significant increase in binding of EGF was observed between cells that express approximately equal amounts of p190 and p170 (EFC-Z, KE, LG) and those expressing more p170 and p190 (CDG), suggesting p190 does not bind EGF.

DISCUSSION

Aberrant expressions of growth factors and their receptors are receiving considerable study to determine their possible roles in tumorigenesis and progression. The EGF-R has been implicated with several types of tumors due to its structural similarity to the v-erb-B oncogene and because of the frequency of aberrant expression in many types of human tumors. Several explanations have been proposed for why aberrant expression of these gene products may be involved in tumorigenesis. An altered gene (eg, the v-erb-B gene) may encode a protein in which the kinase is activated independently of EGF binding. Overexpression of the gene products may result in an increase in the mitogenic response induced by EGF. An autocrine mechanism, such as production of transforming growth factor α (a growth-stimulatory factor related to EGF and which binds EGF-R) might also trigger aberrant cell division [22]. In glial cells, which are differentiated, cell division may be relatively slow. Our studies have indicated that these cells nonetheless produce levels of EGF-R that are comparable with levels observed in dividing fibroblasts. Preliminary data have indicated that EGF receptor maybe differentially expressed on actively dividing glial cells compared to their quiescent counterparts (unpublished observation). This would agree with the cell-cycle variation of EGF-R previously shown [23]. Thus, expression of EGF receptor in these cell lines may correlate with active division of cells and may be a result rather than a cause of tumorigenicity. Amplification and rearrangement of EGF receptor, which has been observed in other cells [11,12], may confer further selective advantage.

An additional protein, designated p190, was also observed in most glial and glioma cells. Several types of evidence suggest that this protein might be the product of, or similar to, the human c-neu proto-oncogene. The neu proto-oncogene has been reported to share structural homology with the EGF-R, but is a distinct gene, located on human chromosome 17 [24], in contrast to the EGF-R gene, which is located on human chromosome 7. Our studies have indicated that the p190 is recognized in immunoprecipitates with the R1 monoclonal antibody to EGF-R as well as in immunoblots with an antiserum to a synthetic v-erb-B peptide. Thus, p190 shares some antigenic determinants with EGF-R. Pulse-chase studies (to be presented elsewhere) have indicated that p190 is not a precursor to p170. In addition, p190 appears to incorporate less carbohydrate by metabolic labeling than does p170, an observation that has been reported for the rat c-neu product. Scatchard analysis, which suggests only one class of EGF binding site for the glioma cells, supports the published observations that the neu gene product does not bind EGF, but may be intimately involved with its activity. Thus, while the possibility that p190 is an aberrant form of EGF-R cannot be eliminated, our current evidence suggests that the former represents a distinct gene product.

The possibility that neu is expressed in glioma cells is intriguing, especially as transfection studies have determined that this gene is activated in glioblastomas as well as in neuroblastomas [24]. Whether the expression of p190 that we observe represents normal expression of the c-neu product, or aberrant expression of the "activated" c-neu gene, or, less likely, the expression of an aberrant form of EGF-R, remains to be determined. Future studies should focus on the significance of p190 to growth regulation in glial and glioma cells.

ACKNOWLEDGMENTS

This research is supported by research grants from the John S. Dunn Foundation and the National Cancer Institutes of Health U.S.P.H.S. R01 CA33027 to W.K.A. Yung. This work was aided by NIH grant No. RR5511-23 and R23 CA39803 to G.E.G. and P.A.S. and by grants from the Clayton Foundation for Research and the James E. Lyan Foundation for Research to J.U.G. The R1 antibody was generously supplied by Michael D. Waterfield.

REFERENCES

1. Carpenter G: Ann Rev Biochem 48:193, 1979.
2. Brown KD, Holley RW: J Cell Physiol 100:139, 1979.
3. Carpenter G, Cohen S: J Cell Biol 71:159, 1976.
4. Pas M, Fox CF: Proc Natl Acad Sci USA 75:2644, 1978.
5. Carpenter G, King LJR, Cohen S: J Biol Chem 254:4884, 1979.
6. Cohen S, Carpenter G, King L: J Biol Chem 225:4834, 1980.
7. Ushiro H, Cohen S: J Biol Chem 255:8363, 1980.
8. Hunter T, Cooper JA: Cell 24:741, 1981.
9. Cohen S, Ushiro H, Sloscheck C, Chimknero M: J Biol Chem 257:1523, 1982.
10. Downeward J, Yarden Y, Mayes E, Scrace G, Totty N, Stockwell P, Ullrich A, Schlessinger J, Waterfield MD: Nature 307:521, 1984.
11. Ozanne B, Shum A, Richards CS, Cassels D, Grossman D, Trent J, Gusterson B, Hendler F: Cancer Cell 3:41, 1985.
12. Libermann TA, Razen N, Bartall AD, Yarden Y, Schlessinger J, Soreq H: Cancer Res 44:753, 1984.
13. Libermann TA, Nusbaum H, Razen N, Kris R, Lax I, Soreq H, Whittle N, Waterfield MD, Ullrich A, Schlessinger J: Nature 313:414, 1985.
14. Heldin CH, Westermark B, Wasteson A: Proc Natl Acad Sci USA 78:3664, 1981.
15. Shapiro JR, Yung WKA, Shapiro WR: Cancer Res 42:992, 1982.
16. Waterfield MD, Mayes ELV, Stroobart P, Bennet PLP, Young S, Goodfellow PN, Banting GS, Ozanne B: J Cell Biochem 20:149, 1982.
17. Kessler SW: J Immunol 115:617, 1975.
18. Laemmli UK: Nature 227:680, 1970.
19. Towbin H, Staehelin T, Gordon J: Proc Natl Acad Sci USA 76:4350, 1979.
20. Gallick GE, Sparrow JT, Single B, Maxwell SA, Stanker LH, Arlinghaus RB: J Gen Virol 66:945, 1985.
21. Liu F, Zinnecker M, Hamoka T, Katz D: Biochemistry 79:690, 1979.
22. Todaro GJ, Fryling C, DeLarco JE: Proc Natl Acad Sci USA 77:5528, 1980.
23. Robinson RA, Branum EL, Volkenart ME, Moseo HL: Cancer Res 42:2633, 1982.
24. Schechter AL, Stein DF, Vaidyanathran L, Decker SJ, Drebin JA, Greene MI, Weinberg RA: Nature 312:513, 1984.
25. Schrechter AL, Hung MC, Vaidyanalter L, Weinberg RA, Yang-Feng TL, Francke U, Ullrich A, Cousseno L: Science 29:976, 1985.

Journal of Cellular Biochemistry 32:11–21 (1986)
Cellular and Molecular Biology of Tumors and
Potential Clinical Applications 35–45

Regulated Expression of the c-*myb* and c-*myc* Oncogenes During Erythroid Differentiation

Ilan R. Kirsch, Virginia Bertness, Jonathan Silver, and Gregory F. Hollis

NCI-Navy Medical Oncology Branch, National Cancer Institute, National Institutes of Health, National Naval Medical Center, Bethesda, Maryland 20814 (I.R.K., V.B., G.F.H.) and Laboratory of Viral Diseases, National Institute of Allergy and Infectious Diseases, National Institutes of Health, Bethesda, Maryland 20205 (J.S.)

We have investigated the expression of the genes c-*myb*, c-*myc*, and alpha globin in murine erythroid cells at different stages of development, in viral-induced erythroleukemias, as well as in two mouse erythroleukemia cell lines that can be induced to terminally differentiate when exposed to dimethylsulfoxide. We find that there is a reciprocal correlation between the cell's production of messenger RNA for c-*myb* and globin. c-*myc* message shows a similar but less dramatic decrease coincident with globin RNA production. Initially with the administration of an inducing agent, dimethylsulfoxide, there is a rapid decrease of *myc* and *myb* mRNA, which is followed by signs of differentiation in the induced culture. We conclude that these oncogenes function in early maturational stages of development of these cells. In the erythroleukemic state these genes are down-regulated by forced differentiation and may play a direct role in influencing the state of differentiation of these cells.

Key words: erythroleukemia, red cell maturation, DMSO

A dedifferentiation or block to normal differentiation often accompanies malignant transformation of cells. Quantitative or qualitative changes in oncogene expression in cancerous tissue has been implicated in causing the malignant phenotype. To understand the relationship of oncogenes to malignant transformation we must obtain a more detailed knowledge of the normal expression and functions of these genes during differentiation. Earlier studies on oncogene expression in human hematopoietic cells concluded that certain of these genes, c-*myb* and c-*myc*, were expressed in the less mature cells of the lymphoid, myeloid, and erythroid lineages, although the "erythroid" cell line screened was derived from a chronic myelogenous leukemia cell line [1,2]. Analysis of avian hematopoietic cells also suggests that these oncogenes are expressed differentially during development [3]. Furthermore, Westin et al dem-

Received February 6, 1986; accepted March 27, 1986.

onstrated that in the case of an acute promyelocytic leukemia cell line, HL60, differentiation led to a diminution of c-*myc* expression. Changes in c-*myc* expression during differentiation have also been noted in murine B cells [4] and murine terato-carcinoma cells [5]. Decreased c-*myb* expression during differentiation has previously been reported by Gonda and Metcalf [6], Craig and Block [7], and Sheiness and Gardinier [8]. Recently a decrease in c-*myc* expression during induced differentiation in a murine erythroleukemia cell line has been observed [9].

In this article we report our analyses of oncogene expression in murine erythroid cells in various stages of maturation in vivo. Then, utilizing murine erythroleukemia cell lines that can be induced to differentiate in vitro we follow oncogene expression as cellular differentiation proceeds. We find a reciprocal relationship between the level of expression of the c-*myb* and c-*myc* oncogenes and extent of cellular maturation.

Futhermore, we report a provocative finding that suggests that sudden transient decreases in the level of transcript of these two oncogenes are either causally related or may serve as markers of movement of these cells into a pathway of progressive differentiation. As an outgrowth of this work, we are also able to arrive at an upper limit of the half-lives of these two oncogene messages in this system.

METHODS
Cell Lines and Induction

The inducible murine erythroleukemia cell lines F4-6 (a polycythemic variant) and 745 (an anemic variant) were kindly supplied to us by Dr. J. Billelo, University of Maryland. The cells were grown in Joklik's modified medium supplemented with 10% fetal calf serum. We observed that induction of the cells varied with the batch of fetal calf serum used. However, we obtained essentially identical results on different occasions with separate lots of serum from three different suppliers.

Induction was accomplished by the addition of dimethylsulfoxide (DMSO:SIGMA) to the culture (10^5 cells/ml) at 1.5% v/v. Measurement of induction is based on amounts of globin message produced but can also be assessed by changes in cellular morphology, hemoglobin, orseillein-aniline blue dye staining for stage of cellular development [10], and most simply by cell pellet color.

Spleen Cells

Spleens were obtained from normal, phenylhydrazine-treated, or erythroleu-kemic spleens from mouse strains NFS, Balb/c, C57B1/6, and DBA/2. No significant difference in strains was observed. Phenylhydrazine provocation of erythroid prolif-eration and splenomegaly was performed as previously decribed [11]. Precent of splenic cells of erythroid lineage was judged following Wright-Giemsa and nonspe-cific esterase [12] staining of splenic touch preps.

DNA Probes

The myb probe used was 1.2-kb linkered Bam HI-Bam HI DNA fragment containing the avian v-*myb* oncogene and was kindly given to us by Dr. E.P. Reddy, NIH, Bethesda, MD. The c-*myc* probe used was a 1.5-kb Cla I-EcoRI fragment containing the third exon of the human c-*myc* oncogene. The human *erb* A1, *erb* A2, and *erb* B probes used were the 2.4-kb EcoRI-Hind III fragment, the 1.9-kb EcoRI fragment, and the 2.5-kb EcoRI-Hind III fragment, respectively, given to us by Dr.

B. Vennstrom, EMBL, Heidelberg, FRG. The *ets* probe used was a 1.28-kb BglI insert in plasmid and was kindly given to us by Dr. M. Nunn, Salk Inst., LaJolla, CA. The murine α-globin probe was a 3-kb SstI fragment prepared from a plasmid kindly supplied to us by Y. Nisihoka, McGill University, Montreal. The $\beta_2$microglobulin probe was a cDNA clone kindly supplied to us by J. Seidman, Harvard University, Boston. The β-actin probe was a 1.9-kb Bam HI to Bam HI approximately full length cDNA for human scleroblast cytoplasmic β-actin kindly supplied to us by L. Kedes via J. Battey.

RNA Preparation

RNA was prepared from the spleens and cell lines essentially as described by Chirgwin et al [13]. Ten micrograms of the total RNA was loaded per lane for the "Northern" blots.

Oncogene Screen

We screened Friend virus induced murine erythroleukemia cells for the coincident expression of non-Friend-virus-related oncogenes [14–16]. The oncogenes analyzed, *myb, myc, erb A, erb B,* and *ets,* have all been cited as contributing to the transformed state of erythroid cells in avian systems when carried by acute transforming viruses [14–16]. Only c-*myc* and c-*myb* showed detectable transcription in this system, being seen in both Friend virus- alone and in Friend complex- (Friend helper plus spleen focus-forming virus, SFFV)-induced erythroleukemias.

In Vivo Studies

We then performed a comparative study of alpha-globin, c-*myb*, and c-*myc* gene expression in normal mouse spleen cells, as well as spleen cells from mice that had been treated with the hemolytic-anemia-promoting agent phenlhydrazine, and the Friend- and Friend complex-induced erythroleukemia mentioned above. The normal spleens, containing approximately 5% erythroid cells showed a strong globin hybridizing RNA species but barely detectable *myb* and *myc* transcripts (Fig. 1). We had chosen to study mice treated with phenylhydrazine because of the marked reactivity of their spleens subsequent to the administration of this drug and the anemia it produces [11]. Following injection of this agent, the spleens are noted to increase in weight five- to ten-fold over the next 4 days. At the time of this analysis, the mice manifested a reticulocytosis of 30–50%, and greater than 95% of the mononuclear cells in the spleen were of erythroid lineage. The pattern and amount of globin, *myb*, and *myc* transcripts in these mice did not vary significantly from that seen in the normal spleens. All strains of mice tested (NFS, Balb/c, C57B1/6, DBA/2) and both adult and 6-wk-old weanlings showed essentially this same pattern except for a slight increase in the amount of *myb* and *myc* transcript seen in the younger mice (data not shown).

The Friend-helper-virus-induced erythroleukemia also yielded a mouse with a massively enlarged spleen of greater than 98% erythroid lineage, but with a reticulocytopenia. In the spleens from these mice, a quite different pattern of expression was seen. Much less globin was produced by the erythroleukemic cells, but much more *myb* and *myc* transcript was present in comparison with either normal or phenylhydrazine-treated spleen cells (Fig. 1). By the criteria of spleen cell morphology, reticulocyte count, and globin RNA production, the normal and phenylhydrazine spleens

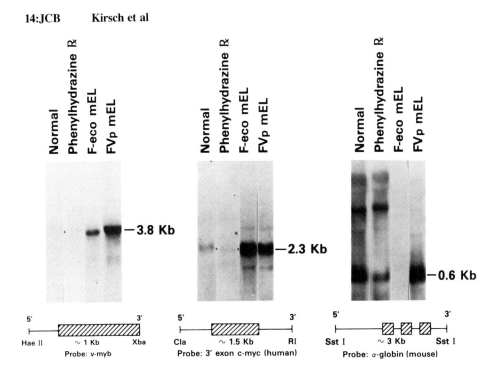

Fig. 1.   RNA transcripts of the *myb* and *myc* oncogenes and a alpha-globin in normal and diseased mouse spleens.

were made up of developmentally more mature erythroid cells than the Friend-virus-induced erythroleukemic spleens. Thus, *myb* or *myc* expression was not increased over the course of the massive erythroid proliferation.

A murine erythroleukemia was also induced by injection of Friend complex, FVp, and RNA was extracted from the spleen cells. In this case, comparatively high amounts of both globin and oncogene transcripts were present (Fig. 1). It is important to note that histologically the Friend complex acute polyclonal erythroleukemic spleen shows a much greater spectrum of erythroid activity (from erythroblasts to reticulocytes) than does the monoclonal, long-latency erythroleukemia induced by Friend virus alone, which demonstrates a narrower spectrum of development dominated by less mature cells.

In Vitro Cell Line Induction

To clarify the relationship between oncogene expression and stage of erythroid development we turned to an inducible murine erythroid cell line system. These widely available cell lines transformed by Friend complex appear to represent cells blocked just prior to terminal differentiation [17,18]. Numerous agents (eg DMSO, hexamethylbisacetamide, hemin, purine, and pyrimidine derivatives) are capable of releasing this block to differentiation [17,18].

Data are shown for analyses performed on a murine erythroleukemia cell line F4-6 induced by a polycythemia (SFFVp) variant of Friend complex. Essentially identical results have been obtained with cell line 745 induced by an anemia (SFFVa) variant of Friend complex. The time course shown represents the results of single experiments. The induction has been performed multiple times with both cell lines and has yielded identical results.

Time zero is the point at which the cells are first exposed to the inducing agent, DMSO, added to give a final concentration of 1.5%. The cells are maintained in the presence of this agent throughout the time course. By day 5, incorporation of ^{3}H-thymidine in the induced cultures was 60% that of control. Cell number in the induced culture was 95% that of control, and viability as measured by trypan blue exclusion was 90–95% in both induced and control cultures.

Alpha-globin messenger RNA, which is barely detectable throughout the experiment in the control culture, shows a steady increase in the induced culture starting at day 1 and reaching a 24-fold increase by day 5 (Fig. 2). In contrast to alpha globin expression, c-*myb* shows a biphasic pattern of expression in the DMSO-induced erythroleukemia cell cultures over the same time course (Figs. 3,4). There is a marked decrease (20-fold) in the amount of c-*myb* RNA by 14 hr after induction (Fig. 3). This result established an upper limit on the half-life of c-myb RNA of 3.5 hr in this system. c-*myb* RNA level begins to increase by 24 hr (greater than 50% of control), peaks around 48 hr (70% of control), then begins a second phase of decrease in the amount of transcript until by day 5 there is 20-fold less c-*myb* RNA than in the control (Fig. 4).

c-*myc* shows a similar dramatic reduction, falling greater than 20-fold by the 4th hr after addition of DMSO in the culture (Fig. 5). This rate of decrease establishes an upper limit on the half-life of c-*myc* RNA in this system to less than 1/2 hr. After this reduction, c-*myc* RNA begins to increase, reaching an amount equivalent to control by 24 hr. The level of c-*myc* RNA then falls gradually during the rest of the experiment, being reduced two-fold below control by day 5 (Fig. 6). These data are summarized graphically in Figure 7.

Detailed studies by others [19–22] have demonstrated that the steroid dexamethasone suppresses the DMSO-induced terminal differentiation of cells in this murine erythroleukemia system. These studies also suggest that this suppression is a posttranscriptional phenomenon. Essential messenger RNA species for terminal differentiation appear to be made in inducer-treated cells but not translated into protein in the presence of dexamethasone.

We examined the expression of the alpha-globin, *myc*, and *myb* messages in our system in the presence of DMSO and 4 μM dexamethasone. The accumulation of alpha-globin mRNA was essentially identical in the induced and "induced plus dexamethasone" treated cultures and not more than three-fold different at 120 hr (Fig. 8). Despite this, only the cells cultured with inducer alone progressed to terminal differentiation and hemoglobin synthesis. Thus, our data are consistent with a post-transcriptional event suppressing evidence of differentiation [19–22]. The messages for the oncogenes *myb* and *myc* showed an identical early shut off at 4 hr in the induced and induced-plus-dexamethasone cultures. However, the cells cultured in the presence of dexamethasone showed an approximately two-fold more rapid rebound accumulation of *myb* and did not show the terminal (hr 120) drop-off seen in the cells cultured with inducer alone.

We wished to determine whether the decrease in message seen from 4 to 14 hr after induction was specific for *myb* and *myc* messages. The baseline alpha-globin message is unaffected at this time, and the beta-actin message shows no decrease over this period relative to control (Fig. 9). Looking at steady-state transcript levels can be

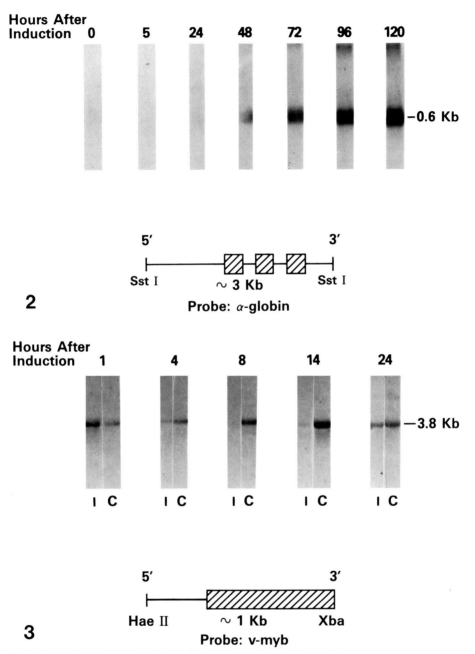

Hours After Induction   0   5   24   48   72   96   120

−0.6 Kb

5′   3′

Sst I   ∼ 3 Kb   Sst I

2   Probe: α-globin

Hours After Induction   1   4   8   14   24

−3.8 Kb

I C   I C   I C   I C   I C

5′   3′

Hae II   ∼ 1 Kb   Xba

3   Probe: v-myb

Fig. 2. Alpha-globin transcripts in a murine erythroleukemia cell line induced to differentiate with DMSO at t = 0. The mouse erythroleukemia cell line F4-6 was grown in Joklik modified medium, 20% fetal calf serum, to 5×10^5 cells/ml then cut back to 10^5 cells/ml and treated with 1.5% DMSO and allowed to continue to grow. Cells were harvested at 0, 5, 24, 48, 72, 96, and 120 hr, and RNA was prepared by the guanidine thicocyanate method [13]. Ten micrograms of total RNA was loaded on a 1% agarose formaldehyde gel and blotted. The blots were hybridized to the nick-translated probe indicated, washed in 15 mM NaCl/1.5 mM sodium citrate, pH 7.0, containing 0.1% NaDodSO$_4$ and visualized by autoradiography.

Fig. 3. c-myb transcripts in a murine erythroleukemia cell line induced to differentiate with DMSO at t = 0. Cells were grown and induced as in Figure 2 and harvested at 1, 4, 8, 14, and 24 hr following induction. Ten micrograms of total RNA was run per lane. The blot was hybridized to the v-myb probe that is diagrammed. Note the sharp decrease in a c-myb transcript occurring between hours 1 and 14. I, induced; C, control.

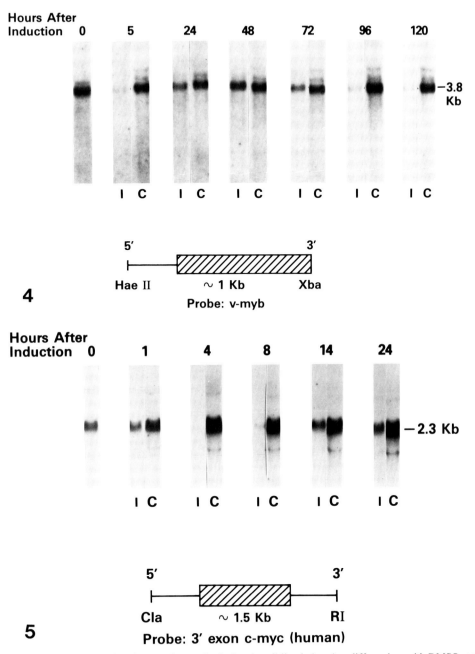

Hours After Induction 0 5 24 48 72 96 120

−3.8 Kb

I C I C I C I C I C I C

5′   3′

Hae II   ∼ 1 Kb   Xba

Probe: v-myb

4

Hours After Induction 0 1 4 8 14 24

−2.3 Kb

I C I C I C I C I C

5′   3′

Cla   ∼ 1.5 Kb   RI

5   Probe: 3′ exon c-myc (human)

Fig. 4. c-*myc* transcripts in a murine erythroleukemia cell line induced to differentiate with DMSO at t = 0. Cells were grown, induced, and harvested and RNA was prepared as in Figure 2. Note the decrease in c-*myb* transcript in the induced culture at hr 5 and 120. I, induced; C, control.

Fig. 5. c-*myc* transcripts in a murine erythroleukemia cell line induced to differentiate with DMSO at t = 0. Cells were grown and induced, and RNA was prepared as in Figure 2. The blot was hybridized to the c-*myc* probe as described. Note the sharp decrease in c-*myc* transcripts in the induced culture of 4 hr following induction. I, induced; C, control.

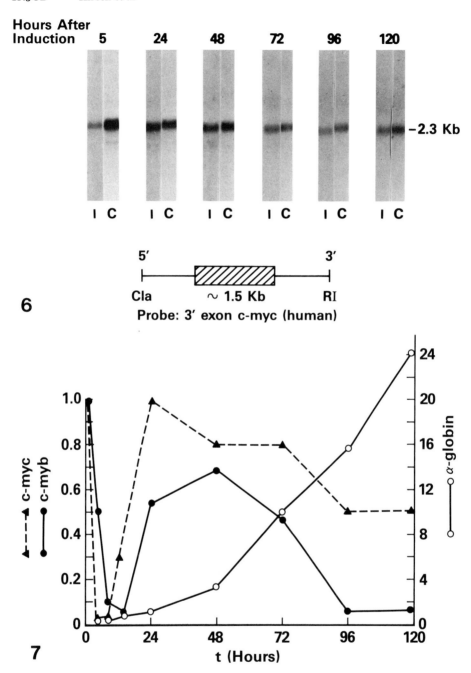

6

7

Fig. 6.   c-*myc* transcripts in a murine erythroleukemia cell line induced to differentiate with DMSO at t = 0. Cells were grown and induced, and RNA was prepared as in Figure 2. I, induced; C, control.

Fig. 7.   Summary of expression of c-*myc*, c-*myc*, and alpha-globin transcripts in murine erythroleukemia cell line F4-6 induced to differentiate with DMSO at t = 0. Densitometric scans were performed on the bands (Fig. 2–6) for each time point. The points on the graph represent the ratio of the density of the band in the induced culture divided by the density of the band in the control culture at each time point.

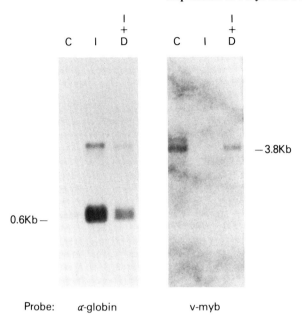

Fig. 8. The effect of dexamethasone on transcript level of alpha globin and c-*myb* in DMSO induced a murine erythroleukemia cell line. Four micromolar dexamethasone was added to an aliquot of the DMSO-induced cells at t = 0. The cells were grown and harvested at t = 120 as described in Figure 2. C, control; I, induced, I + D, induced plus dexamethasone.

deceiving because of differences in the half-lives of the various messages being analyzed. We therefore assessed the level of poly A mRNA transcription in our induced and control cultures during the early phase when the oncogene messages showed such a substantial decrease in the induced cells (hr 3.5–4.5), and then later when the level of transcript was almost that of the control (hr 23.5–24.5). ^{3}H-5 uridine (10μCi/ml) was added for the 1-hr pulses to the induced and control cultures. One hundred μg of labeled total RNA was supplemented with $4,900$ μg of total unlabeled RNA. Poly A mRNA was obtained by three passages of each sample through an oligo dT column as previously described [23]. The RNA was followed by optical density and ethidium-bromide-staining characteristics of the fractions. The counts per minute per microgram of poly A RNA are shown in Table I. The 4 hr induced culture poly A RNA synthesis is at least 59% of the control culture. Given that amount of *myb* and *myc* transcript at 4 hr is less than 5% of the control culture, these data suggest either that DMSO selectively inhibits the RNA polymerase II transcription of certain genes, or that all transcription is shut off equally but that this transiently leads to the disappearance of more short-lived messages. In either case, the effect of this action is a more severe drop in the level of *myb* and *myc* messenger RNA than in messenger RNA with longer half-lives. Despite the continued presence of DMSO in the culture, transcripts of both c-*myb* and c-*myc* have returned practically to baseline level within 24–48 hr.

DISCUSSION

The c-*myb* and *c-myc* oncogenes when inappropriately expressed are capable of contributing to cellular malignant transformation. The normal function(s) of each of

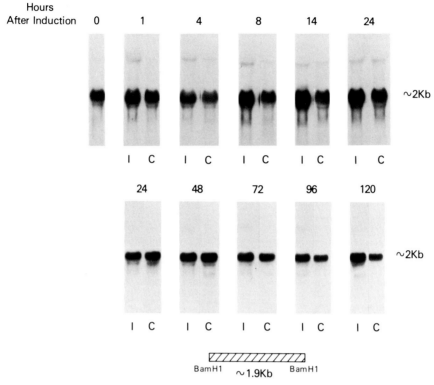

Fig. 9. Beta-actin transcripts in a murine erythroleukemia cell line induced to differentiate with DMSO at t = 0. Cells were grown, induced, harvested, and RNA was prepared as in Figure 2. The blot was prepared as in Figure 2 and hybridized to the human beta-actin probe described. In contrast to alpha-globin, c-*myb*, or c-*myc*, minimal if any changes in beta-actin transcript level is seen during the course of the experiment. I, induced; C, control.

TABLE I. mRNA Synthesis During DMSO Induction

Pulse (hr)	Sample	Oligo dT × 3 μg poly A RNA recovered	^{3}H cpm/μg	Average induced/control (range from two experiments)
3.5–4.5	Control (C)	10.87	1,727	0.59
	Induced (I)	11.66	1,022	(0.56–0.64)
23.5–24.4	Control (C)	14.1	805	1.43
	Induced (I)	5.6	1,155	(1.39–1.46)

these genes remains unclear. Transcripts from these genes are often seen in the presence of cellular proliferation such as that observed by us in the spleen cells of mice with Friend-induced erythroleukemias. But if the net effect of expression of these genes is to stimulate cellular proliferation, it must be a very tightly regulated stimulus as demonstrated by our study of the phenylhydrazine-treated mice. The spleens of these mice were as large on a weight-for-weight basis as their leukemic counterparts, and they had reached that size in a mere 5 days. The percentage of mononuclear cells of erythroid lineage was approximately the same, yet as noted there was a marked discrepancy in oncogene message between these two spleen types.

This observation leads us to consider the possibility that *myc* and *myb* are playing a more fundamental role in determining the differentiated state of erythroid cells. Our data from the studies of the inducible murine erythroleukemic cell lines is consistent with this idea, particularly with respect to c-*myb* whose expression seems to be inversely correlated with the extent of globin production. Unexpectedly, we found a sharp drop in both *myc* and *myb* messages following addition of the inducing agent and prior to any evidence of cellular differentiation. Shortly after the decrease in *myb* and *myc* mRNA, morphologic evidence of differentiation and globin production commences. We cannot say whether DMSO momentarily inhibits all mRNA transcription. At the time of the trough levels of *myb* and *myc* message there is at least 60% the control amount of ^{3}H-uridine incorporation into poly A message. The net effect of any transient inhibition of transcription would be to lower the level of short half-lived messages more than long half-lived messages. Perhaps it will be found that many genes serving important functions for limited times during cellular differentiation will encode mRNAs with relatively short half-lives, making their levels more subject to changes in environmental stimuli.

On the basis of the observations reported in this study, we are currently examining whether the expression of *myb* and *myc* can block differentiation. Our approach is to try and reintroduce these oncogenes into the inducible murine erythroleukemic cells in such a way that we will be able to control the level of their transcription even when an inducing agent is added to the system.

REFERENCES

1. Westin EH, Gallo RC, Arya SK, Eva A, Souza LM, Baluda MA, Aaronson SA, Wong-Staal F: Proc Natl Acad Sci USA 79:2194, 1982.
2. Westin EG, Wong-Staal F, Gelmann EP, Dalla Favera R, Papas TS, Hantenberger JA, Eva A, Reddy EP, Tronick SR, Aaronson SA, Gallo RC: Proc Natl Acad Sci USA 79:2490, 1982.
3. Coll J, Saule S, Martin P, Raes MB, Lagrou C, Graf T, Beng H, Simon IE, Stehelin D: Exp Cell Res 149:151, 1983.
4. McCormack JE, Pepe VH, Kent RB, Dean M, Marshak-Rothstein A, Sorenshein GE: Proc Natl Acad Sci USA 81:5546, 1984.
5. Campisi J, Gray H, Pardee A, Dean M, Sorenshein G: Cell 36:241, 1984.
6. Gonda TJ, Metcalf D: Nature 310:249, 1984.
7. Craig RW, Block A: Cancer Res 44:442, 1984.
8. Sheiness D, Gardinier M: Mol Cell Biol 4:1206, 1984.
9. Lachman HM, Skoultchi AI: Nature 310:592, 1984.
10. Kass L: Am J Clin Pathol 76:302, 1981.
11. Chesebro B, Portis JL, Wesly K, Nishio J: Virology 128:221, 1983.
12. Spivak JL, Marmor J, Dickerman HW: J Lab Clin Med 79:526, 1972.
13. Chirgwin J, Przybyla A, McDonald R, Rutler W: Biochemistry 18:5294, 1979.
14. Ansella J, Geller R, Clarke B, Weeks V, Honoman D: Cell 9:221, 1976.
15. Leprince D, Gegonne A, Coll J, deTaisne C, Schneeberger A, Lagron C, Stehelin D: Nature 306:395, 1983.
16. Graf T, Beug H: Cell 34:7, 1983.
17. Marks PA, Rifkind RA: Annu Rev Biochem 47:419, 1978.
18. Billelo JA, Kuhne J, Warnecke G, Koch G: In Rossi GB (ed) "In Vivo and In Vitro Erythroporiesis: The Friend System." New York: Elsevier North Holland Press, 1980, p 229–238.
19. Chen Z, Banks J, Rifkind RA, Marks PA: Proc Natl Acad Sci USA 79:471, 1982.
20. Murate T, Kaneda T, Rifkind RA, Marks PA: Proc Natl Acad Sci USA 81:3394, 1984.
21. Sheffery M, Marks PA, Rifkind, RA: J Mol Biol 172:417, 1984.
22. Salditt-Georgieff M, Sheffery M, Kranter K, Darnell JE: Rifkind R, Marks PA: J Mol Biol 172:437, 1984.
23. Aviv H, Leder P: Proc Natl Acad Sci USA 69:1408, 1972.

Journal of Cellular Biochemistry 32:23–34 (1986)
Cellular and Molecular Biology of Tumors and
Potential Clinical Applications 47–58

Amplification of RNA and DNA Specific for erb B in Unbalanced 1;7 Chromosomal Translocation Associated With Myelodysplastic Syndrome

Gayle E. Woloschak, Gordon W. Dewald, Rebecca S. Bahn, Robert A. Kyle, Philip R. Greipp, and Robert C. Ash

Mayo Clinic and Foundation, Rochester, Minnesota 55905 (G.E.W., G.W.D., R.S.B., R.A.K., P.R.G.) and Medical College of Wisconsin, Milwaukee, Wisconsin 53226 (R.C.A.)

Previous work has established the presence of an unbalanced chromosome abnormality [+der(1),t(1;7)(p11;p11)] in some therapy-associated myelodysplastic disorders. Recently the EGF receptor has been found to reside at 7p11. Using a probe specific for erb B oncogene, which encodes a truncated form of the EGF receptor, we examined RNA and DNA derived from bone marrow and peripheral blood mononuclear cells from three patients with myelodysplastic syndromes (MDS) and one with acute lymphocytic leukemia (ALL), all bearing an abnormal clone in their bone marrow with a similar unbalanced 1;7 translocation. DNA-excess slot blot hybridization to 5'-32p-labeled cellular RNA revealed from ten- to thirtyfold enhancement in accumulation of mRNA specific for erb B in both peripheral blood and bone marrow cells of the three MDS patients when compared to normal controls. In addition, enhancement of H-ras mRNA accumulation was detected in some, though expression of other genes such as actin, N-ras, myc, src, B-lym, and 20 other genes was not found to be enhanced. Increased erb B expression was not apparent in mononuclear cells from patients with other hematologic disorders such as chronic lymphocytic leukemia, Hodgkin's disease, or lymphoma. Southern blot analysis of restriction-enzyme-cleaved DNA from three MDS patients with an unbalanced 1;7 translocation revealed that erb B gene was amplified at least twentyfold in peripheral blood white blood cells, while levels of actin hybridization were comparable to those of the controls. No such amplification was evident in the ALL patient. Our data suggest that +der(1),t(1;7)(p11;p11) chromosomal anomalies can be specifically associated with amplification of erb B DNA and RNA sequences.

Key words: EGF receptor, oncogene, gene amplification

Chromosomal translocations involving +der(1),t(1;7)(p11;p11) have been found to be associated with myeloproliferative or myelodysplastic syndromes [1–3]. Frequently unbalanced 1;7 translocations of this type are correlated with a history of

Received February 21, 1986; revised and accepted June 3, 1986.

exposure to toxic substances such as alkylating agents, folic acid, environmental agents, or irradiation [1,4,5]. It is of interest that this unbalanced 1;7 translocation involves break and fusion points in chromosomal bands 1p11 and 7p11, and the loss of the 7q arm, centromere, and a small part of 7p arm adjacent to the centromere.

Recent studies have mapped the epidermal growth factor (EGF) receptor gene to 7p11 [6]. Sequence analyses have shown that the erb B oncogene of avian erythroblastosis virus encodes a truncated form of the EGF receptor that is in part responsible for the transforming potential of the virus. The cellular erb B protein product possesses a tyrosine-specific protein kinase activity and is capable of auto- and transphosphorylation [7]. This gene has been shown to be rearranged and/or amplified in a human breast cancer cell line [8], an epidermoid carcinoma cell line [9–10], and human brain tumors of gliomal origin [11]. One recent study, however, demonstrated an enhanced erb B mRNA expression but normal gene copy number in two pancreatic tumor cell lines displaying clonal structural alterations that resulted in overrepresentation of the short arm of chromosome 7 [12]. The similarities between the chromosomal abnormalities reported in pancreatic tumor cell lines and those cells used in this study are unknown.

The experiments described in this report were designed to investigate potential alterations in c-erb B gene structure and expression in cells derived from four patients with hematologic disorders and an abnormal clone containing +der(1),t(1;7)(p11;p11) in their bone marrow. We found amplification of the c-erb B gene as well as enhanced accumulation of erb B-specific mRNA in bone marrow and/or peripheral blood cells of three of these patients.

METHODS
cDNA Probes

pAM91 actin-specific probe was obtained from Dr. A. Minty [13]. c-H-ras, c-K-ras, c-mos, v-src, v-erb A, v-erb B, c-myc, v-fms, N-ras, v-raf, N-myc, and v-fos probes were obtained from American Type Culture Collection. B-lym probe was provided by Dr. G. Cooper, α-tubulin by Dr. C. Veneziale, transferrin receptor by Dr. F. Ruddle, IL2 (interleukin-2) and β-interferon by Dr. Taniguchi, v-fps and v-abl by Dr. A. Balmain, v-rel by Dr. H. Temin, v-bas and v-myb by Dr. R. Scott at the Mayo Clinic, v-fes by Dr. C.J. Sherr, p53 by Dr. Levine, v-sis by Dr. R. Gallo, α-interferon by Dr. C. Weissmann, and ornithine decarboxylase by Dr. Coffino.

Cytogenetics

Chromosome studies were done by using a direct technique for processing of bone marrow aspirates. Slide preparations were stained by GTG-banding or QFQ-banding or both [14]. In each case, 10–40 metaphases were examined.

Southern Blots

Bone marrow or peripheral blood buffy coat cells were obtained from four patients with a +der(1),t(1;7)(p11;p11) in association with hematologic disease (Table I). As a positive control for erb B amplification, the A431 cell line, known to have increased copies of erb B DNA [7], was used. DNA was purified from these cells by extraction in Tris-buffered phenol, precipitation from ethanol, and digestion with 10 μg/ml pancreatic ribonuclease followed by digestion with 50 μg/ml proteinase K [15].

TABLE I. Cytogenetic Data of Patients With an Unbalanced 1;7 Translocation*

Patient	Initial diagnosis	Exposure	Subsequent diagnosis	Specimen	Study	Fraction of metaphases with t(1;7) (karyotype)
1	Primary systemic amyloidosis	Melphalan Prednisone	Primary systemic amyloidosis and MDS	BM	1	27=46,XY/5=46,XY,−7,+der(1),t(1;7)(p11;p11)
					2	24=46,XY/1=46,XY,−7,+der(1),t(1;7)(p11;p11)
2	RARS[a]	Phenylbutazone Anti-inflammatory agents Pyridoxine Folic acid	MDS	BM	1	8=46,XY/8=47,XY,+8/3=46,XY,−7,+der(1),t(1;7)(p11;p11)
					2	17=46,XY/5=46,XY,del(7)(q22q34)/18=47,XY,+8
3	Multiple myeloma	Melphalan Prednisone	MDS	PB	1	20=46,XX
				BM	2	10=46,XX/10=46,XX,−7,+der(1),t(1;7)(p11;p11)
					3	8=46,XX/12=46,XX,−7,+der(1),t(1;7)(p11;p11)
4	ALL[a]	Vincristine Methotrexate Adriamycin Cytoxan L-asparaginase	ALL remission		1	17=46,XY;t(9;22)(q34;q11)
					2	3=46,XY/2=46,XY,t(9;22)(q34;q11)/ 5=46,XY,t(9;22)(q34;q11),+der(1),t(1;7)(p11;p11)

*ALL, acute lymphoblastic leukemia; MDS, myelodysplastic syndrome; RARS, refractory anemia with ringed sideroblasts; BM, bone marrow; PB, peripheral blood.

[a]Fragile site studies on 50 QFQ-banded metaphases revealed the absence of fragile sites.

DNA was digested with the indicated restriction enzymes and subjected to 1.2% agarose gel electrophoresis in E buffer (50 mM boric acid-5 mM $Na_2B_4O_7 \cdot 10H_2O$-10 mM Na_2SO_4-0.1 mM Na_2 EDTA, pH 8.2). In all gels, standard molecular weight markers (Hind III digest of phage λ) were run, and DNA was visualized by staining in ethidium bromide.

DNA was denatured in the gel by incubating for 1 hr at room temperature in 0.5 M NaOH-0.6 M NaCl followed by 1 hr in 1.0 M Tris-HCl (pH 7.4)-1.5 M NaCl at room temperature. DNA from the gel was then transferred to nitrocellulose paper in 20 × SSC (300 mM Na citrate, pH 7.4, 3 M NaCl) for 18–48 hr at 4°C. Blot-bound DNA was hybridized to the appropriate heat-denatured nick-translated DNA probe in Southern hybridization buffer (2.5 μg/ml Poly A, 50 μg/ml herring sperm DNA, 0.1% SDS, 0.2% ficoll, 0.2% bovine serum albumin, 0.2% polyvinylpyrrolidone, 3 × SSC) at 65°C for 18 hr. The blot was then washed three times at 65°C for 1 hr each in 0.1 × SSC [16,17]. Blots were autoradiographed at −70°C to detect erb B-specific sequences.

Slot-Blot Hybridizations

RNA derived from bone marrow or peripheral blood buffy coat cells from each patient was purified in three steps: (1) alkaline phenol extraction, (2) precipitation from 3 M sodium acetate and (3) digestion with RNase-free DNase (Promega Biotec) [18].

Standard slot-blot hybridizations were used to obtain relative estimates of the amounts of specific RNAs within each RNA preparation. The technique of dotting excess clone-specific DNA and hybridizing to ^{32}P-labeled RNA has been used extensively as a means of measuring relative quantities of specific RNAs in a single preparation [19]. In all experiments, 1 μg double-stranded DNA in 1 M ammonium acetate was determined to be DNA excess for the reaction and was used in all experiments reported here. Filters were washed in 4 × SSC and baked in a vacuum oven at 80°C overnight. Prior to hybridization, filters were soaked in 1× Denhardt's solution (0.2% ficoll, 0.2% bovine serum albumin, 0.2% polyvinylpyrrolidine), 3 × SSC (45 mM Na citrate, pH 7.4, 0.45 M NaCl) at room temperature for 1 hr followed by washing for 1 hr at 50°C in hybridization buffer (50% formamide, 1× Denhardt's solution, 10 μg/ml Poly A, 50 μg/ml herring sperm DNA, 3 × SSC).

Poly A$^+$ RNA was 5'-end labeled with ^{32}P as follows: 2 μg RNA were partially hydrolyzed with NaOH. After neutralization of the NaOH with HCl, the RNA was incubated at 37°C for 45 min with T4 polynucleotide kinase and 50 μCi γ-^{32}P-labeled ATP (3,000 Ci/mmol). RNA was separated from unincorporated ATP by Sephadex G50 column chromatography at room temperature in 3 × SSC. Prior to hybridization, RNA aggregates were broken up by heat-shocking the sample for 1 min at 90°C. The RNA was hybridized to the nitrocellulose filters dotted with DNA probes at 50°C for 18 hr. Filters were washed three times for 1 hr each in 3 × SSC at 65°C and three times for 1 hr each in 0.1 × SSC at 65°C. Nitrocellulose filters were set up for autoradiography with X-ray film at −70°C for 24 hr. After autoradiographs were obtained, microdensitometric analysis was performed.

RESULTS
Cytogenetic Studies

Table I summarizes the clinical and cytogenetic data for the four individuals in this study. Each patient had a history of drug therapy prior to the appearance of the clone with an unbalanced 1;7 translocation. Patients 1 and 3 each had an abnormal clone where the only abnormality was a +der(1),t(1;7)(p11;p11). In patient 2 there were at least three different abnormal clones observed; one was trisomy 8, another had a deletion of part of the long arm of a chromosome 7, and the third clone had an unbalanced 1;7 translocation. Patient 4 was studied on two occasions. The first time the only abnormal cells observed were those with a Ph-chromosome. In the second study three of the cells had an apparent unbalanced 1;7 translocation in addition to a Ph-chromosome. Thus, the 1;7 translocation appeared in a subclone of a Ph-chromosome-positive clone. Figure 1 depicts representative karyotypes from bone marrow cells of two of the patients. The fact that these 1;7 translocations are present in only a percentage of the patients' cells and that some patients acquired the t(1;7) translocation after therapy demonstrates that the translocations are somatic, not constitutional.

DNA Studies

Southern blots were performed in order to determine whether t(1;7)(p11;p11) translocations involve amplification of the c-erb B gene. Figure 2 demonstrates amplifications of erb B-specific sequences in peripheral blood lymphocytes from three of four patients bearing a 1;7 translocation. (Similar results were obtained by using bone-marrow-derived DNA from patient 1; data not shown.) Densitometric analyses of these blots revealed levels of erb B-hybridizing sequences enhanced from 20- to 30-fold in three MDS patients compared to placental DNA. This is especially interesting in light of the absence of the 7q arm, the 7 centromere, and a bit of the 7p arm that accompanies the unbalanced 1;7 translocation. One would expect the loss of the chromosome 7p arm to result in decreased copies of c-erb B in the genome if this gene resided on the region of the 7p arm lost in this unbalanced translocation. As depicted in Figure 2, however, this is not the case in at least three of four individuals studied. It should be noted that DNA samples were not derived from cell lines but instead from bone marrow white blood cells taken directly from the patient. (Attempts to establish clonal lines from these individuals were unsuccessful.) Therefore, the cells are a mixture of normal cells and those with a 1;7 translocation. While amplification of c-erb B sequences is evident, it may actually be much higher than observed if experiments could be done with purified cell populations with a 1;7 translocation. Restriction enzyme patterns of erb B sequences from peripheral blood cells of patients with a 1;7 translocation suggest that in some individuals there is selective amplification of specific bands while in others the entire gene is amplified equally. No unusual bands were evident, which implies that amplification occurs over a span of DNA larger than the c-erb B gene itself.

To ensure that equal amounts of DNA were loaded per lane, gels were stained with ethidium bromide prior to transfer. In all cases, relatively equal amounts of DNA were apparent in each lane. In addition, blots were dehybridized overnight in H_2O at $65°C$ and then rehybridized to cDNA probe specific for actin (data not shown). These results established that each lane contained relatively equal amounts of actin-hybridizing DNA.

RNA Studies

Experiments were performed to determine whether the erb B amplification evident in Figure 2 was accompanied by a concomitant enhancement in erb B-specific mRNA accumulation. Total cellular RNA derived from bone marrow and/or periph-

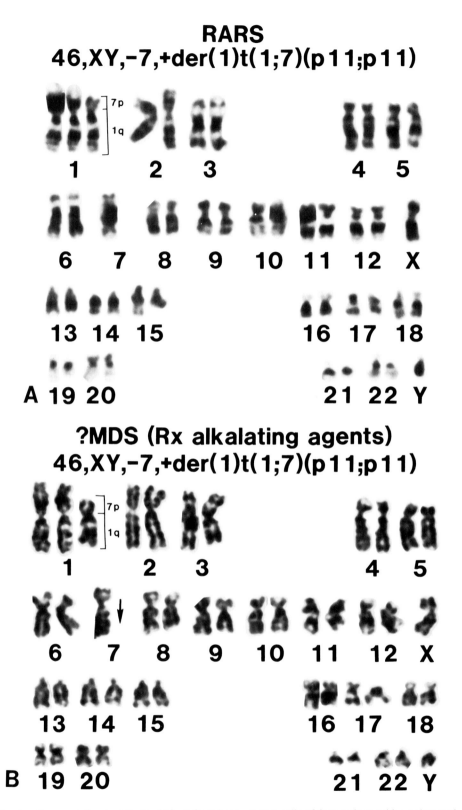

Fig. 1. Representative karyotypes derived from bone marrow cells of four patients with an abnormal clone containing +der(1),t(1;7)(p11;p11). A) Patient 2. B) Patient 3.

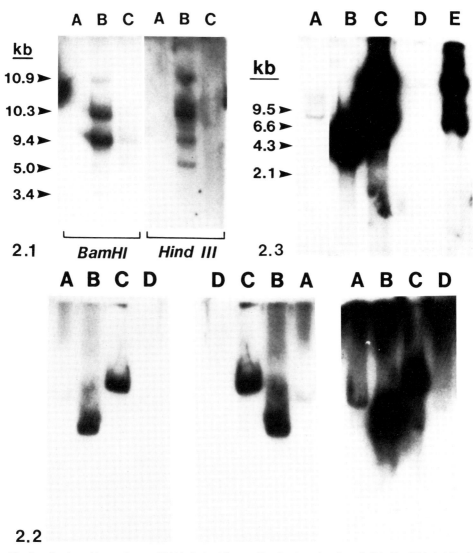

Fig. 2.   Southern blot analyses of DNA derived from cells of patients bearing t(1;7)(p11;p11) hybridized to nick-translated v-erb B DNA. 2.1) DNA from (A) control cells, (B) patient 1, and (C) placenta was digested with Bam HI or Hind III prior to electrophoresis, blotting, and hybridization. 2.2) Bam HI-digested DNA derived from (A) A431 cells, (B) patient 1, (C) patient 2, and (D) placenta hybridized to v-erb B. The left panel represents 12-hr exposure, the middle panel depicts a 24-hr exposure, and the right panel a 48-hr exposure. 2.3) Eco RI digest of DNA derived from (A) patient 4, (B) patient 3, (C) patient 2, (D) placenta, and (E) A431 cells.

eral blood lymphocytes was 5'end-labeled with ^{32}P in a kinase reaction and hybridized to an excess of clone-specific DNA immobilized onto nitrocellulose paper. These dot-blot hybridizations can be used to obtain a relative estimate of the quantity of clone-specific RNA present in the preparation. Figure 3 depicts the results of a representative dot-blot hybridization. The autoradiographs of such blots using equivalent counts and exposure times for each were analyzed by microdensitometry. The results representing three independent observations are listed in Table II. From these it is clear

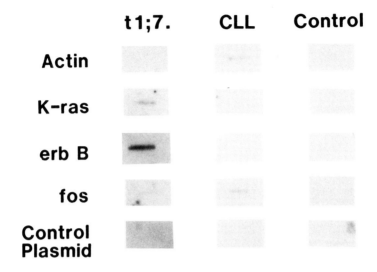

Fig. 3. Autoradiograph of slot blot hybridization of clone-specific DNA to 5'-labeled RNA derived from peripheral blood lymphocytes of t(1;7)(patient 1), control (PHA-activated peripheral blood white blood cells derived from a normal control), and CLL (peripheral blood white blood cells from T-cell chronic lymphocytic leukemia).

that the peripheral blood lymphocytes from three patients with amplified c-erb B DNA (those with MDS) also exhibited increased accumulation of mRNA specific for c-erb B. RNA derived from peripheral blood cells of the Ph-chromosome-positive ALL patient in which no c-erb B amplification was evident also demonstrated no such enhancement in erb B expression. For patients 1 and 4, RNA derived from bone marrow and peripheral blood lymphocytes both demonstrated enhanced erb B mRNA accumulation (data not shown).

Interestingly, studies of other gene sequences also revealed enhanced expression of K-ras, fos, and fes variably in some patients but not others. The significance of this is unclear, though similar enhanced expression of non-amplified c-oncogenes has been detected in many different tumor systems [20,21]. In addition, little change in gene expression was observed in genes associated with chromosome 1, such as B-lym, src, and N-ras.

DISCUSSION

Unbalanced translocations between chromosomes 1 and 7 associated with loss of a small part of a chromosome 7p arm, chromosome 7 centromere, and 7q arm have been correlated with myelodysplastic and myeloproliferative disease; the breakpoints are usually at 1p11 and 7p11. Frequently this chromosomal abnormality is linked with a history of exposure to toxic therapeutic or environmental agents [1–4]. In this study we examined cells from four patients with an abnormal clone in their bone marrow containing an unbalanced t(1;7)(p11;p11). Three of these patients had a history of exposure to cytotoxic drugs (especially alkylating agents) prior to the detection of the translocation. One patient had received a variety of anti-inflammatory agents including phenylbutazone.

TABLE II. RNA Dot Blot Hybridization*

	Control[a]	PBL 1[b]	PBL 2[b]	PBL 3[b]	PBL 4[b]
Actin	1.0	1.1	1.3	1.0	1.1
Transferrin receptor	HND[c]	3.1	HND	HND	10.4
α-tubulin	HND[d]	HND	HND	HND	HND
H-ras	HND	4.7	HND	HND	12.1
K-ras	HND	HND	HND	HND	HND
α-interferon	HND	HND	HND	NT[e]	NT
β-interferon	HND	2.8	HND	NT	NT
B-lym	2.0	1.7	HND	5.1	HND
fes	HND	HND	HND	HND	HND
fps	HND	HND	HND	HND	1.2
pBR322[f]	HND	HND	HND	HND	HND
sis	HND	HND	HND	NT	NT
erb B	HND	14.4	33.7	10.4	HND
myc	HND	HND	HND	HND	HND
mos	HND	3.8	HND	2.1	12.7
myb	HND	HND	21.4	4.3	20.6

*Analysis by microdensitometry. All data reported in arbitary units. All units determined by 1-wk exposure of 3.7×10^5 cpm hybridized per blot. All data reflect mRNA accumulation relative to the amount of actin-mRNA in control cells.
[a]PHA-activated PBL from healthy donors; RNA from tonsillar tissue gave similar results.
[b]Cells from patient bearing an abnormal clone with unbalanced 1;7 translocation.
[c]Hybridization not detected.
[d]Also negative for all cell types: ornithine decarboxylase, p53, abl, raf, fms, N-myc, bas, rel, erb A, N-ras, src.
[e]NT, not tested.
[f]Negative control; parent plasmid.

Since c-erb B gene (EGF receptor gene) has recently been mapped to 7p-11, we examined DNA and RNA derived from cells presumably bearing the chromosomal abnormality. These experiments revealed 20- to 30-fold amplification of c-erb B-specific DNA in three of the four patients. In addition, we found evidence for enhanced erb B mRNA expression in the three patients exhibiting amplified DNA.

Interestingly, the cells from the three patients with a 1;7 translocation and myelodysplastic syndrome displayed amplified c-erb B DNA while cells from the ALL patient with a similar 1;7 translocation showed no such DNA increase. It is possible that c-erb B amplification was not detected in this individual because (1) intensive chemotherapy suppressed or killed cells bearing the 1;7 translocation or (2) cells bearing the 1;7 translocation were present at too low a cell density to detect the amplification. On the other hand, the 1;7 translocation evident in the ALL patient may have involved translocation without amplification of c-erb B sequences.

Our attempts to obtain cell lines from these individuals were unsuccessful. Therefore, all our studies utilized heterogeneous cell samples with less than 50% (as determined by cytogenetics) of cells bearing a 1;7 translocation (see Table I). It is likely that all estimates in this report of levels of erb B gene amplification and mRNA accumulation present in these cells are actually low and reflective of the amount per total cell population rather than per cell bearing a 1;7 translocation.

The 1;7 translocation is accompanied by a loss of a part of chromosome 7p arm and all of the chromosome 7 centromere and 7q arm. Therefore, one may postulate two models for the location of c-erb B gene following a 1;7 translocation: (1) c-erb B gene may be lost with a small part of the 7p arm in the unbalanced chromosomal abnormality or (2) c-erb B gene may be translocated with most of 7p to chromosome 1p11. If the former were true, one would predict the amount of c-erb B-specific DNA to be decreased based on gene dosage [22]. However, since we have detected amplification of c-erb B gene sequences, we favor the latter model associating the translocation with c-erb B gene amplification. In addition, cytogenetic analysis did not reveal the presence of double minutes or homogeneous staining regions to explain this amplification.

7p11 is the site not only for the location of the c-erb B gene but also for a folic acid-sensitive fragile site found in some individuals [23]. Experiments were performed to determine whether these patients also had a fragile site at 7p11 which might affect a predisposition toward a 7p11 breakpoint in response to therapy. Of the two patients tested, fragile sites were not detected in peripheral blood cells cultured in the presence of 5-fluorodeoxyuridine (FUdR; see Table I). This suggests either that the methods needed to detect fragile sites are not sufficiently sensitive or that fragile sites are not necessarily correlated with the origin of such 1;7 translocations.

Recent results by King et al [24] have identified several human tumor cell lines which all display increased c-erb B mRNA expression by three potential mechanisms: (1) gene amplification with rearrangement and altered transcript size, (2) gene amplification without rearrangement and normal mRNA size, and (3) enhanced mRNA expression in the absence of gene amplification. The results presented in this report suggest that the amplified c-erb B gene is associated with 1;7 chromosomal translocation. While the presence of a translocation must involve a genomic rearrangement it is not clear that the c-erb B gene itself is rearranged in all patients. Southern blots (Fig. 2) demonstrated that the 1;7 translocations of patient 1 and patient 3 involved amplification of c-erb B in the absence of erb B rearrangement. This suggests that the amplification event itself involved DNA fragments larger than the c-erb B gene and that the translocation-specific breakpoint on chromosome 7 is located centromeric to c-erb B. On the other hand, Southern blot analyses of DNA derived from patient 2 (Fig. 2.2) demonstrate amplification accompanied by rearrangement within c-erb B gene. Clearly both of these mechanisms can be involved in 1;7 translocations associated with myelodysplastic syndromes.

Many have suggested that drugs that block DNA synthesis cause gene amplification by allowing for local areas of overreplication [25]. The fact that these patients developed a 1;7 translocation associated with c-erb B amplification suggests a potential role for specific therapeutic agents (see Table I) in c-erb B amplification. Moreover, most oncogene amplifications have been associated with aggressive tumors, occurring as late-stage events in oncogenesis [26]. In these patients, MDS represents a preleukemic syndrome with low levels of cellular proliferation. Their subsequent diagnoses of MDS differed from their initially diagnosed diseases. This suggests that gene amplification may also represent an early initial event that later leads to cellular transformation.

It has been hypothesized that specific chromosomal abnormalities highlight areas of active gene transcription in differentiated cells [27]. The data presented in this report suggest that the region of chromosome 7 involved in the translocation encompasses the c-erb B gene. This gene is not normally expressed at a detectable level in bone marrow or peripheral blood cells (Woloschak, unpublished observations). Clearly it is possible that other genes located on chromosome 7 are also involved in the translocation, especially in light of the apparently large size of the amplified DNA. Recent work by Mark et al [28] has isolated another oncogene at 7p11.1 that may also be associated with this and other chromosome 7 abnormalities. The identities of the gene sequences on chromosome 1 that are involved in this translocation are unknown. RNA studies of chromosome 1-associated genes such as src, B-lym, and N-ras revealed little enhancement of expression in patients bearing an abnormal clone with a 1;7 translocation compared to controls (see Table II). Future cloning experiments may help to characterize these genes.

ACKNOWLEDGMENTS

These studies were supported by ACS IM-348, Fraternal Order of Eagles grant 50, and the Mayo Foundation. The authors wish to thank Kathy Jensen for typing the manuscript and Mary Jane Doerge for technical assistance.

REFERENCES

1. Morrison-DeLap SJ, Kuffel DG, Dewald GW, Letendre L: Am J Hematol 21:39, 1986.
2. Smadja N, Krulik M, de Gramont A, Audebert AA, Debray J: Canc Genet Cytogenet 18:189, 1985.
3. Mecucci C, Ghione F, Tricot G, Van Den Berghe H: Canc Genet Cytogenet 18:193, 1985.
4. Sandberg AA, Morgan R, Hecht BK, Hecht F: Canc Genet Cytogenet 18:199, 1985.
5. Scheres JMJC, Hustinx TWJ, Geraedts JPM, Leeksma CHW, Meltzer PS: Canc Genet Cytogenet 18:207, 1985.
6. Merlino GT, Ishii S, Whang-Peng J, Knutsen T, Xu Y-H, Clark AJL, Stratton RH, Wilson RK, Ma DP, Roe BA, Hunts JH, Shimizu N: Mol Cell Biol 5:1722, 1985.
7. Ullrich A, Coussens L, Hayflick JS, Dull TJ, Gray A, Tam AW, Lee J, Yarden Y, Libermann TA, Schlessinger J, Downward J, Mayes ELV, Whittle N, Waterfield MD, Seeburg PH. Nature 309:418, 1984.
8. Filmus J, Pollak MN, Cailleau R, Buick RN: Biochem Biophys Res Commun 128(2):898, 1985.
9. Hunts JH, Shimizu N, Yamamoto T, Toyoshima K, Merlino GT, Xu Y-H, Pastan I: Somat Cell Mol Genet 11:477, 1985.
10. Downward J, Yarden Y, Mayes E, Scrace G, Totty N, Stockwell P, Ullrich A, Schlessinger J, Waterfield MD: Nature 307:521, 1984.
11. Libermann TA, Nusbaum HR, Razon N, Kris R, Lax I, Soreq H, Whittle N, Waterfield MD, Ullrich A, Schlessinger J: Nature 313:144, 1985.
12. Meltzer P, Trent J, Korc M: J Cell Biochem 10A:39, 1986.
13. Minty A, Alonso S, Guenet J-L, Buckingham ME: J Mol Biol 167:77, 1983.
14. Dewald GW: Clin Lab Annual 2:1, 1983.
15. Maniatis T, Fritsch EF, Sambrook J: In: "Molecular Cloning, Cold Spring Harbor Laboratory." 1982, pp 199–206.
16. Southern PJ, Blount P, Oldstone MBA: Nature 312:555, 1984.
17. Southern EM: J Mol Biol 98:503, 1975.
18. Courtney MG, Schmidt LJ, Getz MJ: Cancer Res 42:569, 1982.
19. Foster DM, Schmidt LJ, Hodgson CP, Moses HL, Getz MJ: Proc Natl Acad Sci USA 79:7317, 1983.
20. Seamon DJ, de Kernion JB, Verma IM, Cline MJ: Science 224:256, 1984.
21. Tatosyan AG, Gatetzky SA, Kisseljova NP, Asanova AA, Aborovskaya IB, Spitkowsky DD, Revasova ES, Martin P, Kisseljov FL: Int J Cancer 35:731, 1985.
22. Koprowski H, Herlyn M, Balaban G, Parmiter A, Ross A, Nowell P: Somat Cell Mol Genet 11(3):297, 1985.
23. Michels VV: Mayo Clin Proc 60:690, 1985.

24. King CR, Kraus MH, Williams LT, Merlino GT, Pastan IH, Aaronson SA: Nucleic Acids Res 13:8477, 1985.
25. Mariani BD, Schimke RT: J Biol Chem 259:1901, 1984.
26. Latt S, Shiloh Y, Sakai K, Rose E, Brodeur G, Donlon T, Korf B, Hearlein M, Kang J, Stroh H, Harris P, Bruns G, Seeger R: J Cell Biochem 10A:10, 1986.
27. Alitalo K: Trends Biochem Sci 67:194, 1985.
28. Mark GE, Seeley TW, Shows TB, Mountz JD: submitted, 1986.

Journal of Cellular Biochemistry 32:207–214 (1986)
Cellular and Molecular Biology of Tumors and
Potential Clinical Applications 59–66

A Monoclonal Antibody Reactive With an Activated Ras Protein Expressing Valine at Position 12

W.P. Carney, P. Hamer, D. Petit, H. Wolfe, G. Cooper, M. Lefebvre, and H. Rabin

Biomedical Products Department, E.I. du Pont de Nemours and Company, Inc., North Billerica, Massachusetts 01862 (W.P.C., P.H., D.P., H.R.), Department of Pathology, Dana Farber Cancer Institute (G.C., M.L.), and Tufts University Medical School (H.W.), Boston, Massachusetts 02115

Activated ras transforming genes have been described in a variety of neoplasms and encode 21,000-Dalton (p21) proteins with amino acid substitutions at positions 12, 13, and 61. In this report we describe a monoclonal antibody designated DWP that reacts specifically with synthetic dodecapeptides containing valine at position 12, to a lesser extent with peptides containing cysteine at position 12 and not with peptides containing glycine, arginine, serine, aspartic acid, glutamic acid or alanine at the same position. Western blot and immunoperoxidase studies showed that DWP specifically reacts with activated ras^H or ras^K proteins in NIH cells transformed by DNA from the human carcinoma cells that encode valine at position 12. DWP did not react with normal p21s encoding glycine at position 12, nor with activated p21s encoding aspartic acid, glutamic acid, arginine, serine, or cysteine at position 12. A survey of human tumor cell lines demonstrated that DWP reacted with the human bladder carcinoma cell line T24 but not with human tumor cell lines previously shown to contain other activating mutations at positions 12 or 61. DWP and perhaps additional antibodies that specifically react with alterations at positions 12 or 61 of the ras protein may be valuable in determining the presence and frequency of activated ras proteins in human malignancy.

Key words: monoclonal antibody DWP, activated ras protein reactive antibody, anti-ras antibodies, anti-ras monoclonal antibody

Ras genes homolgous to the Harvey (Ha) and Kirsten (Ki) sarcoma virus oncogenes [1] have been described in a variety of organisms including yeast [2], fruit flies [3], and mammalian cells [4]. In mammalian cells the ras genes encode 21,000-Dalton proteins that are localized to the plasma membrane [5], bind guanine nucleotides [6–8], and mediate GTPase activity [9–12]. DNA transfer experiments have demonstrated that a wide variety of neoplastic cells, including sarcomas, neuroblas-

Received March 10, 1986; revised and accepted July 10, 1986.

tomas, carcinomas, and hematopoietic malignancies [reviewed in 13], contain structurally altered ras genes, which upon transfection into NIH 3T3 cells lead to transformation. These oncogenic ras genes differ from their normal counterparts by point mutations that result in amino acid alterations at positions 12, 13, or 61 of the protein product [14–17]. Since activated ras gene products differ from their normal homologs, we directed our efforts at developing monoclonal antibodies (MOAb) that could discriminate between activated and normal proteins. In a preliminary report [18] we described a MOAb, DWP, that was raised against a ras-related synthetic peptide corresponding to an activated ras protein containing valine at position 12. In this report we extend our investigations and characterizations of DWP to a variety of transformed NIH cells and human carcinoma cells containing either activated or normal ras proteins. Our results demonstrate that DWP reacts specifically with cells having activated ras proteins containing valine at position 12 and not with normal p21s or other activated p21s.

MATERIALS AND METHODS

Hybridoma Production and Selection

To select antibodies specific for activated p21s containing valine at position 12, Balb/c × C57BL/6 mice were immunized with a ras-related synthetic peptide [5]Lys-Leu-Val-Val-Val-Gly-Ala-Val-Gly-Val-Gly-Lys[16] corresponding to positions 5–16 of the activated ras protein in the T24 bladder carcinoma and shown to contain valine at position 12. Peptides were coupled to the carrier protein bovine thyroglobulin (BTG) for immunization and to keyhole limpet hemocyanin (KLH) for screening assays. This strategy avoids selection of antibodies to the BTG carrier protein. Peptides were coupled to carrier proteins using l-ethyl-3-(3-dimethyl amino propyl) carbodiimide hydrochloride as previously described [19]. The immunization schedule consisted of inoculating mice intraperitoneally (ip) on days 1, 14, 28, 42, and 59 with 100–200 μg of conjugate. Inoculations on days 1 and 14 consisted of the peptide carrier-protein conjugate mixed 1:1 with complete Freunds adjuvant whereas the remaining inoculations consisted of conjugate mixed with phosphate buffered saline (PBS). Mouse sera were collected and evaluated by enzyme-linked immunosorbent assay (ELISA) [20] for the presence of antipeptide antibody. Three days prior to fusion mice were inoculated ip with 100 μg of peptide–BTG conjugate. On the day of fusion, spleens were removed and single cell suspensions of immune spleen cells were fused with Sp2/0 cells using polyethylene glycol as previously described [21].

Two to three weeks after cell hybridizations, hybridoma supernatants were evaluated by ELISA for binding to KLH-coupled peptides (500 ng/well) containing either valine or glycine at position 12. The hybridoma secreting the antibody of interest was doubly cloned by limiting dilution, inoculated into Pristane-primed mice, and the resultant ascites fluid used to prepare purified immunoglobulin [22].

Immunohistochemical Staining

Immunoperoxidase studies employed the avidin biotin complex system as previously described [23]. NIH cells and human tumor cell lines were formalin-fixed and embedded in paraffin prior to evaluation. All studies included a class-matched myeloma protein MOPC 141 (Litton Bionetics, Rockville, MD) at identical protein concentrations as DWP.

Cell Cultures

All cells were maintained in Dulbecco's modified Eagle's media supplemented with 5% fetal calf serum.

Production of Nude Tumors

Ten million tissue culture grown cells were resuspended in 0.2ml of PBS and inoculated subcutaneously into nude mice. Tumors were removed 2–4 weeks later and processed as described for the Western blot.

Western Blot

Cell extracts from 10^9 cells were prepared by scraping cells into Triton X-100 lysis buffer and the p21s were concentrated from cell extracts by immunoprecipitation with the broadly reactive anti-ras MOAb, Y13-259 [24,25]. For Western blot analysis, immunoprecipitates were collected, washed, and boiled in sample bufffer containing 2-mercaptoethanol. Immunoprecipitated proteins as well as heavy and light immunoglobulin chains were resolved by SDS-PAGE on 12.5% polyacrylamide gels and transferred to nitrocellulose membranes. After blocking with PBS containing 5% bovine serum albumin (BSA) membranes were incubated for 1 hr with 25 μg/ml of Y13-259, DWP, or MOPC 141. Membranes were washed three times with PBS-NP-40 (0.05%), incubated with either rabbit anti-rat horseradish peroxidase (HRP) to detect Y13-259 or goat anti-mouse HRP for 1 hr to detect DWP and MOPC 141. Membranes were then washed three times with PBS-NP-40, and incubated with 4-chloro-1-napthol substrate to complete the reaction as previously described [26].

RESULTS

Balb/c $\times$ C57B1/6 mice were immunized with a synthetic dodecapeptide corresponding to positions 5–16 of the activated ras protein described in T24 human bladder carcinoma cells. This protein expresses the valine substitution at position 12. Mice that exhibited serum reactivity with the immunogen of greater than 1:50,000 were selected for hybridoma production. Hybridoma supernatants were tested by ELISA for the presence of antibodies that would selectively bind peptides (coupled to KLH) containing valine at position 12 but not peptides containing glycine at position 12. One hybridoma, designated DWP, secreted an antibody with the desired reactivity pattern and was therefore doubly cloned and used to produce purified immunoglobulin from ascites fluid as previously described [22]. Purified DWP was determined by ELISA to be an IgG2b kappa molecule using rabbit antibodies against various classes of mouse immunoglobulins.

DWP was initially characterized by titration on peptides containing either valine or glycine (normal) at position 12. Results presented in Table I show that as little as 5 pg of purifed DWP reacted by ELISA with unconjugated peptide containing valine at position 12, whereas DWP did not react with glycine-position 12 peptides even when as much as 50 μg of peptides was used (data not shown).

To define DWP specificity further, a competition assay was performed using peptides containing a variety of amino acid substitutions at position 12. To do this,

TABLE I. Titration of DWP on RAS-Related Peptides Containing Either Valine or Glycine at Position 12

DWP concentration (ng/ml)	Optical density (488 nm)	
	Peptide-Val-12	Peptide-Gly-12
50	1.8	0
5	1.5	0
0.5	1.0	0
0.05	0.8	0
0.005	0.4	0

Various concentrations of purified DWP were incubated with 100 ng of unconjugated peptides coated onto the surface of microtiter wells. After an overnight incubation at 4°C, plates were washed and the goat anti-mouse horseradish peroxidase conjugate added for 1 hr. Plates were then washed and the substrate o-phenylene-diamine was added to complete the reaction. Colorimetric changes were determined using an ARTEK plate reader at 488 nm.

1.75µg of DWP was mixed wtih various peptides (concentrations ranging from 15.6 –500 ng) and allowed to incubate for 2 hr at 37°C. After the incubation, fluids containing peptides and DWP were incubated with peptides containing valine at position 12 to detect unbound DWP by ELISA. Our results demonstrated that peptides containing glycine, alanine, serine, arginine, aspartic acid, or glutamic acid at position 12 did not bind DWP. In contrast, peptides containing valine at position 12, and to a lesser degree (5–10 X) peptides containing cysteine at position 12, were able to bind DWP.

We next tested the ability of DWP to bind normal or activated cellular ras proteins contained in NIH cells. Several attempts at immunoprecipitating p21 with DWP were unsuccessful and therefore we employed the Western blot procedure. To do this we initially concentrated the ras proteins from cell extracts by immunoprecipitation with the broadly crossreactive anti-ras MOAb Y13-259. Immunoprecipitates were electrophoresed in 12.5% polyacrylamide gels, transferred to nitrocellulose, and tested for reactivity with the positive control Y13-259, the negative control MOPC 141 or DWP. Cell lysates were derived from either NIH cells containing ras proteins with glycine at position 12 or NIH cells transformed by activated ras[H] genes encoding valine at position 12. Results illustrated in Figure 1 show that ras proteins could be identified with the positive control MOAb Y13-259 in cells containing either normal ras proteins (lanes 1, 3) or mutated ras proteins containing valine at position 12 (lane 2,4). Results in Figure 1 show that the migration of the mutated p21 (valine-12) was found to migrate more slowly than normal ras p21 (glycine-12) in accordance with previously published results [24]. DWP reacted with ras proteins containing valine at position 12 (lanes 6,8) but not with normal ras proteins containing glycine at position 12 (lanes 5,7). No specific bands were observed in the p21 range when the MOPC 141 myeloma protein was substituted for DWP (lanes 9–12). Figure 1 also demonstrates that lysates from tissue culture cells (lanes 1, 2, 5, 6) gave results comparable to lysates prepared from nude mouse tumor cells (lanes 3, 4, 7, 8). The immunoblot experiment ilustrated in Figure 2 demonstrates that the positive control Y13-259 was reactive with p21s of all cell lines studied. DWP did not react with p21s from NIH cells (glycine-12) (panel A) but did react with NIH cells transformed by the ras[K] gene from SW480 colon carcinoma cells encoding valine at position 12 of the p21 (panel

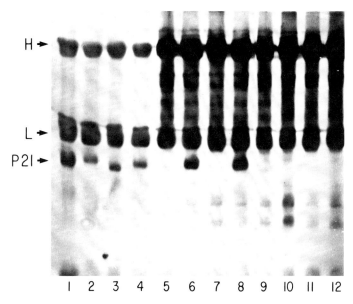

Fig. 1. P21 proteins were concentrated from cell extracts by immunoprecipitation with a broadly crossreactive rat MOAb Y13-259. NIH cells were transformed by either overexpression of the normal human ras[H] gene (glycine at position 12) (lanes 1, 3, 5, 7, 9, and 11), or by the activated ras[H] gene (valine at position 12) (lanes 2, 4, 6, 8, 10, and 12). Lanes 1, 2, 5, 6, 9, and 10 represent cell extracts derived from tissue culture cells whereas lanes 3, 4, 7, 8, 11, and 12 represent cell extracts from solid tumors produced in nude mice. Immunoprecipitates were collected, electrophoresed in 12.5% SDS-PAGE, and transferred to nitrocellulose filters for Western blot analysis. Filters were incubated with a 25 μg/ml of Y13-259 (lanes 1–4), DWP (lanes 5–8), or MOPC 141 (lanes 9–12) for 1 hr. Y13-259 was detected with rabbit anti-rat horseradish peroxidase (Cooper Biomedical Laboratories, Malvern PA), whereas DWP and MOPC 141 were detected with goat anti-mouse horseradish peroxidase (Bio-Rad, Richmond, CA). The p21 protein band is designated by an arrow. The light (L) and heavy (H) chains of immunoglobulins were also reactive with HRP reagents.

B). DWP did not react, however, with activated cellular p21s containing aspartic acid, glutamic acid, arginine, or serine at position 12 (panels C, D, E, and F). Similarly DWP did not react with ras proteins from transformed NIH lines containing cysteine at position 12 (data not shown).

Immunohistochemical analysis of cell lines containing ras proteins with glycine or valine at position 12 were also performed. Prior to incubation with DWP or with the negative control antibody MOPC 141, cells were formalin fixed and embedded in paraffin. Results were consistent with Western blots since positive immunoperoxidase staining as observed with transformed NIH cells containing activated p21s with valine at position 12. NIH cells containing normal p21 (glycine) or activated p21s encoding aspartic acid, glutamic acid, arginine, or serine at position 12 were not reactive by immunoperoxidase staining. An exception was found, however, in that NIH cells transformed by activated by p21s containing cysteine at position 12 were positive by immunoperoxidase.

DWP was also evaluated by Western blot and immunoperoxidase procedures on human bladder carcinoma cell line T24 and human lung adenocarcinoma cell line A549. Figure 3 shows a ras p21 band with the control MOAb Y13-259 in both cell lines. The bladder carcinoma T24 containing the activated ras[H] gene and encoding

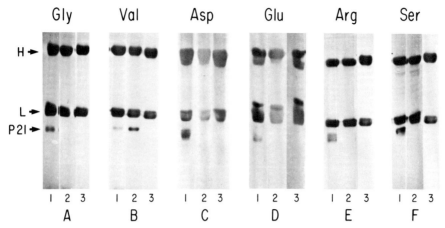

Fig. 2. P21 proteins were concentrated from cell extracts by immunoprecipitation with Y13-259. Cell extracts were derived from NIH cells transformed by overexpression of the normal human ras[H] gene (glycine at position 12) (panel A), by an activated ras[H] gene (valine at position 12) (panel B), by an activated ras[H] gene from the HS0578t carcinosarcoma cell line (aspartic acid at position 12) (panel C), by an activated ras[H] gene (glutamic acid at position 12) (panel D), by the viral ras[H] gene (arginine at position 12) (panel E), or by the viral ras[K] gene (serine at position 12) (panel F). Immunoprecipitates were collected, electrophoresed in 12.5% SDS-PAGE, and transferred to nitrocellulose filters for Western blot analysis. Filters were incubated with 25 μg/ml of Y13-259 (lane 1), DWP (lane 2), or MOPC 141 (lane 3) for 1 hr. Primary antibodies Y13-259, DWP, and MOPC 141 were detected as described in Figure 1.

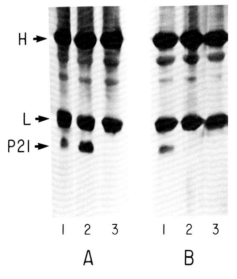

Fig. 3. P21 proteins were concentrated from human tumor cell line extracts T24 bladder carcinoma (panel A) and A549 lung adenocarcinoma (panel B) by immunoprecipitation with Y13-259. Immunoprecipitates were collected, electrophoresed in 12.5% SDS-PAGE, and transferred to nitrocellulose filters for Western blot analysis. Filters were incubated with 25μg/ml of Y13-259 (lane 1), DWP (lane 2), and MOPC 141 (lane 3) for 1 hr. Y13-259, DWP, and MOPC 141 were detected as described in Figure 1.

valine at position 12 was positive with DWP, whereas cell line A549 previously shown not to contain activated p21s [24] was not reactive with DWP. Similarly, human tumor cell lines SW1271 [27] and SK-N-SH [28] containing activated N-ras genes and having position 61 mutations were not reactive with DWP (data not shown).

DISCUSSION

Previous reports have described a rat MOAb, designated Y13-259 that cross-reacts with normal and mutated ras proteins in both yeast and mammalian cells. This antibody has been used to detect elevated levels of ras proteins in colon carcinoma cells. However, because Y13-259 is broadly cross-reactive, it could not be determined whether the elevated level of ras in the colon cells was due to activated or normal ras proteins [29]. MOAbs designated RAP have been shown to react in immunohisto-chemical staining with a high percentage of breast and colon carcinomas, but this antibody has also been reported to cross-react with normal and mutated forms of the ras proteins [30]. An antibody generated to ras-related proteins in rabbits against serine at position 12 has been shown to inhibit GTP binding to ras proteins. However, this antibody has not yet been evaluated for clinical utility [31].

Our objective in this study was to develop an antibody that would specifically react with activated ras proteins containing valine at position 12. In this report we describe a MOAb, DWP, that was raised against a synthetic peptide corresponding to positions 5–16 of the ras protein in T24 bladder carcinoma cells and that specifically reacts by Western blot and immunoperoxidase studies with activated ras proteins containing valine at position 12. DWP did not react by Western blot with normal p21s or activated p21s containing arginine, serine, glutamic acid, aspartic acid, or cysteine at position 12. Immunoperoxidase studies demonstrated, however, that DWP reacted with cells containing ras proteins with valine or cysteine at position 12.

Thus, in human tumors, DWP may allow one to determine the presence and frequency of activated p21s with valine at position 12, a point that we are currently evaluating. DWP and additional antibodies with specificities for activated ras proteins may be valuable in assessing the role of mutated ras in human malignancy.

REFERENCES

1. Ellis R, DeFeo D, Shih T, Gonda M, Young H, Tsuchida N, Lowy D, Scolnick E: Nature 292:506, 1981.
2. DeFeo-Jones D, Scolnick E, Koller R, Dhar R: Nature 306:707, 1983.
3. Shilo B, Weinberg R: Proc Natl Acad Sci USA 78:6789, 1981.
4. DeFeo-Jones D, Tatchell K, Robinson L, Sigal I, Vass W, Lowy D, Scolnick E: Science 228:179, 1985.
5. Willingham MC, Pastan I, Shih TY, Scolnick EM: Cell 19:1005, 1980.
6. Scolnick EM, Papageorge AG, Shih TY: Proc Natl Acad Sci USA 76:5355, 1978.
7. Papageorge AG, Lowy D, Scolnick EM: J Virol 44:509, 1982.
8. Finkel T, Der CJ, Cooper GM: Cell 37:151, 1984.
9. McGrath JP, Capon DJ, Goeddel DV, Levinson AD: Nature 310:644, 1984.
10. Sweet R, Yokoyama S, Kamata T, Feramiso J, Rosenberg M, Gross M: Nature 311:273, 1984.
11. Gibbs JB, Sigal IS, Poe M, Scolnick EM: Proc Natl Acad Sci USA 81:5704, 1984.
12. Manne V, Bekesi E, Kung H: Proc Natl Acad Sci USA 82:376, 1985.
13. Cooper GM, Lane MA: Biochim Biophys Acta Rev 738:9, 1983.
14. Tabin CJ, Bradley SM, Bargmann CI, Weinberg RAM, Papageorge AG, Scolnick EM, Dhar R, Lowy DR, Chang EH: Nature 300:143, 1982.

15. Reddy EP, Reynolds RK, Santos E, Barbacid M: Nature 300:149, 1982.
16. Bos JL, Toksoz D, Marshall CJ, Verlaan-deVries M, Veeneman GH, Vander Eb A, Van Boom JH, Janssen JWG, Steenvoorden ACM, Nature 315:726, 1985.
17. Yuasa Y, Srivastava SK, Dunn CY, Rhim JS, Reddy EP, Aaronson SA: Nature 303:775 1983.
18. Carney WP, Wolfe HJ, Petit D, Bator L, DeLellis R, Tischler AS, Dayal Y, Hamer P, Cooper GM, Rabin H: In Reisfeld RA, Sell S (eds): "Monoclonal Antibodies and Cancer Therapy." Vol. 27, New York: Alan R. Liss, Inc., 1985, p565.
19. Goodfriend TL, Levine L, Fasman GD: Science 144:1344, 1964.
20. Kennett RH, McKearn TJ, Bechal KB (eds): "Monoclonal Antibodies: A New Dimension in Biological Analysis." New York: Plenum Press, 1981.
21. Galfre G, Milstein C, Wright B, Nature 277:131, 1979.
22. Fahey JL: In Wiliams CA, MW Chase, (eds): "Methods in Immunology and Immunochemistry." Vol. I, New York: Academic Press, 1967.
23. Hsu SM, Raine L, Ranger H, Am J Clin Pathol 75:734, 1981.
24. Der CJ, Cooper GM: Cell 32:201, 1983.
25. Furth ME, Davis LJ, Fleurdelys B, Scolnick EM: J Virol 43:294, 1984.
26. Towbin H, Staehelin JG: Proc Natl Acad Sci USA 76:4350, 1979.
27. Yuasa Y, Gol RA, Chang A, Chiu I, Reddy ER, Tronick SR, Aaronson SA: Proc Natl Acad Sci USA 81:3670, 1984.
28. Taparowsky E, Shimizu H, Goldfarb M, Wigler M: Cell 34:581, 1983.
29. Gallick GE, Kurzrock R, Kloetzer WS, Arlinghaus RB: Proc Natl Acad Sci USA 82:1795, 1985.
30. Horan P, Thor A, Wunderlich D, Muraro R, Caruso A, Schlom J: Proc Natl Acad Sci USA 81:5227, 1984.
31. Clark R, Wong G, Arnheim N, Nitecki D, McCormick F: Proc Natl Acad Sci USA 82:5280, 1985.

Journal of Cellular Biochemistry 32:215–222 (1986)
Cellular and Molecular Biology of Tumors and
Potential Clinical Applications 67–74

Somatic Events Unmask Recessive Cancer Genes to Initiate Malignancy

Brenda L. Gallie and Ronald G. Worton

Departments of Ophthalmology, Hematology, and Genetics, Hospital for Sick Children, University of Toronto, Toronto, Canada M5G 1X8

A heritable mutation predisposes an individual to certain childhood malignancies, such as retinoblastoma and Wilms' tumor. The chromosomal locations of the genes responsible for the predisposition are known by linkage with chromosomal deletions and enzyme markers. A study of these tumors in comparison to the normal constitutional cells of the patients, using enzyme and DNA markers near the predisposing genes, has shown that these genes are recessive to normal wild-type alleles at the cellular level. Expression of the recessive phenotype (malignancy) involves the same genetic events that were observed in Chinese hamster cell hybrids carrying recessive drug resistance genes. In both the experimental and clinical situations, the wild-type allele is most commonly eliminated by chromosome loss with duplication of the mutant chromosome. Simple chromosome loss and mitotic recombination have been documented in both systems. In the remaining 30% of cases, inactivation or microdeletion of the wild-type allele are assumed to be responsible for expression of the recessive phenotype. Osteosarcoma is a common second tumor in patients who have had retinoblastoma. Studies with markers in osteosarcoma show that these tumors also result from unmasking of the recessive phenotype by loss of the normal allele at the retinoblastoma locus, whether or not the patient had retinoblastoma. Subsequent chromosomal rearrangements and amplification of oncogenes that occur in these homozygous tumors provide progressive growth advantage. In other malignancies, in which studies have so far focused on oncogene amplification and chromosomal rearrangements, unmasking of recessive mutations may also be the critical initiating events.

Key words: retinoblastoma, recessive, oncogene, somatic

In most cases, comparison of tumor tissue and normal cells does not distinguish initiating events from subsequent progressive changes. By the time tumors are studied in the laboratory, many differences from normal cells are often apparent: Aneuploidy may be obvious on karyotype analysis; oncogenes may be amplified or rearranged, and expression of growth factors may be aberrant. Which events are critical in the genesis of the tumors and which are subsequent changes related to the inherent genetic

Received March 11, 1986; revised and accepted July 10, 1986.

instability of malignant cells, cannot be easily determined. On the other hand, the rare tumors with a hereditary predisposition do allow identification of the earliest genetic abnormality, the premalignant change. Since the majority of the cells predisposed to the malignancy function quite normally in these individuals, the first predisposing mutation is not sufficient for malignancy. Therefore, it was proposed that these mutations might be recessive to the normal wild-type allele [1,2]. Malignancy would only arise following elimination of the dominant wild-type allele.

RETINOBLASTOMA

One of the best studied of the tumors with hereditary predisposition is retinoblastoma. Because surgical cure was possible, the affected individuals lived to reproduce and the inheritance patterns became evident at the beginning of the twentieth century [3,4]. Retinoblastoma occurs in three different genetic situations: 60% of cases develop only one tumor and have no inherited predisposition to the tumor; 40% of cases carry a germline mutation that predisposes them to multiple retinoblastoma tumors and other tumors (mainly osteogenic sarcoma) later in life; and a small number of cases occur in association with deletion of chromosome 13 that includes band q14.1.

Virtually all cases of retinoblastoma are diagnosed before the age of 3 years, strongly suggesting that the target cell for the malignant change must disappear from the retina early in life. When the age of diagnosis is plotted against the logarithm of the proportion of cases not yet diagnosed (100% at birth), the shape of the curve for the unilateral cases (probably nonhereditary) suggests that two or more rate limiting steps are involved in tumor initiation [2]. The shape of the curve for bilateral (hereditary) cases is a decreasing exponential, strongly suggesting that only one rate limiting event is required for the genesis of the tumors in the patients that carry the predisposing mutation. Based on such analysis of clinical data, Knudson et al [5,6] hypothesized that as few as two mutations could lead to retinoblastoma: In hereditary tumors the first mutation occurs in the germline, whereas in nonhereditary tumors the first mutation occurs in the somatic cell that forms the tumor. For both types of retinoblastoma the second mutation occurs in the somatic cell that becomes malignant. Since it is infinitely unlikely for two rare somatic mutations to occur in the same cell in an individual, the nonhereditary retinoblastoma patients have only one tumor. On the other hand, the multiple tumors observed in patients predisposed to retinoblastoma are explained by the relatively high likelihood that the second mutation occurs in more than one retinal precursor cell in an individual. Knudson also predicted that the first and second mutations could be at the same genetic locus: If the inherited predisposing mutation was recessive, tumors would form only when the remaining normal allele was lost by the second event. This second event could then be a second mutation or a "segregation" event that results in loss or inactivation of the second allele allowing expression of the recessive phenotype. Thus the genetic basis for deletion, and hereditary and nonhereditary retinoblastoma could all involve mutations in the same gene.

EXPRESSION OF THE RECESSIVE PHENOTYPE BY
SOMATIC REARRANGEMENTS

Apart from the study of tumor cells themselves we have also utilized an experimental approach to investigate mechanisms for the expression of recessive phenotypes in somatic cells that are heterozygous for a recessive marker. In Chinese hamster cell hybrid lines that were constructed to be heterozygous for a recessive drug resistance gene [7], it had been expected that expression of the recessive (drug-resistant) phenotype might occur by loss of the normal chromosome carrying the wild-type (drug sensitive) allele. This occurred in only about 20% of drug-resistant colonies analyzed [8]. More extensive analysis using hybrids with karyotypically marked chromosomes, revealed that loss of the normal chromosome was often associated with the presence of two copies of the mutant chromosome and this accounted for the majority of drug resistant segregants [9]. Inactivation of the normal allele, probably by DNA methylation, was shown to account for the drug-resistant phenotype in one segregant, in which re-expression of the dominant wild-type gene was documented under demethylating conditions [10]. The fourth mechanism examined in these studies was mitotic recombination. Although no drug resistant lines were found to be the result of mitotic recombination, in other studies with a very similar system including proximal chromosomal markers, mitotic recombination has been observed in 2 of 20 segregants [11].

A variety of segregation mechanisms allowing expression of recessive genes have been documented in mammalian hybrid cells, using a selectable phenotype (drug resistance) and chromosomes distinguishable by markers. A number of other studies have revealed similar mechanisms for the expression of recessive drug resistance markers in near-diploid cells [12]. To test if tumor formation in the hereditary malignancies represents expression of a recessive mutation, markers surrounding the mutant genes were studied.

The chromosomal location of the mutation predisposing the retinoblastoma was suggested to be chromosome 13q14.1 by mapping with rare deletion patients [13]. The ubiquitous enzyme, esterase D (EsD), the only enzyme marker on chromosome 13, was mapped to the same chromosomal band by the observation of hemizygosity in deletion retinoblastoma patients [14]. Studies of families with heritable retinoblastoma without deletion have shown tight linkage of esterase D isoenzymes to the occurrence of retinoblastoma [15–17]. In all informative families reported so far, no meiotic recombination has been observed. Assuming a uniform likelihood of meiotic recombination for any chromosomal region, Mukai et al [17] estimated that the retinoblastoma gene and EsD gene were less than 1,000 kilobase pairs (Kb) apart. One patient with retinoblastoma and a deletion ending in band 13q14.1 has been reported with normal levels of EsD, suggesting that the genes can be separated [18]. Using the recently cloned ESD gene [19], 24 retinoblastoma tumors were found by gene dosage studies to be diploid for EsD with no evidence of DNA rearrangement or deletion. It may be that the region from the EsD gene to the retinoblastoma gene is too large to be homozygously deleted. Since EsD is ubiquitous, total absence of EsD may be lethal to cells. Lack of any EsD rearrangement in 24 retinoblastoma tumors also suggests that the two genes are separated by at least 30 kB (the estimated size of the EsD gene).

In a few tumors, derived from ESD heterozygotes, the isoenzymes of EsD were used as markers for the homologous chromosomes, in a study of segregation events in retinoblastoma tumors involving adjacent regions of chromosome 13 [20]. In 70% of informative tumors, one of the isoenzymes that was present in the constitutional cells, was missing from the tumor cells, suggesting loss or inactivation of this chromosomal region in one homologue. However, two karyotypically normal chromosomes 13 were present. This was the first evidence that segregation mechanisms similar to those observed in Chinese hamster cell hybrids could be involved in retinoblastoma tumor formation.

In order to further analyze chromosomal loss or rearrangement in retinoblastoma tumors, two groups developed restriction fragment length polymorphic (RFLP) markers on chromosome 13 [21,22]. Thus, detailed analysis of chromosomal events around the retinoblastoma locus could be carried out [23,24]. It was observed that in 70% of tumors of informative individuals (heterozygous for chromosome 13 markers), the heterozygous RFLP markers on chromosome 13 were reduced to a homozygous state. Control RFLP's on other chromosomes remained heterozygous in the retinoblastoma tumors. As in the Chinese hamster cell hybrids, the most common mechanism for segregation appeared to be loss of one chromosome 13 with duplication of the homologous chromosome. Subsequent studies with cases of familial retinoblastoma showed that the lost chromosome carried the wild-type allele, while the retained or duplicated chromosome carried the retinoblastoma mutation [25]. Simple loss of the normal chromosome occurred in less than 10% of tumors. In most tumor studies it was not possible to distinguish clearly between loss and duplication of homologous chromosomes on the one hand and mitotic recombination on the other, as both events convert all markers distal to the locus to the homozygous state. In a few cases where both proximal and distal markers were available it was possible to document mitotic recombination events in 10% of tumors [23]. We found that 30% of the tumors did not reduce to homozygosity for informative markers surrounding the retinoblastoma locus. It was presumed that expression from the normal wild-type allele in these cases was eliminatead by mutation, microdeletion, or gene inactivation. Since nonheritable retinoblastoma tumors reduced to homozygosity for chromosome 13q at the same frequency as heritable tumors, the two somatic events leading to nonheritable retinoblastoma appear to be identical to the events in heritable tumors, involving the retinoblastoma locus on chromosome 13.

It has been noticed that the rare deletion retinoblastoma patients generally have fewer tumors than the usual hereditary mutation patients without deletion [26]. This suggested that in the presence of a large deletion around the retinoblastoma locus, the options for segregation of the recessive phenotype were reduced [27]. This can be understood when the mechanisms of segregation of the recessive phenotype are recognized. Loss of the normal and reduplication of the mutant chromosome, mitotic recombination, and simple chromosomal loss would all result in total absence of all the genetic material within a deletion, and would probably be lethal to the cell. Only mutation, gene inactivation, or microdeletion would result in tumor formation. These deletion patients therefore should develop only 30% as many tumors as patients with classical mutations in the retinoblastoma gene. This explains why these deletion patients are unilaterally affected more frequently than expected.

RELATIONSHIP OF THE RECESSIVE, INITIATING MUTATION TO OTHER GENETIC CHANGES IN THE TUMORS

Although the losses and rearrangements documented on chromosome 13 using specific markers are extensive, karyotypic studies of retinoblastoma tumors show only rare cytogenetic abnormalities involving chromosome 13 [28,29]. However all the tumors examined to date do show aneuploidy. Many of the rearrangments are random, but two rearrangements occur with high frequency: Extra copies of chromosome 1q occur in 90% of retinoblastoma tumors; and 70% of tumors carry a marker, isochromosome 6p, that is almost unique to retinoblastoma [29–32].

The oncogene N-*myc* is frequently amplified in neuroblastoma cell lines in association with progressive increase in tumor growth rate and tumor autonomy [33,34]. Similar DNA amplification of N-*myc* has been documented in some retinoblastoma tumors [35–37]. However, in a survey of 18 recently derived retinoblastoma cell lines, N-*myc* DNA amplification was found in only one tumor and the oncogene was expressed in all unamplified retinoblastoma tumors at a level comparable to fetal retina [38]. A later manifestation of the inheritance of the retinoblastoma mutation is a second malignant tumor, most commonly osteosarcoma or soft tissue sarcoma [39]. Although the sarcomas have been shown to be initiated by the retinoblastoma mutation [40], no N-*myc* expression was observed [38]. Although the normal product of the retinoblastoma locus may control or regulate genes related to cell division, there is no evidence to suggest that N-*myc* is the unique target of the retinoblastoma gene product. On the other hand, karyotypic evidence of DNA amplification and the presence of unidentified marker chromosomes has been reported in tumor cells with no amplification of N-*myc* or other known available oncogenes [29]. These unidentified rearrangements could be related to amplification for other genes encoding unknown growth factors.

SEGREGATION OF RECESSIVE ALLELES IN OTHER TUMORS

Osteogenic sarcomas were found to reduce to homozygosity for markers on chromosome 13, both from patients who had previously had retinoblastoma [40] and unassociated with retinoblastoma [40,41]. This suggests a wider role in specific malignancies for the recessive mutation previously associated only with retinoblastoma.

The data for somatic shift to homozygosity in malignant tumors is summarized in Table I. The gene that predisposes to Wilms' tumor was localized to chromosome 11p13 by constitutional deletion, analogous to the localization of the retinoblastoma locus [42]. Study of Wilms' tumor has also shown reduction to homozygosity for markers on chromosome 11p, at a similar frequency and with similar mechanisms to retinoblastoma [43–46]. Hepatoblastoma and rhabdomyosarcoma were also studied with markers on 11p, since these tumors may occur in the rare Beckwith–Widemann Syndrome, characterized by specific congenital anomalies. Both tumor types were found to reduce to homozygosity for 11p markers [47]. In Ewing's sarcoma, on the other hand, neither chromosome 11p nor 13q reduces to homozygosity. Markers on chromosome 13 and other chromosomes do not change in the tumors thought to be induced by a recessive tumor gene on chromosome 11p.

Transitional cell carcinoma of the bladder, linked to Wilms' tumor only because it may arise in a similar embryological tissue, has also been shown to reduce to homozygosity for chromosome 11p markers [48]. However, the frequency of homozygosity demonstrated was not as high as in Wilms' tumor, and other chromosomes also became homozygous at low frequency. Random aneuploidy, developing subsequent to the initiating reduction to homozygosity, can presumably occasionally result in homozygosity of other chromosomes.

TABLE I. Frequency of Reduction to Homozygosity in Tumors

Tumor type	Chromosome		Other chromosomes (chromosomes tested)	References
	13q	11p		
Retinoblastoma	11/18[a]	0/11	0/11 (1,3,10,12,15,17,18,20)	23,24
Osteosarcoma				
with retinoblastoma	2/3	0/3	0/3 (2,3,5,6,20,22)	40
without retinoblastoma	4/10	0/4	0/4 (3,6,17,20,22)	40,41
Wilms' tumor	0/6	12/22	0/7 (1,5,6,14,17,18,21)	42–45
Hepatoblastoma	0/3	2/3	0/3 (6,14,20,22,)	47
Rhabdomyosarcoma	0/3	2/3	0/3 (6,14,20,22)	47
Transitional cell carcinoma of bladder	0/12	5/12	3/12 (1,2[b],3,12,14[b],15,17,18,20)	48

[a]Tumors homozygous/informative tumors tested.
[b]Homozygosity shown for these chromosomes.

DISCUSSION

The genes documented to lead to malignancy by segregation of the recessive tumor forming phenotype, are tissue specific and may be developmentally regulated. Patients with the retinoblastoma germline mutation develop hemopoietic malignancies at the same frequency as the normal population, although we would expect that the segregation events involving 13q occur randomly in all tissues, not only in retinal cells. Therefore, the retinoblastoma gene and its mutations must be irrelevant in hemopoietic tissues. Somatic loss of the gene product in specific tissues may be the critical factor in tumor formation.

The only difference between hereditary and nonhereditary retinoblastoma is the timing of the first mutation, which occurs in the germline in hereditary cases and in the somatic cell that becomes malignant in nonhereditary cases. The first mutation leading to retinoblastoma is a rare (estimated 10^{-6} events per cell division) [2] deletion, microdeletion, or point mutation in a tissue-specific gene localized at 13q14. The mutation is recessive, and as long as the normal allele is present no cellular growth abnormality is detected in the tissue. The second mutation may be a more frequent segregation event. In experimental situations, similar segregation events, usually an abberrant chromosome disjunction that results in loss of the wild-type allele and duplication of the mutant allele, occur at an estimated frequency of 10^{-3} per cell division [11]. Since the number of retinal cells in which the retinoblastoma gene product is relevant is unknown, the frequency of the segregation event resulting in the tumors can not be estimated.

In retinoblastoma, both the first and the second events are rate limiting for the occurrence of the tumor. However, many tertiary mechanisms are available to increase growth advantage subsequently. Oncogenes can be amplified or rearranged, presumably providing an augmentation of growth factors. A single tumor type appears to use more than one tertiary mechanism, for example isochromosome 6p, extra copies of chromosome region 1q and N-amplification all occur in retinoblastoma tumors. Different tumor types also can use the same tertiary mechanism, for example amplification of N-*myc* occurs in both retinoblastoma and neuroblastoma.

ACKNOWLEDGMENTS

This work was supported by grants from Medical Research Council of Canada, National Cancer Institute of Canada, and Fight-for-Sight, Inc., New York City.

REFERENCES

1. Comings DE: Proc Natl Acad Sci USA 70:3324, 1973.
2. Knudson AG: Proc Natl Acad Sci USA 68:820, 1971.
3. Vogel F: Hum Genet 52:1, 1979.
4. Musarella MA, Gallie BL: In Renie WA (ed): "Golberg's Genetic and Metabolic Eye Disease." Boston: Little, Brown and Co, 1986, p 423.
5. Knudson AG, Hethcote HW, Proc Natl Acad Sci USA 75:2453, 1978.
6. Knudson AG: Cancer 35:1022, 1975.
7. Campbell CE, Worton RG: Somatic Cell Genet 6:215, 1980.
8. Worton RG, Duff C, Campbell CE: Somatic Cell Genet 6:199, 1980.
9. Campbell CE, Worton RG: Mol Cell Biol 1:336, 1981.
10. Worton RG, Grant SG, Duff C: In Pearson ML, Sternberg NL (eds): "Gene Transfer and Cancer." New York: Raven Press, 1984, p 265.
11. Wasmuth JJ, Hall LV: Cell 36:697, 1984.
12. Worton, RG and Grant, SG: In Gottesman MM (ed): "Molecular Cell Genetics." New York: John Wiley and Sons, 1985, p 831.
13. Ward P, Packman S, Loughman W, Sparkes M, Sparkes R, McMahon A, Gregory T, Ablin A: J Med Genet 21:92, 1984.
14. Sparkes RS, Sparkes MC, Wilson MG, Towner JW, Benedict W, Murphree A, Yunis JJ: Science 208:1042, 1980.
15. Connolly MJ, Payne RH, Jonhson G, Gallie BL, Alderdice PW, Marshall WH, Lawton RD: Hum Genet 65:122, 1983.
16. Sparkes RS, Murphree AL, Lingua RW, Sparkes MC, Field LL, Funderburk SJ, Benedict WF: Science 219:971, 1983.
17. Mukai S, Rapaport JM, Shields JA, Dryja T: Am J Ophthalmol 97:681, 1984.
18. Sparkes RS, Sparkes MC, Kalina RE, Pagon RA, Salk DJ, Disteche CM: Hum Genet 68:258, 1984.
19. Squire J, Dryja TP, Dunn J, Goddard A, Hofmann T, Musarella M, Willard HF, Becker AJ, Gallie BL, Phillips RA: Proc Natl Acad Sci USA, 83:6573, 1986.
20. Godbout R, Dryja TP, Squire J, Gallie BL, Phillips RA: Nature 304:451, 1983.
21. Cavenee W, Leach R, Mohandas T, Pearson P, White R: Am J Hum Genet 36:10, 1984.
22. Dryja TP, Rapaport JM, Weichselbaum R, Bruns GAP: Hum Genet 65:320, 1984.
23. Cavenee WK, Dryja TP, Phillips RA, Benedict WF, Godbout R, Gallie BL, Murphree AL, Strong LC, White RL: Nature 305:779, 1983.
24. Dryja TP, Cavenee W, White R, Rapaport JM, Petersen R, Albert DM, Bruns GAP: N Engl J Med 310:550, 1984.
25. Cavenee WK, Hansen MF, Nordenskjold M, Kock E, Maumenee I, Squire JA, Phillips RA, Gallie BL: Science 228:501, 1985.
26. Strong LC, Riccardi VM, Ferrell RE, Sparkes RS: Science 213:1501, 1981.
27. Knudson AG: Prog Nucleic Acid Res Mol Biol 29:17, 1983.
28. Gardner HA, Gallie BL, Knight LA, Phillips RA: J Cancer Genet Cytogenet 6:201, 1982.
29. Squire J, Gallie BL, Phillips RA: Hum Genet 70:291, 1985.
30. Kusnetsova LE, Progogina EL, Pogosianz HE, Belkina BM: Hum Genet 61:201, 1982.
31. Gallie BL, Phillips RA: Birth Defects 18:689, 1982.
32. Squire J, Phillips RA, Boyce S, Godbout R, Rogers B, Gallie BL: Hum Genet 66:46, 1984.
33. Schwab M, Ellison J, Busch M, Rosenau W, Varmus HE, Bishop M: Proc Natl Acad Sci USA 81:4940, 1984.

34. Brodeur GM, Seeger RC, Schwab M, Varmus HE, Bishop JM: Science 224:1121, 1984.
35. Kohl NE, Gee CE, Alt FW: Science 226:1335, 1984.
36. Sakai K, Kanda N, Shiloh Y, Donlon T, Schreck R, Shipley J, Dryja T, Chaum E, Chaganti RS, Latt S: Cancer Genet Cytogenet 17:95, 1985.
37. Lee W-H, Murphree AL, Benedict WF: Nature 309:456, 1984.
38. Squire J, Goddard AD, Canton M, Becker A, Phillips RA, Gallie BL: Nature 322:555, 1986.
39. Abramson DH, Ellsworth RM, Kitchin FD, Tung G: Ophthalmology 91:1351, 1984.
40. Hansen MF, Koufos A, Gallie BL, Phillips RA, Fodstad O, Brogger A, Gedde-Dahl T, Cavenee W: Proc Natl Acad Sci USA 82:6216, 1985.
41. Dryja TP, Rapaport JM, Epstein J, Goorin AM, Weichselbaum R, Koufos A, Cavenee WK: Am J Hum Genet 38:59, 1986.
42. Riccardi VM, Sujansky E, Smith AC, et al: Pediatrics 61:604, 1978.
43. Reeve AE, Housiaux PJ, Gardner RJM, Chewings WE, Grindley RM, Millow LJ: Nature 309:174, 1984.
44. Koufos A, Hansen MF, Lampkin BC, Workman ML, Copeland NG, Jenkins NA, Cavenee WK: Nature 309:170, 1984.
45. Orkin SH, Goldman DS, Sallan SE: Nature 309:12, 1984.
46. Fearon ER, Vogelstein B, Feinberg AP: Nature 309:176, 1984.
47. Koufos A, Hansen MF, Copeland NG, Jenkins NA, Lampkin BC, Cavenee WK: Nature 316:330, 1985.
48. Fearon ER, Fineberg AP, Hamilton SH, Vogelstein B: Nature 318:377, 1985.

Journal of Cellular Biochemistry 32:247–259 (1986)
Cellular and Molecular Biology of Tumors and
Potential Clinical Applications 75–87

Human A673 Cells Secrete High Molecular Weight EGF-Receptor Binding Growth Factors That Appear to be Immunologically Unrelated to EGF or TGF-α

Kurt Stromberg, W. Robert Hudgins, Charlotte M. Fryling, Parul Hazarika,
John R. Dedman, Robert L. Pardue, William R. Hargreaves, and
David N. Orth

Frederick Cancer Research Facility, National Cancer Institute, Frederick, Maryland 21701-
1013 (K.S., W.R.H., C.M.F.), Departments of Physiology and Cell Biology, University of Texas
Medical School, Houston, Texas 77225 (P.H., J.R.D., R.L.P.), Biotope, Inc., Seattle,
Washington 98109 (W.R.H.), and Division of Endocrinology, Vanderbilt University, Nashville,
Tennessee 37232 (D.N.O.)

Extracts of serum-free conditioned medium from human rhabdomyosarcoma A673 cells contain high molecular weight (HMW) transforming growth factors (TGFs) that can be partially purified by Bio-Gel P-100 and carboxymethyl (CM)-cellulose chromatography (Todaro et al: Proc Natl Acad Sci USA 77:5258, 1980). Reverse-phase high performance liquid chromatography (HPLC) revealed a principal peak of epidermal growth factor (EGF) radioreceptor assay (RRA) activity and anchorage-independent growth (AIG) activity that coeluted with 25–26% acetonitrile. If a trailing shoulder of EGF RRA activity from the CM-C chromatography was included in the material for HPLC analysis, additional active fractions were observed at 21–22% acetonitrile. Importantly, both active regions from HPLC failed to compete in radioimmunoassays under reduced and denatured conditions for human EGF (hEGF), human TGF-α (hTGF-α), or rat TGF-α (rTGF-α) and failed to give positive signals in Western blots under conditions in which TGF-α was readily detected when using an antisera raised against the 17 C-terminal amino acids of rTGF-α. Nonreducing sodium dodecyl sulfate polyacrylamide gel electrophoresis (SDS-PAGE) revealed EGF RRA and AIG activities in gel slices corresponding to M_r 15,000 and 22,000 in the 25–26% acetonitrile eluate and M_r 15,000, 20,000, 27,000, and 48,000 in the 21–22% acetonitrile eluate. The presence of multiple forms of EGF-receptor-binding peptides produced in vitro suggest size heterogeneity and possible immunologic diversity among high molecular weight members of the EGF/TGF-α family of growth-promoting polypeptides.

Charlotte M. Fryling's present address is Meloy Laboratories, Inc., Springfield, VA 22151.

Received March 18, 1986; accepted October 9, 1986.

Key words: epidermal growth factor, transforming growth factors, NRK colony formation

Transforming growth factors (TGFs) are acid-stable growth regulatory polypeptides that confer anchorage-independent growth (AIG) on normal rat kidney (NRK) fibroblasts [1,2]. Epidermal growth factor (EGF) radioreceptor assay activity (RRA) and AIG activity were first identified in extracts of conditioned medium from cells transformed by a murine sarcoma virus [3]. Two classes of TGFs were subsequently defined depending on their ability to bind to the EGF membrane receptor and their AIG activity in NRK cells [4–6]. Unlike TGF-α, TGF-β does not compete with EGF for receptor binding sites and requires EGF or TGF-α to induce AIG in NRK cells in semisolid media [6,7]. The original active factor secreted by these cells was found to consist of both polypeptides [8]. The prototype, extracellular low molecular weight forms of TGF-α have been purified from human [9], rat [10,11], and mouse [12,13] transformed cell lines, and rTGF-α has been synthesized [14] and consists of single-chain polypeptides of approximately M_r 5,600 (5.6K), which are about 30% homologous with human EGF (hEGF) and mouse EGF (mEGF) [12,13]. TGF-β has been purified to homogeneity from normal human [15] and bovine [16] tissues, human tumor cells [17], and retrovirus-transformed rat cells [18] and consists of a dimer of 25K that on reduction yields two identical chains of 12.5K. Nucleotide sequences of complementary DNAs encoding mEGF [19,20], hTGF-α [21], rTGF-α [22], and human TGF-β [23], indicate that the functional low molecular weight form of each peptide is synthesized from a much larger precursor. Consequently, high molecular weight (HMW) forms of these growth factors might be found in vitro and in vivo.

Urine from patients with disseminated cancer appears to have increased concentrations of a HMW growth factor of approximately 30–35K with NRK AIG activity and EGF RRA activity [24,25]. When characterized from the urine of patients with malignant brain tumors, this tumor-associated HMW TGF appears to be a HMW form of hEGF and is present at a fourfold higher level than in the urine of normal individuals [26]. Both a low molecular weight form and HMW (>10K) forms of TGF-α-like growth factors have been described in conditioned medium from several human tumor cell lines [27–29], in a retrovirus-transformed rat cell line [30], in the urine of human tumor-bearing athymic mice [31], and in extracts of the same human tumor cells [17]. These latter two studies utilized human rhabdomyosarcoma cell line A673 [32], which unlike most human tumor cells line in long-term culture, release relatively large amounts of HMW growth factors with EGF RRA and AIG activities. In an effort to clarify the relationship between the HMW TGFs present in urine [24,25,31] and conditioned medium [27–30], and to compare these extracellular forms with the intracellular [17] form of HMW TGF-α, this report describes chromatographic properties, apparent molecular weights, and immunologic characteristics of HMW peptides with EGF-receptor-binding activity in the conditioned medium of human A673 cells.

MATERIALS AND METHODS
Conditioned Medium

Human rhabdomyosarcoma A673 cells [32] were grown as described [27] in roller bottles (850 cm^2; polystyerene, CORNING, Corning, NY) in 50 ml of DMEM with 10% fetal bovine serum (GIBCO, Grand Island, NY). Confluent monolayers were rinsed twice with serum-free DMEM and incubated in 50 ml of serum-free Waymouth's medium for 8 hr. The medium was aspirated, and the A673 cells in each roller bottle were incubated in a second 50 ml of serum-free Waymouth's medium for 48 hr. The medium (conditioned medium) from several roller bottles was pooled, 1 μg per ml of phenylmethylsulfonyl fluoride (Sigma Chemical Co., St. Louis, MO) was added, and the medium was centrifuged (10,000g for 30 min) and stored at −20°C. Thawed medium was concentrated 25-fold using a hollow fiber concentrator (DC-2; Amicon, Lexington, MA) extensively dialyzed (spectraphor tubing, molecular weight cutoff 3500, Spectrum Medical Industries, Inc., Los Angeles, CA) against 1% acetic acid (HOAc), lyophilized, and stored at −70°C.

Soft Agar Growth Assay

Aliquots of column eluate fractions or extracts of gel slices were examined for AIG activity in semisolid medium (Agar Noble, Difco Laboratories, Detroit, MI) [27] in DMEM containing 10% calf serum. Purified TGF-β (kindly provided by Dr. Michael B. Sporn), was added at 2 ng per ml over a 0.5% agar base layer in 35-mm dishes (Cat. No. 3001, Falcon, Oxnard, CA), and 1 ml of 0.3% agar was added, which contained the test sample in the presence of 3×10^3 NRK cells, clone SA$_6$, (kindly provided by Dr. Joseph E. DeLarco). On day 5 the dishes were overlaid with medium containing 0.3% agar, and incubation at 37°C in a humidified 5% CO_2 atmosphere continued until day 14. The number of colonies containing at least 20 cells or 50 cells or more in eight low-power fields were counted on day 14. SA$_6$ NRK cells, used between passages 12 and 16, do not form colonies in 0.3% agar except in the presence of clonogenic growth-promoting factors.

EGF Radioreceptor Assay

Samples were assayed for EGF RRA activity in 16-mm multiwell tissue culture plates (Linbro/Flow Labs, Hamden, CT) containing 10^4 A431 cells per well and highly purified mEGF as the ^{125}I-labeled tracer and reference standard [27]. More recently, a more rapid and convenient EGF RRA that uses isolated A431 cell membranes was employed [33]. Each assay included a standard curve of graded quantities of unlabeled mEGF with which to calculate the EGF equivalents in the test samples. Half-maximal inhibition of ^{125}I-mEGF binding to isolated A431 cell membranes is observed with 2–4 ng of competing unlabeled mEGF. In these two RRAs, hEGF and mEGF are equivalent.

Gel Filtration, Ion-Exchange, and Reverse-Phase High Performance Liquid Chromatography

Procedures for Bio-Gel P-100 (Bio-Rad Laboratories, Richmond, CA) and CM-cellulose (CM-52, Whatman, Clifton, NJ) chromatography were performed [27]. Lyophilizates of 100 L (pool A) or 250 L (pool B) of conditioned medium stored at −70°C were reconstituted in 10 ml of 1 M HOAc and centrifuged (10,000g for 30 min), and the supernate was subjected to chromatography on a Bio-Gel P-100 (100–200 mesh) column (5 × 82.5 cm), equilibrated, and eluted with 1 M HOAc at 4°C; 12.4-ml fractions were collected.

Biologically active eluate fractions from the P-100 column (M_r approximately 15,000–20,000) were pooled, lyophilized, resuspended in 1 M HOAc, dialyzed (molecular weight cutoff 3,500) overnight against 5 mM ammonium acetate, pH 4.5, at 4°C, and centrifuged at 100,000g for 30 min. The supernate was applied to a CM-cellulose column (1.5 × 3 cm) equilibrated with 5 mM NH_4OAc, pH 4.5 (starting buffer). A linear elution gradient formed of 200 ml of starting buffer and 200 ml of limit buffer (0.5 M NH_4OAc, pH 6.8) in a two-chamber, constant-level mixing device was applied at a flow rate of 80 ml per hr at 22°C. Fractions of 10 ml were adjusted to 1 M with respect to HOAc, and aliquots were concentrated by lyophilization prior to assay of biological activity.

Reverse-phase HPLC was performed with a C_{18}-μBondapak column (10-μm particle size, 0.39 × 30 cm, Waters Associates, Milford, MA) in a Waters Associate Liquid Chromatograph system equipped with two Model 6000 M solvent delivery pumps, a Model 660 solvent programmer, and a Model 450 variable wave-length UV detector set at 206 nm. A linear elution gradient of 18–35% acetonitrile in 0.05% trifluoroacetic acid was applied over 120 min at a flow rate of 0.7 ml per min at 22°C.

Protein concentration was determined by the method of Lowry et al [34] using bovine serum albumin as standard, or by amino acid analysis of hydrolyzed samples [35].

Sodium Dodecyl Sulfate (SDS) Polyacrylamide Gel Electrophoresis (PAGE)

Samples were subjected to SDS-PAGE on 15% polyacrylamide slab gels according to the method of Laemmli [36] and sliced into 2-mm sections in a mechanical gel slicer (Model 190, Bio-Rad, Richmond, CA). Prestained molecular weight standards (Bethesda Research Labs, Gaithersburg, MD) were ovalbumen (43K), chymotrypsinogen (25.7K), β lacto-globulin (18.4K), lysozyme (14.3K), aprotinin (6.2K), and the β subunit of insulin (3.0K). Each test sample lane was bracketed by lanes of prestained standards to assist slicing and determination of molecular weight. For assay for biological activity, materials in individual SDS-PAGE slices were extracted by adding 1 ml of 1 M HOAc containing 100 μg of bovine serum albumin as carrier, crushing the gel slice in a conical tube with a glass rod, and incubating them for at least 24 hr at 4°C to permit polypeptides to leach out of the gel matrix. Following a 5-min centrifugation (Microfuge B, Beckman, Palo Alto, CA), 0.7 ml of supernate was aspirated and stored at either 4°C or −70°C prior to assay.

Radioimmunoassays for hEGF and TGF-α

Homologous hEGF radioimmunoassay (RIA) was performed by modifications [37] of a method [38] that uses an antiserum raised to highly purified hEGF that was generously provided by Dr. Yukio Hirata, National Cardiovascular Institute Research Center, Osaka, Japan. Highly purified hEGF [39] was used as ^{125}I-labeled tracer and reference standard. TGF-α RIA was performed using a commercial kit (Biotope, Inc., Seattle, WA), and as described [40], with bioactive synthetic rTGF-α (Peninsula Laboratories, Belmont, CA) used as radioiodinated tracer and reference standard. Antisera to the C-terminal 17-amino acid fragment (C17A) of rTGF-α were raised either in rabbits (Biotope, Inc.) or as an affinity-purified antiserum raised in sheep [40]. Half-maximal competition is observed in the Biotope system with about 0.5–1.0 ng native or reduced TGF-α. A noncommercial assay (Biotope, Inc.) with similar sensitivity was also used employing rabbit antiserum raised against synthetic human TGF-α (residues 1–50). All TGF-α RIAs using either rabbit or sheep antisera detected hTGF-α and rTGF-α equally well. Western immunoblots [40] for TGF-α were carried out on the two biologically active HPLC components; the technique detected 50–75 ng of either rTGF-α or hTGF-α as reference standards. Synthetic hTGF-α was the gift of Dr. J.E. Tam, Rockefeller University (New York, NY).

RESULTS

The column eluate of Bio-Gel P-100 chromatography of 100 L of conditioned medium from A673 cells contained a 13–20K region of AIG and EGF RRA activity (Fig. 1). The elution profiles of both the 100-L pool and the 250-L pool (data not shown) of conditioned medium suggested the presence of at least two M_r species. The trailing shoulder with AIG and EGF RRA activities has previously been noted in medium from A673 cells [27, 41].

Column fractions comprising the entire region of TGF activity of the 100-L and 250-L pools were separately pooled, concentrated, and applied to a CM-cellulose column. There again appeared to be two components with EGF RRA activity in both the 100-L (Fig. 2, upper panel) and 250-L (Fig. 2, lower panel) pools, but neither was adequately resolved. Consequently, the earlier-eluting fractions 22–31 (Fig. 2,

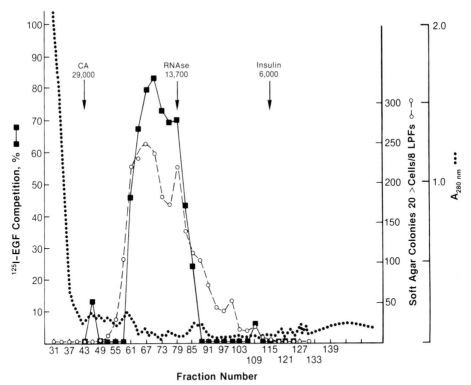

Fig. 1. Gel filtration chromatography of concentrated conditioned medium (100 L) from A673 cells. The lyophilized sample was dissolved in 1 M HOAc and centrifuged to remove insoluble material, and the supernate was applied to a Bio-Gel P-100 column (5 × 82.5 cm, 100–200 mesh), equilibrated, and eluted with 1 M HOAc in 12.4-ml fractions. Protein was determined by absorbance at 280 nm (.....). A 100-μl aliquot of every third fraction was assayed for binding to EGF receptors (■ --- ■), and a 50-μl aliquot was assayed for NRK clonogenicity in semisolid medium (○ --- ○) [27]. Molecular weight markers were carbonic anhydrase, 29K; ribonuclease, 13K; and insulin, 6K.

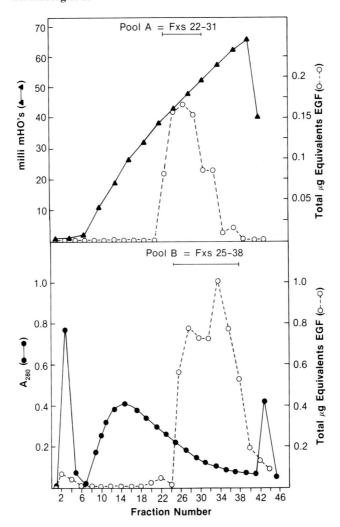

Fig. 2. Ion exchange chromotagraphy of pooled Bio-Gel P-100 fractions with TGF activity from 100-L (upper panel) (fractions 61–85, Fig.1) or 250 L (lower panel) (P-100 chromatograph not shown) of A673 conditioned medium. The pooled fractions were lyophilized, reconstituted, dialyzed, applied to, and eluted from a column of CM-cellulose as described in "Materials and Methods." In the upper panel, conductivity (▲ -- ▲) is shown as a measure of the linearity of the pH elution gradient, while in the lower panel, absorbance at 280 nm (● -- ●) is a measure of protein concentration. RRA activity (○--○) was determined by competition of 200-μl aliquots from each 10-ml fraction with ^{125}I-EGF for binding to isolated A431 membranes as described [33]. Fractions containing the major peak of TGF activity in the upper panel (fractions 22–31, designated pool A) and all TGF activity in the lower panel (fractions 25–38, designated pool B) were pooled and lyophilized.

upper panel) from the 100-L pool were combined (pool A) and compared with all the TGF active fractions 25–38 (Fig. 2, lower panel) from the 250-L pool (pool B) by reverse-phase HPLC (Fig. 3). Pools A and B both contained a component with TGF activity that eluted with 25–26% acetonitrile (fractions 25–27, upper panel and fractions 20–22, lower panel, Fig. 3). Fractions 25–27 from pool A generated a linear dose-response curve in the EGF radioreceptor assay (inset, upper panel, Fig. 3). The

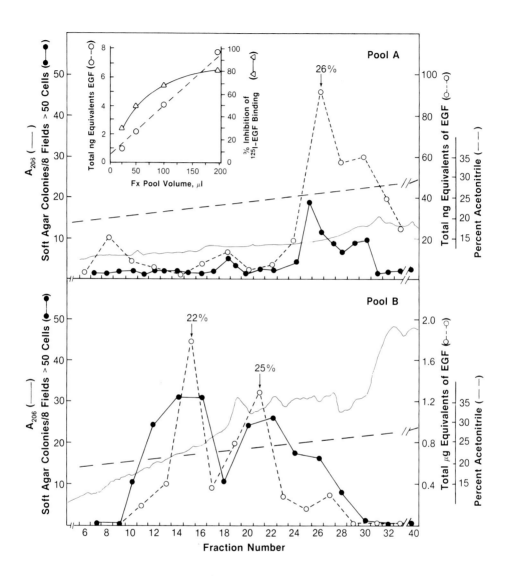

Fig. 3. Reverse-phase HPLC of Pool A (fractions 22–31) and Pool B (fractions 25–38) from CM-cellulose (Fig. 2). Each pool was lyophilized, resuspended in 0.05% trifluoroacetic acid, and subjected to HPLC; 100-μl aliquots of alternate fractions (1.8 ml total volume) were assayed in duplicate for EGF RRA activity (○ -- ○), and 50-μl aliquots were assayed for NRK AIG activity (● -- ●), as described in "Materials and Methods." Fractions 25–27 of pool A (upper panel) were pooled to evaluate the dose-response relationship in the EGF RRA assay (inset, upper panel). The arrows and percentages above the peaks of TGF activity indicate acetonitrile elution.

inclusion in pool B of the trailing shoulder of the larger peak of TGF activity from CM-cellulose chromatography generated an additional peak of AIG and RRA activity, which eluted with 21–22% acetonitrile (fractions 14–16, Fig. 3, lower panel). Because this latter activity was not observed in pool A, it appeared that it might represent components eluting in CM-C fractions 32–38 (Fig. 2, lower panel).

Aliquots of fractions 25–27 from pool A, which had the highest AIG and EGF RRA activity (Fig. 3, upper panel), were combined and subjected to SDS-PAGE under nonreducing conditions. Two TGF species of M_r 15,000 and 22,000 were identified by coincident peaks of AIG activity, EGF RRA activity, and mitogenic activity [41] (data not shown). An identical result (Fig. 4, upper panel) was obtained after SDS-PAGE of the peak activity fractions 20–22 from pool B. Comparable

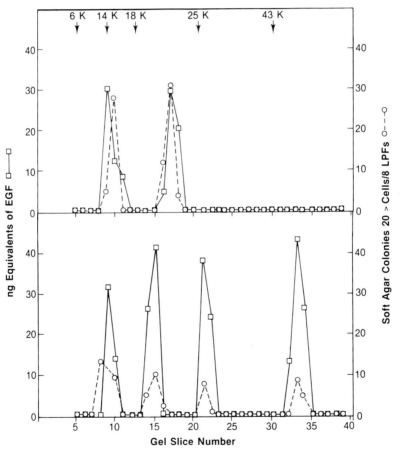

Fig. 4.   SDS-PAGE of two peaks of TGF activity from pool B HPLC (Fig. 3, lower panel). Equal aliquots of fractions 14–16, representing the 21–22% acetonitrile elution region (lower panel),and fractions 20–22 from the 25–26% acetonitrile elution region (upper panel) were analyzed on 15% polyacrylamide slab gels under nonreducing conditions, and gel slices were eluted, as described in "Materials and Methods." A 200-μl aliquot of each 0.7-ml eluate was assayed for AIG activity (○ -- ○), and 500 μl was assayed in duplicate for EGF RRA activity (□ -- □). Prestained molecular weight standards were ovalbumin (43K), chymotrypsinogen (25.7K), β lactoglobulin (18.4K), lysozyme (14.3K), aprotinin (6.2K), and the β subunit of insulin (3.0K).

analysis of the more hydrophilic region of activity (fractions 14–16) from pool B revealed four peaks of coincident EGF RRA and AIG activity (Fig. 4, lower panel).

Pool B of A673 conditioned medium contained the most EGF equivalents (Figs. 2 and 3, lower panels). Aliquots of the two HPLC peaks of TGF activity from pool B were evaluated for their immunological relatedness to TGF-α [9–14] by RIAs and Western immunoblots (Table I). In both Biotope TGF-α RIAs using antisera raised in rabbits against either the C17A fragment of rTGF-α or the entire synthetic hTGF-α, and adding up to 100 ng of antigen as measured by the EGF RRA activity, neither of the HPLC peaks displaced ^{125}I-labeled rTGF-α from the antibodies. The same result using an affinity-purified shccp antisera raised against the synthetic C17A fragment of rTGF-α is shown in Figure 5. In this system, the TGF-α RIA detected hTGF-α activity in conditioned medium of human melanoma cells A-2058 [40]. Synthetic hTGF or synthetic rTGF-α in either its C-terminal (residues 34–50) or full length form (residues 1–50) did react fully [40] (Fig. 5), whereas highly purified hEGF did not react at all. Moreover, both of the HPLC peaks with AIG and EGF RRA activities failed to react in a sensitive RIA for hEGF [37,38]. Furthermore, as summarized in Table I, neither HPLC peak of AIG activity (added in an amount of 200 ng EGF equivalents by RRA) was detected by Western immunoblots under conditions in which 50–75 ng of synthetic rTGF-α or hTGF-α were clearly detected [40].

DISCUSSION

The A673 human cell line is unusual in its continued secretion of HMW forms of growth-promoting polypeptides with TGF-α-like biological activity even at a high

TABLE I. Immunologic Characterization of Partially Purified HMW TGFs Secreted by A673 Cells

	Immunologic assay		
	RIA		Western immuno-blot
Growth factor	hEGF[a]	rTGF-α[b]	rTGF-α[c]
hEGF[d]	+	−	−
hTGF-α[e]	−	+	+
HPLC fraction[f]			
21–22% MeCN	<0.01 ng	<0.1 ng	−
25–26% MeCN	<0.01 ng	<0.1 ng	−

[a]hEGF RIA [37,38] in which detectability (10% displacement) is 0.1 ng highly purified hEGF reference standard [39], and 50% displacement occurs with 0.5 ng hEGF under reduced and denatured conditions.
[b]rTGF-α RIAs (Biotope, Inc., Seattle, WA) utilizing rabbit antisera against both C17A fragment of rTGF-α or entire synthetic hTGF-α. Detectability (10% competition) is 0.3 ng synthetic rTGF-α reference standard and in which 50% competition occurs with 0.5 ng competing synthetic rTGF-α or hTGF-α under reduced and denatured conditions.
[c]rTGF-α immunoblot [40] sensitive to detection of 50–75 ng of synthetic rTGF-α or hTGF-α.
[d]Highly purified hEGF [39].
[e]Synthetic hTGF was biologically active prior to testing.
[f]Equal aliquots of active HPLC fractions 14–16 (21–22% MeCN elution) or active HPLC fractions 20–22 (25–26% MeCN elution), as shown in Figure 3, lower panel, were combined to provide 30 ng of EGF RRA equivalents [33] for hEGF RIA, 100 ng of EGF RRA equivalents for either of the rTGF-α RIAs (see "Methods"), and 200 ng EGF RRA equivalents for Western immunoblots [40]. Both rTGF-α and hTGF-α were included at 75 ng as positive controls in each Western immunoblotting experiment.

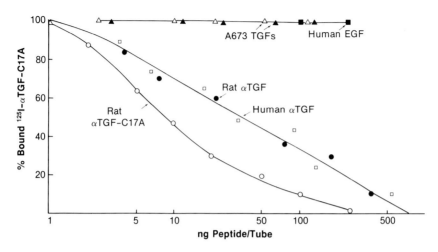

Fig. 5. Rat TGF-α RIA [40] for synthetic C17A fragment (○) and complete (●) rat TGF-α [14] and human TGF-α (□), purified [39] hEGF (■), and the two peak regions of TGF activity from HPLC (Fig. 3, lower panel) of A673 conditioned medium (△, ▲). The amount of A673-derived TGF-α activity added per RIA tube is expressed as ng equivalents of mEGF as measured in the EGF RRA. Each sample was reduced and denatured and was competed against ^{125}I-labeled rTGF-α (C-terminal 17-amino acid fragment) in the presence of affinity-purified sheep antisera raised against the same fragment of rTGF-α [40].

passage number. Accordingly, this human tumor line was selected to evaluate HMW polypeptides as a potential model for processing of TGF-α precursor species. Immunologic reagents developed against the C-terminal 17 amino acids of rTGF-α, a low molecular weight (5.6K) polypeptide [14], were reported in Western immunoblots to detect species of 22K, 42K, and 44K in medium conditioned by feline sarcoma virus-transformed rat cells [30]. Similarly, an affinity-purified sheep antiserum raised against the same C-terminal rTGF-α fragment detected a 20–22K TGF-α-like peptide in medium conditioned by the same transformed rat cell line in immunoblots [40]. More recently, an 18K intracellular form of hTGF-α-like biological activity was reported as the predominate species in A673 cell extracts, but was not immunologically characterized [17]. Other HMW species of extracellular peptides with TGF-α-like activity from tumor cells have been reported [28,29], but these too have not been immunologically characterized.

Fractionation of medium conditioned by A673 cells by sequential gel filtration, cation exchange, and reverse-phase high performance liquid chromatography revealed two components with TGF-α-like activity by assays for binding to EGF cell membrane receptors and NRK cell colony formation in soft agar. Immunological comparison to TGF-α by RIA and estimation of molecular weight by SDS-PAGE revealed a lack of immunological relatedness and size heterogeneity in both components. Besides failing to compete in RIAs under reduced and denatured conditions for hEGF or rTGF-α, neither active components from HPLC was detected in Western immunoblots under conditions in which rTGF-α and hTGF-α at about one-third the concentration were readily detected. Moreover, neither of these two active peaks in HPLC was detected in an ELISA assay for hTGF-α (R. Derynck and T.S. Bringman, unpublished data). Finally, precursor-specific antipeptide antibodies directed against the carboxy terminal amino acids of the rTGF-α precursor [22] were unable to immune precipitate any peptides from ^{35}S-cysteine-labeled A673 cell cultures, in contrast to a readily detectable 14–17 K protein found in retroviral-transformed Fisher rat embryo cells (L.E. Gentry et al, submitted for publication).

Nonreducing SDS-PAGE of these two HMW growth-promoting components revealed EGF RRA and NRK cell AIG activities at 15K and 22K in the relatively hydrophobic materials eluting in HPLC with 25–26% acetonitrile, and 15K, 20K, 27K, and 48K in the relatively hydrophilic materials that eluted in HPLC with 21–22% acetonitrile. In addition to the major 18K species, growth factors of various molecular weights with TGF-α-like activity were also described in A673 cell extracts [17]. Thus, size heterogeneity of HMW EGF-receptor-binding growth factors may be characteristic of A673 cells. The predominant extracellular HMW forms that we observed were 15K and 20–22K. Our extracellular 20K form may correspond to the 18K moiety previously described in cell extracts [17], and the extracellular 15K species may result from glycosidase cleavage of the 20K species. Virally transformed rat cells contain a bioactive 17–19K TGF-α precursor, which after elastase treatment is converted to mature TGF-α, and after endoglycosidase treatment becomes a 14K moiety in Western immunoblots using an antisera raised against the synthetic rTGF-α C-terminal 20 amino acids ([42] and J. Massague, personal communication). In addition, tunicamycin treatment converts an 18K moiety of TGF-α produced by CHO cells transfected with a TGF-α expression vector into a 14K immunoreactive TGF-α species (R. Derynck, personal communication). The larger 27K and 48K species observed in nonreducing SDS-PAGE gels may represent HMW precursor forms or artifacts that are due to protein binding or aggregation of smaller species, as has been described for mEGF [43]. Similarly, in addition to secreted HMW TGF-α of 20K [30,40], 42K and 44K forms have also been observed in Western immunoblots of extracts of medium conditioned by feline sarcoma virus-transformed rat cells [30].

The urine of athymic mice bearing A673 cells is reported to contain a tumor-associated 20K complex of growth factors, which after resolution by HPLC includes a more hydrophilic component than mEGF that reacts with an antiserum raised against the C-terminal 17-amino acid fragment of rTGF-α [31]. Two RIAs using an antisera raised to the same antigen [40] (Biotope, Inc., Seattle, WA) detected HMW TGF-α-like factors in conditioned medium of the human breast carcinoma cell line MCF-7 (S. Bates and M.E. Lippman, personal communications) and in extracts of human milk and human mammary tumor tissue (D.S. Salomon and W.R. Kidwell, personal communications). In addition, we have detected hTGF-α in the urine of patients with disseminated breast carcinoma using the Biotope antiserum in a TGF-α RIA (K. Stromberg et al., submitted for publication). The fact that we have not detected similar HMW forms of immunoreactive TGF-α in A673 conditioned medium, even in an RIA using antisera raised against the entire low molecular weight hTGF-α, suggests several possibilities. First, it is possible that more specific immunologic reagents may be required to detect human HMW TGF-α-like growth factors of nonbreast origin. Second, the immunoreactive TGF-α-like component in athymic mouse urine [31] may be a murine growth factor, perhaps produced in response to the tumor. Third, the conditions under which A673 cells grow (ie, in vivo in the athymic mouse versus in vitro in cell culture) may influence the forms or relative amounts of the growth factors they produce. Fourth, there may be tissue-specific differences in the kinds of growth factors that are produced. Fifth, the inability of the antiserum to react may be due to sequestration of critical epitopes within these possible TGF-α precursor molecules. The antiserum may also require the free C-terminal amino acid residue of TGF-α for reactivity, as has been described for other antisera [44,45] which are sometimes referred to as "wraparound" antisera. In support of this hypothesis, the synthetic hTGF-α C-terminal 17-amino acid fragment [14] that has a C-terminal residue blocked by an amide group is recognized only poorly by the Biotope antiserum (W.R. Hargreaves, unpublished data). Thus, hTGF-α precursors with C-terminal extensions [21,22] would probably not react with the Biotope antiserum. RIAs using antisera raised against various precursor forms of hTGF-α might identify the EGF-receptor-binding HMW growth factors secreted by A673 cells as immunologically related to hTGF-α. Alternatively, A673 cells may secrete HMW growth factors more closely related to the EGF-receptor-binding glycosylated growth factor of 23K released into conditioned medium of vaccinia virus-infected cells [46]. Last, and least likely, perhaps A673 cells produce immunologically distinct forms of HMW growth factors of the EGF/TGF-α family.

ACKNOWLEDGMENTS

We thank P.A. Johnson, S. Vargo, L. Dorman, G. Harris, B.J. Sherrell, and C.D. Mount for technical assistance, and Drs. Rik Derynck and Timothy S. Bringman of Genentech, Inc., and L.E. Gentry of Oncogen, Inc. for immunologic assay of HMW growth factors from A673 cells or conditioned medium.

REFERENCES

1. Todaro GJ, Marquardt H, Twardzik DR, Reynolds FH Jr, Stephenson JR: In Weinstein IB, Vogel HJ (eds): "Genes and Proteins in Oncogenesis." New York: Academic Press, 1983, pp 165–182.
2. Sporn MB, Anzano MA, Assoian RK, De Larco JE, Frolik CA, Meyers CA, Roberts AB: In Levine AJ, Van de Woude GF, Topp WC, Watson JD (eds): "The Transformed Phenotype." Cold Spring Harbor, NY: Cold Spring Harbor Laboratory, 1984, pp 1–4.
3. De Larco JE, Todaro GJ: Proc Natl Acad Sci USA 75:4001, 1978.
4. Frolik CA, Dart LL, Sporn MB: Fed Proc Fed Am Soc Exp Biol 41:855, 1982.
5. Anzano MA, Roberts AB, Meyers CA, Komoriya A, Lamb LC, Smith JM, Sporn MB: Cancer Res 42:4776, 1982.
6. Roberts AB, Anzano MA, Lamb LC, Smith JM, Frolik CA, Marquardt H, Todaro GJ, Sporn MB: Nature 295:417, 1982.
7. Sporn M, Roberts A, Shull J, Smith J, Ward J, Sodek M: Science 219:1329, 1983.
8. Anzano MA, Roberts AB, Smith JM, Sporn MB, De Larco JE: Proc Natl Acad Sci USA 80:6264, 1983.
9. Marquardt H, Todaro GJ: J Biol Chem 257:5220, 1982.
10. Twardzik DR, Todaro GJ, Marquardt H, Reynolds FH, Stephenson JR: Science 216:894, 1982.
11. Massague J: J Biol Chem 258:13606, 1983.
12. Marquardt H, Hunkapiller MW, Hood LE, Twardzik DR, De Larco JE, Stephenson JR, Todaro GJ: Proc Natl Acad Sci USA 80:4684, 1983.
13. Marquardt H, Hunkapiller MW, Hood LE, Todaro GJ: Science 233:1079, 1984.
14. Tam JP, Marquardt H, Rosberger DF, Wong TW, Todaro GJ: Nature 309:376, 1984.
15. Frolik CA, Dart LL, Meyers CA, Smith DM, Sporn MB: Proc Natl Acad Sci USA 80:3676, 1983.
16. Roberts AB, Anzano MB, Meyers CA, Wideman J, Blacher R, Pan YCE, Stein S, Lehrman SR, Smith JM, Lamb LC, Sporn MB: Biochemistry 22:5692, 1983.
17. Dart LL, Smith DM, Meyers CA, Sporn MB, Frolik CA: Biochemistry 24:5925, 1985.
18. Massague J: J Biol Chem 259:9756, 1984.
19. Gray A, Dull TJ, Ullrich A: Nature 303:722, 1983.
20. Scott J, Urdea M, Quiroga M, Sanchez-Pescador R, Fong N, Selby M, Rutter WJ, Bell GI: Science 221:236, 1983.

21. Derynck R, Roberts AB, Winkler ME, Chen EY, Goeddel DV: Cell 38:287, 1984.
22. Lee DC, Rose TM, Webb NR, Todaro GJ: Nature 313:489, 1985.
23. Derynck R, Jarrett JA, Chen EY, Eaton DH, Bell JR, Assoian RK, Roberts AB, Sporn MB, Goeddel DV: Nature 316:701, 1985.
24. Twardzik DR, Sherwin SA, Ranchalis J, Todaro GJ: J Natl Cancer Inst 69:793, 1982.
25. Sherwin SA, Twardzik DR, Bohn WH, Cockley KD, Todaro GJ: Cancer Res 43:403, 1983.
26. Stromberg K, Hudgins WR, Dorman LS, Henderson LE, Sowder RC, Sherrell BJ, Mount CD, Orth DN: Cancer Res (in press).
27. Todaro GJ, Fryling CM, De Larco JE: Proc Natl Acad Sci USA 77:5258, 1980.
28. Van Zoelen EJJ, Twardzik DR, Van Oostwaard TMJ, Van der Saag PT, De Laat SW, Todaro GJ: Proc Natl Acad Sci USA 81:4085, 1984.
29. De Larco JE, Pigott DA, Lazarus JA: Proc Natl Acad Sci USA 82:5015, 1985.
30. Linsley PS, Hargreaves WR, Twardzik DR, Todaro GJ: Proc Natl Acad Sci USA 82:356, 1985.
31. Twardzik DR, Kimball ES, Sherwin SA, Ranchalis JE, Todaro GJ: Cancer Res 45:1934, 1985.
32. Giard DJ, Aaronson SA, Todaro GJ, Arnstein P, Kersey JJ, Dosik HK, Parks WP: J Natl Cancer Inst 51:1417, 1973.
33. Kimball ES, Warren TC: Biochim Biophys Acta 771:82, 1984.
34. Lowry OH, Rosebrough NJ, Farr AL, Randall RJ: J Biol Chem 193:265, 1956.
35. Cohen SA, Tarvin TL, Bidlingmeyer T: Am Lab 16:48, 1984.
36. Laemmli UK: Nature 227:680, 1970.
37. Oka Y, Orth DN: J Clin Invest 72:249, 1983.
38. Dailey GE, Kraus JW, Orth DN: J Clin Endocrinol Metab 46:929,1978.
39. Mount CD, Lukas TJ, Orth DN: Arch Biochem Biophys 240:33, 1985.
40. Hazarika P, Pardue R, Lorenzo I, Sawada T, Earls R, Dedman JR:(in press).
41. Iwata KK, Fryling CM, Knott WB, Todaro GJ: Cancer Res 45:2689, 1985.
42. Ignotz RA, Kelly B, Davis RJ, Massague J: Proc Natl Acad Sci USA 83:6307, 1986.
43. Taylor JM, Mitchell WM, Cohen S: J Biol Chem 249:2188, 1974.
44. Wilson, RE, Orth DN, Nicholson WE, Mount CD, Bertagna XY: J Clin Endocrinol Metabol 53:1, 1981.
45. Orth DN: "Methods of Hormone Radioimmunoassay," 2nd Ed. New York: Academic Press, 1979, pp 245–293.
46. Stroobant P, Rice AP, Gullick WJ, Cheng DJ, Kerr IM, Waterfield MD: Cell 42:383, 1985.

Journal of Cellular Biochemistry 33:87–94 (1987)
Cellular and Molecular Biology of Tumors and
Potential Clinical Applications 89–96

Viral *P21* Ki-RAS Protein: A Potent Intracellular Mitogen That Stimulates Adenylate Cyclase Activity in Early G$_1$ Phase of Cultured Rat Cells

Douglas J. Franks, James F. Whitfield, and Jon P. Durkin

Cell Physiology Group, Division of Biological Sciences, National Research Council of Canada, Ottawa, Ontario, Canada K1A OR6 (D.J.F., J.F.W., J.P.D.), and Department of Pathology, Faculty of Health Sciences, University of Ottawa, Ottawa, Ontario, Canada K1H 8M5 (D.J.F.)

Rat kidney (NRK) cells infected with a temperature-sensitive mutant of the Kirsten sarcoma virus were arrested in the G$_0$/G$_1$ phase of their cell cycle by incubation in serum-deficient medium at a *p21*-inactivating temperature of 41°C. These quiescent *ts* K-NRK cells were then stimulated to transit G$_1$ and initiate DNA replication by lowering the temperature to 36°C, which rapidly reactivated *p21*. Reactivating the viral Ki-RAS protein by temperature shift led to an increase in adenylate cyclase activity in early G$_1$ phase. The Ki-RAS protein increased the sensitivity of adenylate cyclase to guanyl nucleotides by a mechanism that seemed to involve inactivation of the enzyme's inhibitory G$_1$ regulatory protein.

Key words: c-AMP, G-proteins, Ki-*ras* oncogene, proliferation, transformation

RAS genes may control the G$_1$ transit of the yeast *Saccharomyces cerevisiae* by increasing adenylate cyclase activity. Thus the yeast cell needs the product of at least one of its two RAS genes to transit G$_1$ [1,2]. Yeast cell proliferation is also dependent upon adenylate cyclase activity and cyclic AMP-dependent protein kinase [3–5]. These needs appear to be linked by the fact that both of the RAS gene products stimulate yeast adenylate cyclase, although the RAS2 (SC2) protein is by far the better stimulator [6]. Furthermore, the inhibition of G$_1$ transit in RAS$^-$ mutants can be overcome by the *bcy*1 mutation that permanently raises cyclic AMP-dependent protein kinase activity by preventing the synthesis of the cyclic AMP-dependent protein kinase regulatory (R) subunit [6].

It would be reasonable to expect that the smaller, though still closely related, mammalian RAS proteins are also adenylate cyclase stimulators that may be responsible for the transient burst of adenylate cyclase activity that normal (but not all

Received September 18, 1986; revised and accepted September 21, 1986.

neoplastic) cells appear to require in order to complete G_1 transit and initiate DNA replication [7]. At first sight this possibility seems to have been ruled out by Beckner et al [8] and Broek et al [9] who showed that one mammalian *ras* gene product, the *p21* Ha-RAS protein, neither stimulates nor inhibits mammalian adenylate cyclase. However, extending these results obtained with the Ha-RAS protein to include the Ki-*ras* gene product is clearly premature because the two genes are structurally distinct [10], and their patterns of expression during the cell cycle are different [11]. Thus, the Ha-*ras* and Ki-*ras* genes may function differently. A relation between the Ki-RAS protein and mammalian adenylate cyclase is suggested by the facts that a burst of cellular Ki-*ras* gene transcription coincides with the burst of adenylate cyclase activity that occurs in both regenerating rat liver and BALB/c 3T3 cells as they near the G_1/S transition [7,11,12] and that an oncogenic viral Ki-*ras* protein does affect adenylate cyclase in BALB/c 3T3 cells [13].

Using a temperature-sensitive mutant of the Kirsten sarcoma virus we have shown recently that activation of the Ki-*ras* protein in quiescent, synchronous *ts* K-NRK cells leads to an early increase in adenylate cyclase activity [14]. Here we present further evidence suggesting that a stimulation of adenylate cyclase might be one of the early events in the G_1 transit of NRK cells that is triggered by the oncogenic viral Ki-RAS and that the mechanism of the adenylate cyclase stimulation may involve inactivation of the Gi regulatory protein (inhibitory G protein) of adenylate cyclase.

METHODS
Cell Lines

NRK cells and *ts* K-NRK cells were generous gifts from Dr. E.M. Scolnick (Merck, Sharpe and Dhome, West Point, PA). The *ts* K-NRK cells were derived by infecting normal NRK cells with a temperature-sensitive, transformation-defective mutant (ts 371) of Kirsten sarcoma virus that produces an abnormally thermolabile *p21* Ki-RAS protein [15].

Cell Culture

Cells were routinely cultured in a complete medium consisting of 85% Dulbecco's modification of Eagles medium (DMEM) containing gentamicin and 15% bovine serum (Colorado Serum Co., Denver, CO) and maintained at 36°C in a humidified atmosphere of 95% air and 5% CO_2. Before each experiment, cells were detached by a brief exposure to 0.25% trypsin in phosphate-buffered saline (PBS). They were then plated in 100-mm dishes at a density of 1.5×10^3 cells/cm^2 in 15 ml of complete medium and incubated at 40°C. After 48 hr the cells were arrested at G_0/G_1 by a further 48-hr incubation at 41°C in DMEM-F12 (1:1) medium containing 10 mM Hepes (pH 7.2) and 0.2% bovine serum [16].

Adenylate Cyclase Assay

Cells were washed twice with PBS and scraped off the dish in 2 ml of PBS using a rubber policeman. The cells were sedimented by centrifugation at 500 g for 3 min and washed once with 5 ml of PBS. After centrifugation, the cell pellet was frozen at −90°C. The thawed cell pellets were homogenized in 0.5 ml of a buffer consisting of 50 mM Tris (pH 7.4), 330 mM sucrose, 1 mM MgCl$_2$, and 1 mM dithiothreitol (DTT). Cells were homogenized in a motor-driven teflon/glass homogenizer (10 strokes, 10,000 rpm). The homogenizer was rinsed with a further 0.5 ml of homogenizing buffer, and the combined homogenate (1 ml) was centrifuged at 20,000g for 20 min. The supernatant fluid was discarded, and the pellet was dispersed in a small volume of homogenizing buffer using a small Dounce homogenizer. This dispersed pellet was the source of adenylate cyclase.

Adenylate cyclase activity was determined by measuring the conversion of α [^{32}P]-ATP to [^{32}P]-cyclic AMP as previously described [17]. The reaction mixture (0.1 ml) contained 50 mM Tris buffer (pH 7.4), 10 mM MgCl$_2$, 2 mM DTT, 2 mM cyclic AMP + 0.01 μCi [^{3}H]-cyclic AMP, 0.5 mM ATP-Mg + 0.5 μCi α [^{32}P]-ATP, 0.15% bovine serum albumin, an ATP regenerating system consisting of 5 mM phosphocreatine and 0.4 mg/ml phosphocreatine kinase, and 20–50 μg of enzyme protein in a total volume of 0.1 ml. The reaction was started by adding the enzyme preparation, and it was allowed to proceed for 10 min at 37°C. The reaction was stopped by adding 0.1 ml of 10 mM ATP and diluting the reaction mixture to 0.6 ml with water. Cyclic AMP was isolated by sequential Dowex and alumina chromatography as described previously [17]. The reaction was linear with time and protein concentration under the conditions used. All assays were performed in triplicate. Protein concentration was determined by the method of Bradford [18].

DNA Synthesis

DNA synthetic activity was assessed autoradiographically by exposing cells, which had been grown on 25-mm round plastic coverslips, to [^{3}H] thymidine (5 μCi/ml of medium: Sp Act. 20 Ci/mole: New England Nuclear, Boston, MA), immediately after lowering the incubation temperature to 36°C. The coverslips were processed as previously described [19], and the percentage of labeled nuclei was determined by examining at least 1,000 cells.

RESULTS

Incubation at 41°C inactivated the *p21* product of the Ki-ras gene in *ts* K-NRK cells and caused the cells to become proliferatively quiescent in a G_0/G_1 state in medium containing 0.2% serum instead of the normal 15% serum [16]. Reactivating *p21* by dropping the temperature to 36°C caused the cells to transit G_1 and initiate DNA replication, despite the serum deficiency (Fig. 1). Uninfected NRK cells were also arrested in a G_0/G_1 state by incubation in the serum-deficient media at 41°C, but they were not stimulated to transit G_1 by dropping the temperature to 36°C (data not shown).

The *p21*-activating 41°C to 36°C temperature shift also caused a GTP-dependent increase in adenylate cyclase activity in crude membrane preparations from *ts* K-NRK cells that became significant (P < .001) 5 hr after the *p21*-activating temperature shift (Fig. 1). By contrast, dropping the incubation temperature from 41°C to 36°C slightly (15%) decreased the adenylate cyclase activity in crude membrane preparations from uninfected NRK cells (data not shown). Moreover, concentrations of the nonhydrolysable GTP analogue GMPPNHP between 0.01 and 100 μM stimulated adenylate cyclase activity in crude membrane preparations obtained from *ts* K-NRK cells 5 hours after a 41°C to 36°C shift to a significantly greater extent than the enzyme in membranes from *ts* K-NRK cells held at 41°C (Fig.

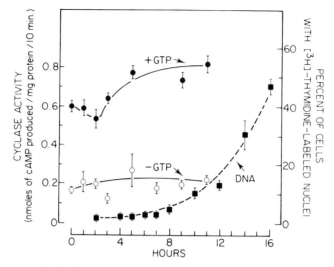

Fig. 1. Time course of adenylate cyclase activity and DNA synthesis in *ts* K-NRK cells. Adenylate cyclase was assayed in absence (open circles) and presence (solid circles) of 10 μM GTP. Cells were rendered quiescent by incubation in serum-deficient medium for 48 hr at 41°C. Cells were harvested at the time points indicated, and adenylate cyclase activity was measured in crude membrane preparations as described in "Materials and Methods." The points are means ± SEM of at least 18 determinations. DNA synthesis was determined by autoradiography as described in "Materials and Methods."

2A). This increased sensitivity to GMPPNHP did not occur in normal NRK cells that had been shifted from 41°C to 36°C for the same time period (Fig. 2B).

The viral *p21* protein might have stimulated the adenylate cyclase catalytic subunit. If this were the case, a potent catalytic subunit stimulator, such as forskolin [20], should override *p21* action. To test this, the stimulation of adenylate cyclase by 10 μM GMPPNHP and 10 μM forskolin was compared in membranes prepared from normal NRK cells and *ts* K-NRK cells held at 41°C and 5 hr after shifting them to 36°C. The 41°C to 36°C temperature shift did not alter the ability of either agent to stimulate the adenylate cyclase of normal NRK cells (Fig. 3). By contrast, the adenylate cyclase of *ts* K-NRK cells at 36°C was more sensitive to stimulation by both GMPPNHP and forskolin than was the enzyme of *ts* K-NRK cells that had been held at 41°C (Fig. 3). In addition, forskolin did not override the effect of *p21* reactivation; hence, it is probable that the viral protein affected one of the adenylate cyclase's regulatory components.

Since adenylate cyclase activity is regulated by both stimulatory (Gs) and inhibitory (Gi) G proteins [21], *p21* could have increased the enzyme's activity either by activating the Gs protein or by inactivating the Gi protein. To determine which of the two regulatory proteins was affected by *p21*, we took advantage of the fact that the Gs and Gi proteins have different Mg^{2+} requirements [22]. The two activities cannot easily be separated in the presence of high Mg^{2+} concentrations (ie, the 10 mM Mg^{2+} used in the experiment and shown in Fig. 2). However, at lower Mg^{2+} levels (eg, 1 mM) that are suboptimal for Gs but optimal for Gi, it is possible to detect changes in Gi activity. Therefore, adenylate cyclase was assayed in the presence of 1 mM Mg^{2+} in membranes from quiescent *ts* K-NRK cells at 41°C in serum-deficient medium and in the same cell 5 hours after a *p21*-activating shift to 36°C.

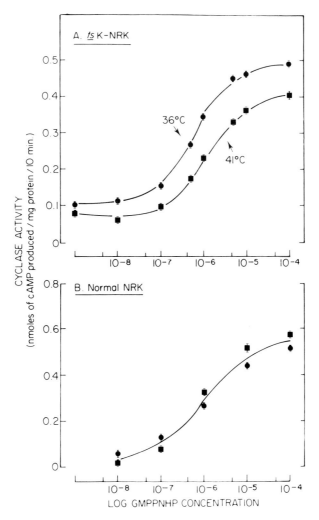

Fig. 2.   Sensitivity to GMPPNHP of adenylate cyclase in membranes from *ts* K-NRK cells at 41°C and after 5 hours at 36°C. Adenylate cyclase activity was determined as described in "Materials and Methods." Values are means ± SEM of three determinations. Identical experiment, but using membranes from normal NRK cells that were shifted to 36° for the same time period.

The nonhydrolysable GTP analogue GTPγS was used as the enzyme stimulator at concentrations ranging from 0.001 to 50 μM. There was significant inhibition of the adenylate cyclase from *ts* K-NRK cells held at 41°C by GTPγS concentrations higher than 5 μM, but there was no inhibition of the enzyme from *ts* K-NRK cells that had been shifted to 36°C (Fig. 4). Hence, it would appear that reactivating *p21* somehow interferes with the inhibitory action of Gi on the adenylate cyclase.

DISCUSSION

Reactivation of the temperature-sensitive, oncogenic viral Ki-RAS protein in quiescent serum-deficient *ts* K-NRK cells caused these cells to transit G_1 and replicate

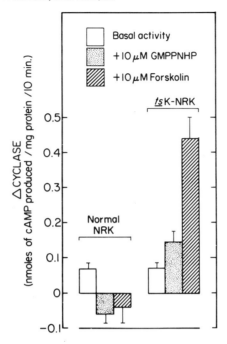

Fig. 3.   Comparison of effect of 10 μM GMPPNHP and 10 μM forskolin on adenylate cyclase in normal NRK cells and *ts* K-NRK cells. Adenylate cyclase activity was determined as described in "Materials and Methods." $\triangle$ cyclase represents the *increase* in enzyme activity in membranes from cells 5 hr after a 41°C to 36°C temperature shift, relative to the activity in membranes from cells held at 41°C. Values are means $\pm$ SEM of three determinations.

DNA [16]. The reactivated RAS protein also stimulated adenylate cyclase activity. At first sight, it might seem that the present observations conflict with the finding that the mammalian Ha-RAS protein does not directly stimulate mammalian adenylate cyclase [8], although it does stimulate yeast adenylate cyclase [9]. However, the viral Ki-RAS protein does stimulate adenylate cyclase in *ts* K-NRK cells [14], but we do not know whether it does so directly or indirectly. The viral *p21* might have affected the action of the distantly related Gs or Gi proteins, or it may have mimicked the action of the Gs protein by directly stimulating the enzyme's catalytic component. A direct, Gs-like stimulation of the catalytic component is unlikely, since a powerful stimulator of the catalytic component, such as forskolin, was unable to override or mask the *p21*-induced activation. However, the fact that the cyclase's biphasic response to a nonhydrolysable guanyl nucleotide in the presence of a low Mg^{2+} concentration at 41°C was eliminated by reactivating *p21* at 36°C indicates that *p21*, either directly or indirectly, inactivated the Gi protein or dissociated it from adenylate cyclase.

The slowness of the stimulation of adenylate cyclase activity by *p21* reactivation suggests that its effect on the Gi protein is indirect. It appears that *p21* activation stimulates phosphatidylinositol degradation [23]. The fact that phosphatidylinositol degradation activates protein kinase C [24] suggests a possible mechanism of the *p21*-induced adenylate cyclase stimulation, since protein kinase C is known to increase adenylate cyclase activity in platelets [25] and pituitary cells [26] by inactivating the Gi protein.

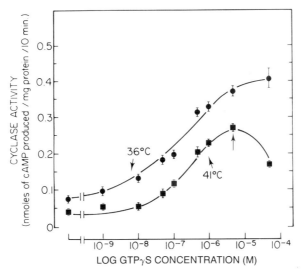

Fig. 4.   Sensitivity to GTPγS of adenylate cyclase in membranes from *ts* K-NRK cells at 41°C and after 5 hours at 36°. Adenylate cyclase activity was determined as described in "Materials and Methods," but the enzyme was assayed at 1 mM Mg^{2+} instead of 10 mM Mg^{2+}. The arrow indicates the GTPγS concentration at which inhibition of adenylate cyclase occurs. Values are means ± SEM of three determinations.

Since the viral Ki-RAS protein does cause a burst of adenylate cyclase activity, similar to that which is required for G_1 transit of normal mammalian cells, and since a burst of cellular Ki-*ras* gene transcription coincides with the late G_1 burst of adenylate cyclase activity in regenerating rat liver cells and mouse 3T3 cells [11,12], it is tempting to speculate that it is the cellular Ki-RAS protein that causes this burst of adenylate cyclase activity. It is also tempting to speculate that the mitogenic, and ultimately the oncogenic, capability of the viral Ki-RAS protein is due at least in part to a stimulation of adenylate cyclase.

ACKNOWLEDGMENTS

This study was supported in part by a grant (MA-8922) from the Medical Research Council of Canada. The authors thank Ms. K. Prokai, Ms. S. Soder, and Ms. L. Aasheim for excellent technical assistance, and Dr. D.J. Gillian for preparing the illustrations.

REFERENCES

1. Kataoka T, Powers S, McGill C, Fasano O, Strathern J, Broach J, Wigler M: Cell 37:437–445, 1984.
2. Tatchell K, Chalell D, Defeo-Jones D, Scolnick E: Nature 309:523–527, 1984.
3. Matsumoto K, Uno I, Oshima Y, Ishikawa T: Proc Nat Acad Sci USA 79:2355–2359, 1982.
4. Matsumoto K, Uno I, Ishikawa T: Cell 32:417–423, 1983.
5. Uno I, Matsumoto K, Ishikawa T: J Biol Chem 257:14110–14115, 1982.
6. Toda T, Uno I, Ishikawa T, Powers S, Kataoka T, Broek D, Cameron S, Broach J, Matsumoto K, Wigler M: Cell 40:27–36, 1985.
7. Boynton AL, Whitfield JF: Adv Cyclic Nucleotide Res 15:193–294, 1983.

8. Beckner SK, Hattori S, Shih TY: Nature 317:71–72 1985.
9. Broek D, Samiy N, Fasano O, Fujiyama A, Tamanoi F, Northrup J, Wigler M: Cell 41:763–769, 1985.
10. Shih TY, and Weeks MO: Cancer Invest 2:109–123, 1984.
11. Goyette M, Petropoulos CJ, Shank PE, Fausto N: Mol Cell Biol 4:1493–1498, 1984.
12. Campisi J, Gray HE, Pardee AB, Dean M, Sonnenshein G: Cell 36:241–247, 1984.
13. Saltarelli D, Fischer S, Gacon G: Biochem Biophys Res Comm 127:318–325, 1985.
14. Franks DJ, Whitfield JF, Durkin JP: Biochem Biophys Res Comm 127:318–325, 1985.
15. Scolnick EM, Goldberg, RJ, Parks WP: Cold Spring Harbor Symp Quant Biol 39:885–895, 1974.
16. Durkin JP, Whitfield JF: Mol Cell Biol 6:1368–1392, 1986.
17. Franks DJ, Plamondon J, Hamet P: J Cell Physiol 119:41–45, 1984.
18. Bradford M: Anal Biochem 72:248–254, 1979.
19. Durkin JP, Whitfield JF: J Cell Physiol 120:135–145, 1984.
20. Seamon KB, Daly JW: J Cyclic Nucleotide Protein Phosphor Res 7:201–204, 1981.
21. Rodbell M: Nature 284:17–22, 1980.
22. Jakobs KH, Aktories K, Minuth M, Schultz G: Adv Cyclic Nucleotide Protein Phosphorylation Res 19:137–150, 1985.
23. Fleishman LF, Chahwala SB, Cantley L: Science 231:407–410, 1986.
24. Takai YK, Kikkawa U, Kaibuchi K, Nishizuka Y: Adv Cyclic Nucleotide Protein Phosphorylation Res 18:119–158, 1984.
25. Katada T, Gilman AG, Watanabe Y, Bauer S, Jacobs KH: Eur J Biochem 151:431–437, 1985.
26. Summers ST, Cronin MJ: Biochem Biophys Res Comm 135:276–281, 1986.

Journal of Cellular Biochemistry 33:257–266 (1987)
Cellular and Molecular Biology of Tumors and
Potential Clinical Applications 97–106

Myc Family of Cellular Oncogenes

Ronald DePinho, Lisa Mitsock, Kimi Hatton, Pierre Ferrier,
Kathy Zimmerman, Edith Legouy, Abeba Tesfaye, Robert Collum,
George Yancopoulos, Perry Nisen, Ronald Kriz, and Frederick Alt

Department of Biochemistry and Biophysics, Columbia Presbyterian Medical Center,
Columbia University, New York, New York 10032 (R.D., K.H., P.F., K.Z., E.L., A.T., R.C.,
G.Y., F.A.), Department of Pediatrics, Schneider Children's Hospital of LI Jewish Medical
Center, New Hyde Park, New York 11042 (P.N.), and Genetics Institute, Cambridge,
Massachusetts 02138 (R.K., L.M.)

The myc family of cellular oncogenes contains three well-defined members: c-myc, N-myc and L-myc. Additional structural and functional evidence now suggests that other myc-family oncogenes exist. The overall structure and organization of the c-, N-, and L-myc genes and transcripts are very similar. Each gene contains three exons: encoding a long 5' untranslated leader and a long 3' untranslated region. The proteins encoded by these myc genes share several stretches of significant homology. The conservation of sequences at the carboxy-terminus of the L-myc protein suggests that it is also a DNA-binding, nuclear-associated protein. Each myc gene will cooperate with an activated Ha-ras oncogene to cause transformation of primary rat embryo fibroblasts. Characteristics of several new myc-family members are described.

Key words: myc-related genes, nucleotide sequence, transformation

The characterization of multiple myc-related oncogenes has extended our understanding of the fundamental structural and functional properties that define this important class of oncogene. Assignment of a gene to the myc family is based upon specific architectural features of the gene and its transcript, the presence of conserved myc homology regions, nuclear targeting and DNA-binding capacity, and equivalent oncogenic activity in the cotransformation assay [1,2]. Although the myc-family genes display remarkable conservation in both structure and function, they exhibit very distinctive patterns of expression during normal development [3]. While the function of myc-family genes in normal cells is not known, the expression and amplification of myc oncogenes in a wide variety of tumors has fueled speculation that myc genes are intimately involved in tumorigenesis and tumor progression. The mechanisms by which these genes act and their specific role in carcinogenesis are not yet understood.

Received September 25, 1986; revised and accepted November 11, 1986.

THE c-MYC GENE

The characterization of transforming genes (v-myc) from several different strains of avian retroviruses [4] and the search for a cellular counterpart of such transforming sequences have led to the discovery of the first and most thoroughly studied member of this family, the c-myc gene [5,6]. Structurally, c-myc is composed of three exons with the coding region located solely on exons 2 and 3; the remainder of the gene is untranslated, encoding a transcript with large 5' and 3' untranslated regions [7,8]. The c-myc gene product is a nuclear-associated phosphoprotein that has a strong, albeit nonspecific, affinity for DNA and chromatin [9]. It is widely thought that c-myc is involved in cellular differentiation and proliferation and that "activated" c-myc expression can induce cellular proliferation and can interfere with differentiation processes in vitro [10–17]. In systems in which tumors can be induced to differentiate in culture, the level of c-myc expression decreases rapidly following treatment with inducing agents [14] and reappears later in a cell-cycle-restricted manner [15] at the point of commitment to terminal differentiation [16]. Moreover, the ability of constitutive c-myc expression to block DMSO-induced differentiation in mouse erythroleukemic cells suggests that c-myc can drastically influence the processes leading to terminal differentiation [17]. A role for c-myc in oncogenesis is strongly suggested by the presence of chromosomal translocations, proviral insertions, or gene amplifications involving the c-myc locus in a wide variety of tumors (reviewed in reference 18), as well as by the cooperation between a transfected c-myc gene with an activated ras gene to produce malignant transformation in cell culture [19].

The c-myc gene was originally thought of as a unique member of a particular class of oncogene. Recently, however, the identification and characterization of several other genes that share significant structural and functional properties with c-myc have clearly indicated that the c-myc gene can no longer be considered an isolated entity but is, in fact, a member of a larger myc oncogene family. At present, the myc family contains three well-defined members: c-myc, N-myc, and L-myc, and is likely to extend to several other genes which we have termed R-myc, L-myc ψ, and p-myc (Fig. 1) [1,2]. The discovery and isolation of additional members of the myc gene family were based upon the presence of highly conserved amino acid

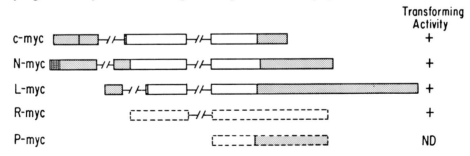

Fig. 1.   Structure and organization of the myc-family genes. Exons are indicated by boxes: open boxes represent translated regions: shaded areas are untranslated regions. Vertical lines in exon 1 locate some of the multiple transcriptional initiation sites identified by S1 nuclease and primer extension assays. Dashed boxes represent regions of cross-hybridization to known myc exon 2 and 3 probes. Myc-related clones were isolated from complete EcoR1 human genomic library in Charon 35A and 16A as described previously [24].

sequences found across all of the myc genes. These sequences are sufficiently conserved at the nucleotide level to permit detectable cross-hybridization under nonstringent conditions, especially in tumors with amplification and overexpression. These features facilitated the discovery of N-myc in neuroblastomas [20,21] and L-myc in small-cell lung carcinomas [22]. As described below, each of these genes and their products have strikingly similar structures and display functional similarities in the context of development and cancer.

THE N-MYC GENE

The detailed structural characterization of the N-myc gene in both mouse [23] and human [24,25] led to the concept that the myc family extended beyond the c-myc gene. The complete nucleotide sequence of N-myc revealed a gene organization very similar to c-myc. Both genes have three exons, 5' and 3' untranslated regions flanking the coding domain, and highly related gene products with an abundance of basic amino acids at the carboxy terminus. The positive charges in this region may account for the affiliation of the protein with DNA and chromatin [23]. The nuclear localization of the N-myc protein has been confirmed by anti-N-myc specific antibody studies [26,27]. Thus, like c-myc, the N-myc gene appears to encode a nuclear-associated, DNA-binding protein product.

Though the normal physiological function of N-myc during cellular growth and development is not known, a role in cellular differentiation is suggested by a significant decrease in the expression of N-myc prior to retinoic-acid-induced morphological differentiation of human neuroblastomas [28]. The participation of N-myc in normal development is also supported by its tissue- and developmental stage-specific pattern of expression; this pattern of expression is distinct from the generalized transcriptional activity seen with c-myc during the pre- and postnatal development of the mouse [3,29]. A striking example of differential myc-family gene expression occurs during the immunodifferentiation program of B lymphoid cells in which pre-B cells express both N- and c-myc, but only c-myc is expressed at later stages of B cell development [3].

A casual role for N-myc in the genesis and/or progression of tumors is suggested by its frequent amplification and/or overexpression in certain tumors, such as neuroblastoma [20, 21, 30], Wilms tumor [31], small-cell lung carcinoma [32,33], and retinoblastoma [30, 34, 35]. Furthermore, the degree of N-myc gene amplification in primary neuroblastomas correlates well with tumor stage, metastatic potential, prognosis [36,37], and ability of these tumors to adapt to culture as established cell lines [36]. Most notably, N-myc has been shown to encode oncogenic activity indistinguishable from c-myc in the rat embryo fibroblast (REF) cotransformation assay [39,40].

We have previously characterized in detail the murine [23] and human [24,25] N-myc genes and demonstrated the existence of multiple highly conserved blocks of homology across each of the known myc-related genes: v-myc, and N-myc. Such regions could represent domains that confer "generalized" myc functions. Based on this assumption, we expected that, if other unidentified myc genes existed, then they might conserve at least some of these same conserved regions. Preliminary low-stringency hybridization Southern and Northern analyses, using N-myc- and c-myc-derived probes from exons 2 and 3, suggested that additional myc family members indeed existed [2]. Under the same experimental conditions, we screened mouse and human genomic libraries and thereby identified and isolated many independent myc-related clones. Some of the clones that cross-hybridized with probes from several regions of individual myc genes are evolutionarily conserved in both mouse and human genomes. Moreover, the presence of homology to several different myc probes made it unlikely that these signals represented random low-stringency hybridization artifacts. One of these clones has now been characterized in detail and has been found to be a true functional myc gene, ie, the L-myc gene [3,22].

THE L-MYC GENE FAMILY

Probes from the newly isolated genes also allowed identification of additional homologous sequences. In particular, probes from the second and third exons of the newly isolated L-myc gene detected several L-myc-related bands which clearly possessed homology to more than one region of L-myc. In particular, a 3' untranslated probe identified a 12-kb band referred to as R-myc, an 8.3-kb band referred to as L-myc ψ, and a 5.1 kb-band referred to as p-myc. Each of these bands was considered to harbor a true myc-gene because all hybridized to multiple probes from L-myc. The EcoR1 fragments containing each of these L-myc-related genes have been isolated, and an extensive characterization has begun.

The L-myc gene was isolated by two independent methods. L-myc was first detected as a myc-related sequence found to be amplified in a subset of human small-cell lung carcinomas [22]. Using second- and third-exon myc homology probes derived from N-myc and c-myc, L-myc was also isolated from unamplified human and mouse genomic libraries on the basis of cross-hybridization. In a manner similar to N-myc [1–3], L-myc gene expression appears to be tissue-specific and developmentally regulated [3]. Tumor and developmental expression patterns, coupled with significant cross-hybridization to known myc homology box probes, suggested that L-myc would likely be a functional myc-family member [3,22].

L-Myc Gene Structure and Organization

We have isolated a 10.6-kb EcoR1 human genomic clone, pR11.1, which contains a complete copy of the L-myc gene [1,2]. Comparison of the nucleotide sequence of this clone with the sequences of the murine L-myc clone pmL-myc and the highly related human L-myc-processed pseudogene clone pR1.3 (corresponds to the 8.3-kb EcoR1 L-myc ψ described above) indicates that the L-myc gene is organized into the same three exon-two intron pattern characteristic of c- and N-myc genes. This proposed organization is based on several lines of evidence. A computer analysis comparing the human L-myc and L-myc ψ gene sequences shows that they share three regions of significant homology and that each region of homologous sequence is separated by large stretches of unrelated sequence [2]. At each of the boundaries between conserved (putative exons) and divergent sequence (putative introns), there exists a typical donor or acceptor splice consensus recognition sequence [38] (Fig. 2). The boundaries of the 3' end of exon 2 and the 5' border of exon 3 are also suggested by sequence comparisons with the murine L-myc gene: the murine organization was confirmed by S1 nuclease protection experiments (Mitsock, Zimmerman, Legouy, Kriz, and Alt, in preparation). Most notably, a highly conserved myc homology region spanning the exon 2/3 interface in each of the known myc genes is also present in the L-myc genes.

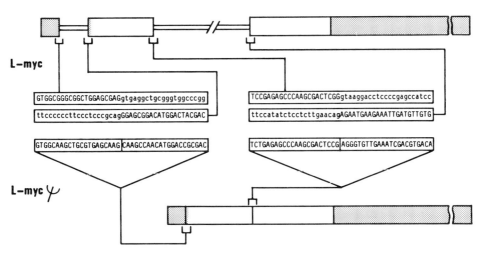

Fig. 2.   Structural relationships between L-myc and an L-myc Pseudogene. Nucleic acid sequence was determined by the partial chemical degradation method as previously described [23]. Exons are represented by boxes, introns as double lines. The origin of the sequences spanning the noted junctional regions is indicated.

The 5′ border of exon 2 and the existence of exon 1 were confirmed by end-labelled oligonucleotide-primed RNA sequencing from the 5′ region of exon 2 into the first exon as well as by hybridization of the putative first exon to the L-myc message [2]. The existence of an additional 5′ boundary for exon 2 has not been ruled out. Preliminary primer extension data reveal as many as 15–20 distinct initiation sites which span 140–510 bp 5′ to the exon 1/2 boundary [2]. At the 3′ end of the gene, the location of the adenylation signal was determined by sequence comparison between the human genomic sequence and the corresponding 3′ terminus of the processed L-myc pseudogene, L-myc ψ. The position of this adenylation signal is conserved in man and in mouse.

The L-Myc Transcript

The complete L-myc message measures approximately 3.8 kb; the mRNA size agrees well with the predicted measurements based on the proposed exon organization discussed above. The first ATG sequence of a long open reading frame occurs approximately 10 bp downstream from the 5′ boundary of exon 2; beginning at this position the open reading frame extends 1,089 nucleotides to an in-phase terminator in exon 3 [2]. The location of this coding domain corresponds precisely to the coding region defined in the mouse L-myc sequence (Kriz, Zimmerman, Legouy, and Alt, in preparation). The mouse sequence contains minor in-phase insertions in two regions of exon 3 coding domain, not involving conserved regions. Analysis of the corresponding region in the L-myc ψ reveals multiple deletions and basepair changes that result in terminators in all three reading frames. Thus, the mature 3.8-kb human L-myc transcript consists of (1) a 5′ untranslated leader of varying length (approx. 150–520 bp) encoded by the first exon and the 5′ portion of exon 2, (2) a 1.1-kb coding domain spanning exons 2 and 3, and (3) a large (approx. 2.2 kb) 3′ untranslated region encoded by the downstream portion of exon 3.

The function of both 5′ and 3′ untranslated regions of myc genes is not known; that they may serve some important regulatory role is underscored by the remarkable degree of nucleotide sequence conservation in regions that are not under any selective pressure at the protein level. For any given myc gene, evolutionary conservation between mouse and human ranges from 80% to 90%. In contrast, sequence comparisons of the untranslated regions between different myc family members (eg, c-myc vs N-myc vs L-myc) reveals complete divergence. This sequence divergence in these potential regulatory regions is not surprising given the differential patterns of expression seen among different myc-family genes [23].

MYC GENE PRODUCTS

The putative L-myc transcript could encode a protein of 362 amino acids. An amino acid homology computer analysis reveals clusters of amino acids that are highly conserved across all myc proteins (Fig. 3), including two clusters previously noted in the 5' portion of the coding domain in exon 2 [20,22] and two additional ones identified in the coding domain in exon 3 [23–25]. The remarkable conservation of these myc homology boxes in all three proteins suggests that they are essential for some general aspect of myc gene function such as transforming capacity and targeting to the nucleus. The putative L-myc protein also contains a highly conserved C-terminus containing basic amino acids, which suggests DNA-binding ability. Additional sequences are found conserved between only two of the myc-family genes (wavy lines, Fig. 3); these regions are less likely to be important for general myc properties.

THE MYC FAMILY OF CELLULAR ONCOGENES

Several new genes can now be classified within the myc family of cellular oncogenes: L-myc and R-myc. This assertion is based on a number of similarities with respect to structure and function that these genes have with c-myc and N-myc genes and gene product. Specifically, we have shown L-myc is a structurally related gene which encodes a related gene product. In addition, both L-myc and R-myc possess similar transforming activity in the rat embryo fibroblast cotransformation assay, as noted below. Several additional members of the myc family have been characterized; one is a pseudogene and the functional activity of at least one other

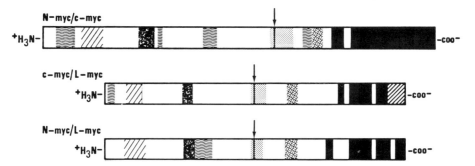

Fig. 3. Comparison of putative myc-family proteins. Each shaded box represents 70% or greater amino homology between the genes indicated. Boxes containing wavy lines identify regions that are homologous between only two but not all three of the myc genes. Arrows locate sequence encoded by the splice between exons 2 and 3.

(p-myc) has been suggested but not confirmed [1, 2]; preliminary nucleotide sequence analysis of the human p-myc gene has revealed extensive regions of significant homology with the human L-myc gene and expression during a narrow window of murine development (Ferrier, DePinho, and Alt, unpublished data). Additional evolutionarily conserved myc-related clones which bear multiple myc homologies are currently being analyzed. Preliminary evidence suggests that the myc family of oncogenes probably contains additional members.

MYC GENE-TRANSFORMING ACTIVITY

Deregulated expression of myc family genes has been noted in many different tumors, suggesting that aberrant myc gene expression can contribute to the development of neoplasia. The oncogenic potential of c-myc and N-myc has been examined [19,39,40]. Both c-myc [19] and N-myc [39,40] can play a direct role in tumor formation. Expression constructs containing the c-myc or N-myc genes can cooperate equally well with an activated Ha-ras oncogene to malignantly transform normal embryonic fibroblasts. The human L-myc gene has a similar myc-like oncogenic activity. A vector which contained the L-myc gene in the same transcriptional orientation as flanking long terminal repeats (LTRs) (designated pV11.1A) was not able to transform REFs alone but was able to cooperate with the mutant Ha-ras gene in the REF assay to produce dense foci that overgrew the normal monolayers (Fig. 1). The pV11.1-transformed REFs also demonstrated anchorage-independent growth in soft agar and the ability to cause tumors in young syngeneic rats. The morphological appearance of L-myc-transformed REFs was indistinguishable from the N-myc and c-myc controls. Northern blot analysis of c-myc-, N-myc-, or L-myc-transformed REFs confirmed the presence of high-level expression of both the transfected myc gene construct and the ras gene [2]. Thus, the L-myc gene possesses transforming potential comparable to that of c-myc and N-myc genes. Similar analyses of LTR-R-myc expression vectors in the cotransformation assay have indicated that R-myc has a transforming activity equivalent to that of other myc-family genes [2].

DEVELOPMENTAL EXPRESSION PATTERNS PREDICT TUMOR
EXPRESSION PATTERNS: N-MYC EXPRESSION IN WILMS TUMOR

We have demonstrated that high-level expression of N-myc and L-myc genes is very restricted with respect to tissue and developmental stage, while expression of c-myc is more generalized. The restricted tissue-specific expression patterns of N-myc and L-myc seem to correlate with the restricted types of tumors in which these genes are amplified and/or overexpressed. For example, N-myc expression, which is extremely high in the developing brain, is amplified and overexpressed in neuroblastomas [3,30], whereas L-myc expression in the developing lung correlates well with its potential role in lung carcinoma [3,22]. In contrast, the more generalized pattern of c-myc expression parallels c-myc overexpression in a wide range of tumors.

High-level N-myc expression was also observed in the developing mouse kidney; this observation prompted us to analyze myc expression and myc-gene-copy number in normal developing human kidney and Wilms tumor [31]. Wilms tumor is a frequent childhood kidney carcinoma that arises from embryonal cells. We also assayed for myc expression in various other human tumors including a set of neoplasms which also arise from primitive or undifferentiated cells, eg, hepatoblastoma and medulloblastoma. In general, enhanced N-myc expression was characteristic of tumors which derive from certain primitive cell lineages [31]. In particular, almost all of the Wilms tumor examined expressed greatly elevated levels of N-myc [31]. Notably, in contrast to high-level expression of N-myc in neuroblastomas, which is generally associated with N-myc gene amplification [30,31], all tested Wilms DNA samples demonstrated single-copy N-myc levels. Thus, greatly enhanced expression of the N-myc gene in Wilms tumors occurs in the absence of gene amplification [31]. The level of N-myc expression per gene copy in such tumors is 20- to 30-fold greater than that of human neuroblastoma N-myc expression per gene copy [31]. It is not yet clear whether such expression reflects a property of the normal progenitor cell or is directly related to tumorigenesis.

CROSS-REGULATION AMONG MYC FAMILY MEMBERS

Analysis of the relative level of c-myc expression appeared to be inversely correlated with relative N-myc expression levels in Wilms tumors and human neuroblastomas [31] and in REFs which expressed very high levels of cotransfected LTR-N-myc vector (1) and in preliminary experiments, a co-transfected LTR-L-myc construct [2]. Numerous 3T3 or L cell transformants which expressed the LTR-N-myc construct at low (baseline) levels also expressed the c-myc gene (Zimmerman and Alt, unpublished results). Low-level coordinate expression of multiple myc members has been seen in normal cells and tumors [3]. Our preliminary analyses suggest that relatively high-level expression of N-myc or L-myc is necessary to cross-regulate c-myc expression [1].

WHAT IS THE ROLE OF MYC GENES?

Although current studies suggest that the differential or combinatorial expression of myc family genes plays a fundamental role in cellular differentiation processes, the function(s) of myc-family genes in normal tissues is not known. The myc-gene products may have a direct role in regulating the expression of other genes is suggested by (1) their probable DNA binding capability, (2) the possibility that c-myc expression has positive regulatory activity on other genes [41] and negative autoregulatory activity on itself [42–44], and (3) the phenomenon of cross-regulation whereby elevated N-myc or L-myc expression may down-regulate c-myc expression [31]. The mechanism(s) by which cross-regulation occurs remains to be determined, and an interesting possibility is that products of one member of this gene family might be capable of directly influencing the expression of other family members. In this way, myc genes may conceivably act in an orchestrated manner, temporally and spatially, to affect the expression patterns of each other as well as other developmentally regulated genes and thereby control a specific differentiation pathway.

As discussed, the distinct patterns of myc-family gene expression patterns in normal tissues have helped to predict the types of tumors in which they are expressed or activated. The activated expression of myc-family genes in tumors is often the result of gene amplification [30]. The genetic events which lead to myc gene amplification and the role that amplification has in the genesis of certain cancers are poorly understood. Several studies have now addressed the latter issue by examining the expression and gene copy number of N-myc in the context of neuroblastoma clinical staging. Significantly, these investigations clearly documented a strong correlation between N-myc amplification and more advanced stages of neuroblastoma (stages 3 and 4) [36,37,45], and further demonstrated that at any stage of the disease, N-myc amplification and neuroblastoma stage were associated with a worse prognosis [37]. Thus, assuming that the more progressive forms of neuroblastoma derive from the less progressive ones, amplification of N-myc appears involved with tumor progression: early stages express N-myc at low levels and have no gene amplification, later stages demonstrate increased N-myc copy number and resultant overexpression. By analogy to methotrexate-resistance gene amplification studies [46], one could thus imagine a scenerio whereby N-myc amplification was not a primary event in the generation of a neuroblastoma, but that increased amounts of the N-myc gene product, secondary to amplification of the N-myc gene, conferred a selective advantage to those cells.

N-myc clearly plays an oncogenic role in tumors which have high-level N-myc expression from amplified genes. It is unclear, however, whether N-myc expression in unamplified tumors plays a role in tumorigenesis or simply reflects the inherent expression profile of the cell from which the tumor is derived [1,3]. Given that myc-family genes are developmentally regulated, it is possible that the continuous expression of N-myc locks these precursor embryonal cells in a dedifferentiated, proliferating state—just as constitutive c-myc expression blocked DMSO-induced differentiation of myeloid erythroleukemia cells [15]. The N-myc gene would thereby be a candidate for amplification as selective growth pressures prevailed. The basic question then becomes: What is responsible for the deregulated expression of N-myc which freezes N-myc expression at an early embryonic expression pattern? One model of oncogenesis in certain embryonal tumors with a genetic predisposition (eg, retinoblastoma and Wilms tumor) has focused on recessive "anti-oncogenes" which encode a function that regulates the expression of a transforming gene (eg, N-myc) during embryogenesis [1,47,48]. The loss of an anti-oncogene via an inherited and/or spontaneous event would then result in the continual expression of the transforming gene and the inability of that cell to enter the normal developmental program and terminally differentiate.

ACKNOWLEDGMENTS

This work was supported by NIH grants CA23767-06 and CA42335, ACS grant CD-269, and a Searle Scholars Award to F.A. and by the Rosalind and Sol Chaikin Institute for Childhood Cancer Research of the Schneider Children's Hospital. F.A. is an Irma T. Hirschl Career Scientist and Malinckrodt Scholar. E.L. and P.F. are recipients of EMBO fellowships. R.D. is a recipient of the NIH Physician Scientist Award, AI-00602-03.

REFERENCES

1. Alt FW, DePinho RA, Zimmerman K, Legouy E, Hatton K, Ferrier P, Tesfaye A, Yancopoulos CD, Nisen P: Cold Spring Harbor Symp Quant Biol, in press.
2. DePinho RA, Hatton KS, Ferrier P, Tesfaye A, Alt FW: Submitted.
3. Zimmerman KA, Yancopoulos GD, Collum RG, et al: Nature 319:780–783, 1986.

4. Coffin JM, Varmus HE, Bishop JM, Essex M, Hardy WD, Martin GS, Rosenberg NE, Scolnick EM, Weinberg RA, Vogt PK: J Virol 40:953–957, 1981.
5. Sheiness DK, Hughes SH, Varmus HE, Stubblefield E, Bishop JM: Virology 105:415–424, 1980.
6. Sheiness D, Bishop JM: J Virol 31:514–521, 1979.
7. Battey J, Moulding C, Taub R, Murphy W, Stewart T, Potter H, Lenoir G, Leder P: Cell 34:779–787, 1983.
8. Stanton LW, Farlander PD, Tesser PM, Marcu KB: Nature 310:423–425, 1984.
9. Persson H, Leder P: Science 225:718–721, 1984.
10. Gonda TJ, Metcalf D: Nature 310:249–251, 1984.
11. Grosso LE, Pitot HC: Cancer Res 45:847–850, 1985.
12. Dony C, Kessel M, Gruss P: Nature 317:636–639, 1985.
13. Coppola JA, Cole MD: Nature 320:760–763, 1986.
14. Lachman HM, Skoultchi AI: Nature 310:592–594, 1984.
15. Lachman HM, Hatton KS, Skoultchi AI, Schildkraut CL: Proc Natl Acad Sci USA 82:5323–5327, 1985.
16. Lachman HM, Cheng G, Skoultchi AI: Proc Natl Acad Sci USA 83:6480–6484, 1986.
17. Dmitrovsky E, Kuehl WM, Hollis GF, Kirsh IR, Bender TP, Segal S: Nature 322:748–750, 1986.
18. Rabbitts, TH: Trends Genet 1:327–331, 1985.
19. Land H, Parada LF, Weinberg RA: Nature 304:596–601, 1983.
20. Schwab M, Alitalo K, Klempnauer L, Varmus H, Bishop J, Gilbert F, Brodeur G, Goldstein M, Trent J: Nature 305:245–248, 1983.
21. Kohl NE, Kanda N, Schreck RR, Bruns G, Latt SA, Gilbert F, Alt FW: Cell 35:359–367, 1983.
22. Nau M, Brooks B, Battey J, Sausville E, Gasdar A, Kirsh I, McBride O, Bertness V, Hollis G, Minna J: Nature 318:69–73, 1985.
23. DePinho RA, Legouy E, Feldman LB, Kohl NE, Yancopoulos GD, Alt FW: Proc Natl Acad Sci USA 83:1827–1831, 1986.
24. Kohl N, Leguoy E, DePinho R, Smith R, Gee C, Alt FW: Nature 319:73–77, 1986.
25. Stanton LW, Schwab M, Bishop JM: Proc Natl Acad Sci USA 83:1772–1776, 1986.
26. Ikegaki N, Bukovsky J, Kennett RH: Proc Natl Acad Sci USA 83:5929–5933, 1986.
27. Slamon DJ, Boone TC, Seeger RC, Keith DE, Chazin V, Lee HC, Souza LM: Science 232:768–772, 1986.
28. Thiele CJ, Reynolds CP, Israel MA: Nature 313:404–406, 1985.
29. Jakobovits A, Schwab M, Bishop JM, Martin GR: Nature 318:188–191, 1985.
30. Kohl NE, Gee CE, Alt FW: Science 226:1335–1337, 1984.
31. Nisen PD, Zimmerman KA, Cotter SV, Gilbert F, Alt FW: Cancer Res 46:6217–6222, 1986.
32. Nau MM, Brooks BJ, Carney DN, Gazdar AF, Battey JF, Sausville EA, Minna JD: Proc Natl Acad Sci USA 83:1092–1096, 1986.
33. Wong, AJ, Ruppert JM, Eggleston J, Hamilton SR, Baylin SB, Vogelstein B:Science 233:461–464, 1986.
34. Lee WH, Murphee AL, Benedict WF: Nature 309:458–460, 1984.
35. Squire J, Goddard AD, Canton M, Becker A, Phillips RA, Gallie BL: Nature 322:555–557, 1986.
36. Brodeur GM, Seeger RC, Schwab M, Varmus HE, Bishop JM: Science 224:1121–1124, 1984.
37. Seeger R, Brodeur G, Sather H, Dalton A, Siegel S, Wong K, Hammond O: N Engl J Med 313:1111–1119, 1985.
38. Mount SM: Nucleic Acids Res 10:459–472, 1982.
39. Yancopoulos GD, Nisen PD, Tesfaye A, Kohl NE, Goldfarb MP, Alt FW: Proc Natl Acad Sci USA 82:5455–5459, 1985.
40. Schwab M, Varmus HE, Bishop JM: Nature 316:160–162, 1985.
41. Kingston R, Baldwin A, Sharp P: Nature 312:280–282, 1984.
42. Klein G: Nature 294:313–318, 1981.
43. Kelly K, Cochran B, Stiles C, Leder P: Cell 35:603–610, 1983.
44. Adams J, Harris A, Pinkert C, Corcoran L, Alexander W, Cory S, Palmiter R, Brinster R: Nature 318:533–538, 1985.
45. Schwab M, Varmus H, Bishop JM, Grzeschik K-H, Naylor S, Sakaguchi A, Brodeur G, Trent J: Nature 308:288–291, 1984.
46. Alt FW, Kellems RE, Bertino JR, Schimke RT: J Biol Chem 253:1357–1371, 1978.
47. Knudson AG, Strong LC: J Natl Cancer Inst 48:313–323, 1972.
48. Comings D: Proc Natl Acad Sci USA 70:3324–3327, 1973.

Journal of Cellular Biochemistry 33:267–288 (1987)
Cellular and Molecular Biology of Tumors and
Potential Clinical Applications 107–128

Oncogene Amplification and Chromosomal Abnormalities in Small Cell Lung Cancer

J.M. Ibson, J.J. Waters, P.R. Twentyman, N.M. Bleehen, and P.H. Rabbitts

Ludwig Institute for Cancer Research (J.M.I., P.H.R.), MRC Clinical Oncology and Radiotherapeutics Unit, MRC Centre (P.R.T., N.M.B.), Department of Cytogenetics, Addenbrooke's Hospital (J.J.W.), Cambridge, CB2 2QH England

Twelve cell lines isolated from patients with small cell lung cancer have been studied for amplification of the three characterised members of the myc proto-oncogene family (c-myc, N-myc, and L-myc) and for abnormalities of chromosome 3. Ten of these lines were being studied for the first time. Ten of the 12 small cell lung cancer cell lines had amplification of one member of the myc proto-oncogene family. Amplification of c-myc was observed in only one small cell lung line—a "morphological variant." One "classic" small cell lung cancer line expressed c-myc but had no obvious amplification of the gene. N-myc and L-myc were more commonly amplified than c-myc. Chromosomal abnormalities (mainly deletions) in chromosome 3 were observed in all small cell lung carcinoma cell lines examined. When the small cell lung carcinoma lines were grouped according to "classic" or "variant" characteristics, it was found that the "classics" had deletions of the short arm of chromosome 3, whereas the "biochemical variants" had deletions of the long arm of chromosome 3. The extent of the deletions varied between cell lines. For the deletion in the short arm of chromosome 3 the minimum common region of overlap was assigned to bands 3p23–3p24.

Key words: c-myc, N-myc, L-myc, chromosome 3, oncogene amplification, chromosomal abnormalities, small cell lung cancer

In a significant number of tumour types, the activation of a proto-oncogene is associated with a chromosomal abnormality—a translocation, inversion, or deletion [for review, see ref 1]. Examples of consistent chromosomal abnormalities are the translocations in Burkitt's lymphoma involving the c-myc gene on chromosome 8 [2] and the Philadelphia chromosome in acute myeloid leukaemia involving the c-abl gene on chromosome 9 [3]. The proto-oncogene mapping to the chromosomal abnormality may not be the only activated oncogene in the tumour, however: in in vitro transformation experiments, oncogenes have been shown to be required to act synergistically to bring about transformation [for recent review, see ref 4]. Wilm's tumour

Received August 11, 1986; revised and accepted October 29, 1986.

and retinoblastoma provide likely in vivo examples of more than one gene being involved in the transformed phenotype [5,6]. The two genes may be activated by different mechanisms—mutations in the coding or regulatory regions of the gene or amplification of the gene are two possible mechanisms other than chromosomal rearrangement.

Some cell lines isolated from patients with small cell lung cancer (SCLC) exhibit amplified genes from the myc gene family [7–12] and some show chromosomal abnormalities—most notably a deletion in the short arm of chromosome 3 (3p$^-$) [13–18]. The purpose of this present study was to characterise the same set of cell lines (mainly isolated from patients in Cambridge, UK) with respect to both amplification and 3p$^-$ status. These 2 abnormalities may be independent or synergistic factors in the transformed phenotype of SCLC cell lines.

Dr. J. Minna and his coworkers have developed a classification of SCLC cell lines based on certain in vitro morphological and biochemical criteria [19]. The biomarkers include the expression of the lung APUD (amine precursor uptake and decarboxylation) enzyme L-3,4-dihydroxyphenylalanine decarboxylase (DDC), neurone-specific enolase (NSE), the brain isoenzyme of creatine kinase (CK-BB), and bombesin-like immunoreactivity (BLI, a gastrin-releasing peptide hormone). All SCLC cell lines exhibit elevated levels of CK-BB and NSE. Two subtypes can be distinguished, however—"classic" and "variant." "Classic" cell lines, accounting for 70% of SCLC cell lines, grow as tightly packed floating aggregates, have high levels of all four biomarkers, and possess neuroendocrine tissue-related dense-core vesicles. The "variant" cell lines (30% of all SCLC cell lines) do not express DDC or BLI but can be further subdivided into "biochemical" and "morphological" subclasses on a morphological basis [11]. The "biochemical variants" have "classic" morphology, while the "morphological variants" show less differentiated morphology than "classic" lines (they resemble undifferentiated large cell lung carcinoma [LCLC], having more cytoplasm and one or more prominent nucleoli, and grow as loose-floating aggregates).

The "morphological variant" SCLC cell lines have increased tumorigenicity in nude mice and are more resistant to X-rays compared with "classic" cell lines [20–22]. It seems likely that these cell lines are the in vitro correlate of the mixed SCLC/LCLC histogenic subtype [9]. Patients with such tumours have poorer prognosis than patients with histologically pure SCLC [23,24]. "Morphological variant" SCLC cell lines either express their phenotype at the onset of culture or acquire it in vitro with the loss of APUD marker expression and the development of c-myc amplification [9]. The "morphological variants" may therefore represent a form of tumour progression, perhaps in association with amplification of the c-myc gene [7,11,25]. In neuroblastoma, N-myc amplification and/or overexpression correlates with progression toward more malignant stages [25–28]. This study of myc family amplification is therefore interesting in the light of the SCLC subclass phenotypes; gene amplification may have important implications for diagnosis and treatment of patients with SCLC.

MATERIALS AND METHODS
Cell Lines: Origin, Establishment, and Culture

Controls for molecular studies. The following cell lines were used as controls: JI (Burkitt's lymphoma cell line (t2;8) expressing c-myc RNA) [29], COLO

320 HSR (colon carcinoma cell line with amplified copies of the c-myc gene associated with homogeneously staining regions) [30], Kelly (neuroblastoma line with amplification and expression of the N-myc gene) [31].

SCLC cell lines (classified as detailed above). The SCLC cell lines used were as follows: from the USA—NCI N417 ("morphological variant," established from a nude mouse heterotransplant of an untreated tumour sample) [19]; NCI H69 ("classic," established from a patient receiving prior therapy) [19]; from Sutton, UK—MAR, POC, FRE ("classics," cultured directly from a surgically treated patient, from a xenografted tumour from a chemotherapy-treated patient, and directly from a chemotherapy-treated patient, respectively), MOR (adenocarcinoma). The following lines were established in Cambridge, UK, by the authors (see Table I): NCI H69-LX4 (a multi-drug-resistant variant of NCI H69 [32]); COR-L42, -L47, -L51, -L88 ("classics"); COR-L27, -L24, -L103 ("biochemical variants," COR-L24 and -L103 coming from the same patient before and after chemotherapy, respectively). All COR lines were established directly in culture from pleural effusion, lymph node, or marrow aspirate samples from untreated patients (except COR-L103) in Cambridge [33].

All cell lines were routinely passaged in RPMI 1640 medium plus 10% foetal calf serum and the antibiotics penicillin and streptomycin. NCI H69-LX4 had 0.04 μg ml^{-1} adriamycin added to the growth medium. Kelly, COR-L88, and COR-L23 were passaged using trypsin treatment. All remaining lines grew as floating aggregates and were subcultured by being allowed to settle out, all but a small volume of medium being removed and replaced with fresh medium. Aggregates were mechanically dispersed on subculturing.

TABLE I. Properties of Cell Lines Established in Cambridge (UK) [32]

Line no.	Cytology[a]	L-dopa decarboxylase[b]	Ck-BB[c]	NSE[d]	Months in culture[e]
COR-L23	LCLC	−0.16	2.8; 0.0	9.7	3
COR-L42	SCLC	−0.09; +0.04; +0.05; 0.76	>543; >366	18.5	24
COR-L51	SCLC	+1.73; +3.04	500; >714	16.0	6
COR-L88	SCLC	+2.92; +5.66; +1.27	>312; >565	NA	9
COR-L47	SCLC	+2.14; +0.97; +1.18	52.4; >680	21.5	9
COR-L24	SCLC	+0.06; +0.15; 0.09	280; 253	18.1	18
COR-L27	SCLC	−0.17; +0.04	>700	16.3	12

[a]As kindly classified by Dr. A. Gazdar: LCLC, large cell lung carcinoma; SCLC, small cell lung cancer.
[b]All sample and control values are expressed as cpm mg^{-1} protein. The human SCLC cell line NCI H69 and the mouse tumour line EMT6 served as positive and negative controls, respectively. Values given (V) were calculated as follows: $V = (Z−Y/X−Y)$, where X = cpm mg^{-1} NCI H69 control; Y = cpm mg^{-1} protein EMT6 control; Z = cpm mg^{-1} protein test cells. (A negative value indicates a lower activity for the test cells than for EMT6.)
[c]Values given are ng mg^{-1} protein.
[d]Values are % specific binding of NSE by the monoclonal antibody B12/A6, calculated as (cpm bound by McAb − cpm bound by P3NSO spent medium/input cpm × 100). P3NSO is a nonsecreting mouse myeloma. Values represent the mean of triplicate determinations, from within a single experiment, which varied by less than 5%. Binding of B12/A6 to nonpulmonary cell lines is low, eg, T lymphoblastoid (target cell Molt 4) = 1.5% specific binding. (Data reproduced with kind permission of Dr. J. Reeve [49].) NA, not available.
[e]Estimated times for non-Cambridge lines (NCI H69, MAR, POC, FRE) = >18 months.

Isolation of DNA

Logarithmically growing stock cultures of cells in suspension or in trypsinised monolayers were pelleted, resuspended in 10 mM Tris, 5 mM ethylenediamine tetraacetic acid (EDTA), pH 8, and lysed by the addition of 1% lithium dodecyl sulphate. The mixture was then subjected to four phenol-chloroform extractions and DNA precipitated from the final aqueous phase with 0.2 M sodium acetate and ethanol. The DNA was dissolved and stored in sterile distilled water at $-20°C$.

Preparation of Total Cellular RNA

Cells in log phase were pelleted and resuspended in a drop of medium before adding 6 M guanidine hydrochloride, 0.2 M sodium acetate, pH 5.5 (20 ml per 5 × 10^7 cells), and vortexing. The DNA was sheared with a VirTis homogenizer. RNA was precipitated by addition of a half volume of ethanol and placed at $-20°$ overnight. The RNA was pelleted by centrifugation and resuspended by vigorous homogenisation in 7 M urea, 0.35 M NaCl, 50 mM Tris pH 7.5, 1 mM EDTA, 0.2% sodium dodecyl sulfate (SDS). After a single phenol-chloroform extraction, RNA was recovered by ethanol precipitation.

Preparation of Cytoplasmic RNA

Pelleted log phase cells were resuspended in 0.9% saline, lysed with a 0.5% NP40 buffer (0.14 M NaCl, 1.5 mM MgCl$_2$, 10 mM Tris, pH 8.6), then layered onto a sucrose cushion (0.14 M NaCl, 1.5 mM MgCl$_2$ 10 mM Tris, pH 8.6, 1% NP40, 24% sucrose). After centrifugation at 3,000 rpm, 4°C, for 25 min, the upper layer was removed, and an equal volume of PK buffer (0.2 M Tris pH 7.5, 0.3 M NaCl, 0.025 M EDTA, 2% SDS, 400 μg/ml Proteinase K) was added and incubated at 37°C for 30 min, followed by incubation at 65°C for 3 min. After a single phenol-chloroform extraction, RNA was recovered by ethanol precipitation.

Filter Hybridisation

DNA. Fifteen micrograms of genomic DNA was completely digested with EcoRI at 37°C and size fractionated in 0.8% agarose gels, using as size markers λDNA digested with HindIII and end labeled with [α^{32}P]-dCTP and Klenow polymerase. The DNA was denatured and transferred to nylon (Hybond^{TM}-N, Amersham) according to Southern [34]. Filters were treated with ultraviolet light for 2–5 min.

RNA. Ten-microgram samples of total cellular RNA were glyoxylated [35] and size fractionated in 1.4% agarose gels. λDNA digested with HindIII and end labeled with [α^{32}P]-dCTP and Klenow polymerase was glyoxylated and run as size markers. RNAs were transferred to nylon (Hybond^{TM}-N, Amersham) by Northern blotting, and filters were baked for 2 hr at 80°C.

Filters with RNA or DNA were treated identically. After 1 hr at 65°C in hybridisation solution (6 × SSC, 0.2% polyvinylpyrrolidone, Ficoll 400, and bovine serum albumin, 0.1% sodium dodecyl sulphate, 50 μg/ml sonicated denatured salmon sperm DNA, 5% dextran sulphate), denatured nick-translated probe [36] (specfic activity at least 10^8 cpm/μg) was added to a final concentration of 10^6 cpm/ml. The probes were restriction enzyme fragments purified from agarose gels. Hybridisation was overnight at 65°C. Filters were washed free of unhybridised probe at 65°C using 0.1 × SSC, 0.1% SDS, prior to autoradiography.

Probe removal prior to rehybridising with a second probe was achieved by incubating DNA filters at 45°C for l30 min in 0.4 M NaOH followed by a 30-min incubation in 0.1 × SSC, 0.1% (w/v) SDS, 0.2 M Tris-HCl, pH 7.5. RNA filters were washed for 2 hr at 65°C in 0.005 M Tris-HCl, pH 8.0, 0.002 M Na_2 EDTA, 0.002% w/v polyvinylpyrrolidone, Ficoll 400, and bovine serum albumin. Filters were autoradiographed overnight to assess the effectiveness of probe removal.

G-Banding

Cells growing in log phase were treated with 0.05 μg/ml of colcemid 1½ and 3 hr before harvesting by centrifugation. The pelleted cells were swollen in 0.075 M KCl for 5 min, fixed twice in 3:1 methanol-acetic acid; then stored for up to 18 hr at −20°C. G-banding was performed by the trypsin method [37].

RESULTS
myc Gene Amplification in SCLC Cell Lines

Southern filter hybridisation analysis was used to evaluate the copy number of each of the characterised members of the myc gene family (c-myc, N-myc, and L-myc) in the SCLC cell lines, using placenta DNA as a single-copy control. Filters were hybridised first with a myc gene probe and second with an immunoglobulin k-chain constant region gene probe [38], which acted as an internal control for the amounts of DNA transferred to the filter. The results are summarised in Table II. A very high proportion of the SCLC cell lines studied—ten out of 12—showed amplifi-

TABLE II. myc Gene Amplification and Chromosome 3 Abnormalities

Cell line	myc amplification	Chromosome 3 abnormalities
Classic SCLC		
NCI H69[a]	N-myc × 80	del in 3p, del 3pq
NCI H69-LX4[b]	N-myc × 80	del 3p
FRE[c]	N-myc × 50	del 3p
MAR[c]	N-myc × 90	del 3p, del 3pq
POC[c]	N-myc × 100	del 3p
COR-L42[b]	?	del 3p
COR-L51[b]	—	t(3;11)(p14;p15.2) iso 3q
COR-L88[b]	L-myc × 15	del 3p
COR-L47[b]	L-myc × 25	del 3p
Variant SCLC[d]		
COR-L24[b] (BV)	L-myc × 10	Normal 3p, del 3q
COR-L103[b] (BV)	L-myc × 10	Normal 3p, del 3q
COR-L27[b] (BV)	L-myc × 10	Normal 3p, del 3q or iso 3q
NCI N417[a] (MV)	c-myc × 50	Normal 3p, 3q+
Large cell lung carcinoma		
COR-L23[b]	c-myc × 30	Complex rearrangements
Adenocarcinoma		
MOR[c]	c-myc × 2	N.D.

[a]From U.S.A.
[b]From Cambridge, UK.
[c]From Sutton, UK.
[d]BV, "biochemical variant"; MV, "morphological variant."

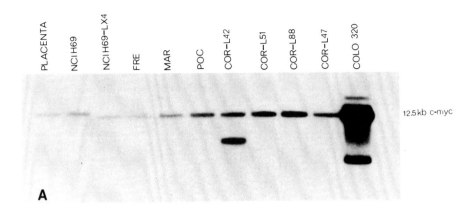

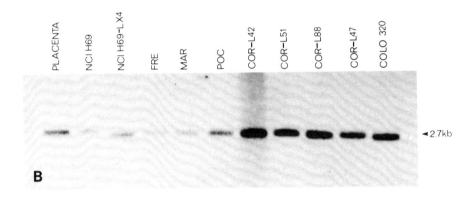

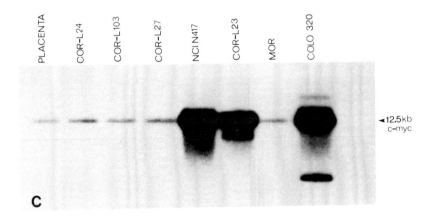

Figure 1 (Continued on following page)

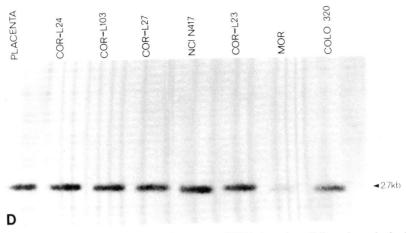

D

Fig. 1.   Amplification of c-myc gene. Ten micrograms of DNA from the cell lines shown in the figure was digested with EcoRI and fractionated in 0.8% agarose gels. After transfer to nylon, the filters were hybridised first with a c-myc exon 1 probe (see text) (**A,C**) and, following autoradiography and removal of the signal, reprobed with an immunoglobulin K-chain constant region gene probe (**B,D**) (A and B therefore represent the same filter as do C and D). The c-myc probe hybridises to a 12.5-kb EcoRI fragment, the immunoglobulin probe to a 2.7-kb EcoRI fragment. Fragment sizes were estimated by coelectrophoresis of bacteriophage lambda DNA digested with HindIII.

cation of c-myc, N-myc, or L-myc. No cell line had amplification of more than one member of the myc gene family (Figs. 1–3) as reported by Dr. J. Minna's laboratory [7–9,12].

From analyses of metaphase spreads it was found that all the SCLC cell lines showing myc gene amplification, with the single exception of COR-L47, had chromosomal markers of gene amplification—double minutes (DM) or homogeneously staining regions (HSR)—previously shown to be the location of amplified c-myc [30] and N-myc [31] genes. NCI H69 and NCI N417 had an HSR on chromosomes 12 and 1, respectively. Chromosome 1p+ markers in COR-L88, -L24/-L103, and -L27 were probable HSRs. DMs were observed in NCI H69-LX4, MAR, FRE, POC, and the LCLC cell line COR-L23. The lines COR-L42 and COR-L51, with no apparent myc gene amplification, had no visible HSR or DM.

Our c-myc probe (Sp65 myc HS1 #31) was a 3-kilobase-pair (kb) HindIII-SacI fragment of exon 1/intron 1 that did not cross-hybridise with N- or L-myc (the three characterised myc genes do not have exon 1 sequence homology [39,8,40]). In all DNAs studied the c-myc probe detected a 12.5-kb EcoRI fragment (Fig. 1A,C) which represents the germline c-myc gene [41,42]. Amplification of c-myc was observed only in the "morphological variant" SCLC cell line NCI N417, in the LCLC cell line COR-L23, possibly in the adenocarcinoma MOR (Fig. 1C,D shows that although MOR appears to have single-copy c-myc, the filter has less MOR DNA, and other filters show 2–3 copies of c-myc in this cell line), and in our positive control COLO 320 HSR. COR-L23 and COLO 320 HSR also showed unique amplified EcoRI fragments with the c-myc probe (Fig. 1C) in several DNA preparations. Such fragments are consistent with possible c-myc rearrangements that may have occurred prior to amplification. This phenomenon is not manifest at the RNA level (see below and Fig. 4C). The novel fragments may alternatively represent polymorphisms of the

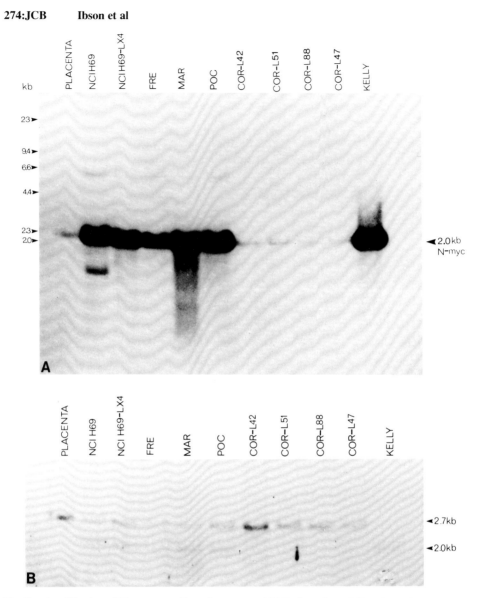

Fig. 2. Amplification of N-myc gene. Ten micrograms of DNA from the cell line shown in the figure was digested with EcoRI and filters prepared as for Figure 1. The two filters were probed first with the Nb-1 probe (see text) (**A,C**) and second with the immunoglobulin gene probe (**B,D**). The Nb-1 probe hybridises to a 2.0-kb EcoRI fragment. Note that in B and D the Nb-1 signal has not been completely removed from those lines with amplification of the N-myc gene. (Continued on following page)

c-myc gene, which are as yet unreported. The novel fragment of ~8.5 kb in COR-L42 (Fig. 1A) is interesting; no RNA species of this line hybridised to the c-myc probe (Fig. 4A), nor were N- or L-myc found to be amplified or expressed in it (Figs. 2A, 3A, 5A, 6A). As both N-myc and L-myc were originally identified by their limited sequence homology to exons 2 and 3 of c-myc, COR-L42 may have amplification of some other myc-related gene.

The N-myc probe Nb-1 (ATCC No: 41011, a 1-kb EcoRI-BamHI fragment), which represents 318 base pairs of intron 1 and 679 base pairs of exon 2 of the N-

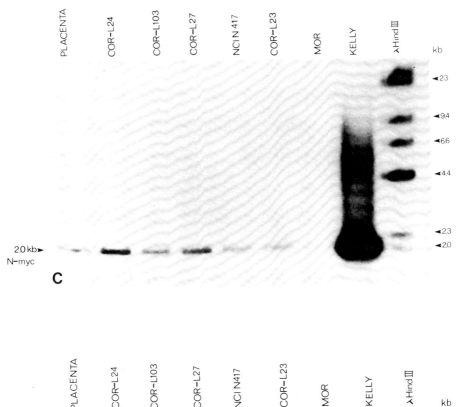

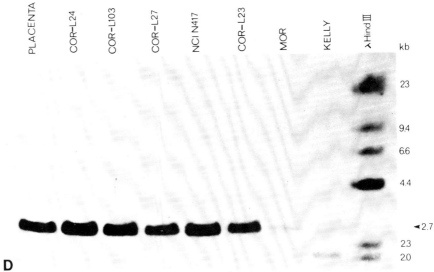

Figure 2 Continued

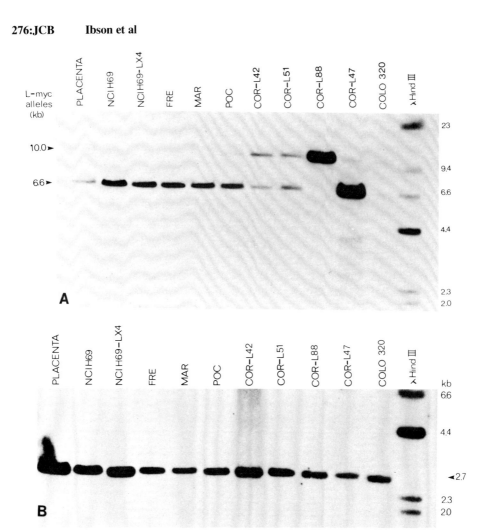

Fig. 3. Amplification of the L-myc gene. Ten micrograms of DNA from the cell lines shown in the figure was digested as for Figure 1. The two filters were probed first with the L-myc probe (see text) (**A,C**) and second with the immunoglobulin gene probe (**B,D**). The L-myc probe hybridises to the two L-myc EcoRI polymorphic fragments of 10.0 and 6.6 kb. D is a very short exposure. (Continued on following page)

myc gene, detected a 2-kb EcoRI germline N-myc gene fragment, amplified in four of the classic lines and none of the four "variant" SCLC cell lines (Fig. 2A,C). Only NCI H69 showed a novel slightly amplified fragment of ~1.3 kb (Fig. 2A), which may represent a rearrangement of the N-myc gene (although there is no evidence of such at the RNA level, Fig. 5A).

The L-myc probe, a 1.8-kb SmaI-EcoRI fragment [8] detected a 10.0-kb and/or a 6.6-kb EcoRI fragment(s), which represented the germline L-myc gene in its two EcoRI restriction site polymorphic forms (Fig. 3A,C). In heterozygous cells, only one of the two alleles is amplificd; COR-L47 is an example (Fig. 3A). Amplification of L-myc occurred in both "classic" and "variant" SCLC subtypes. The L-myc gene in COR-L47 may be amplified as a relatively short unit, of which there were no visible manifestations in metaphase spreads. COR-L47 did, however, show a rear-

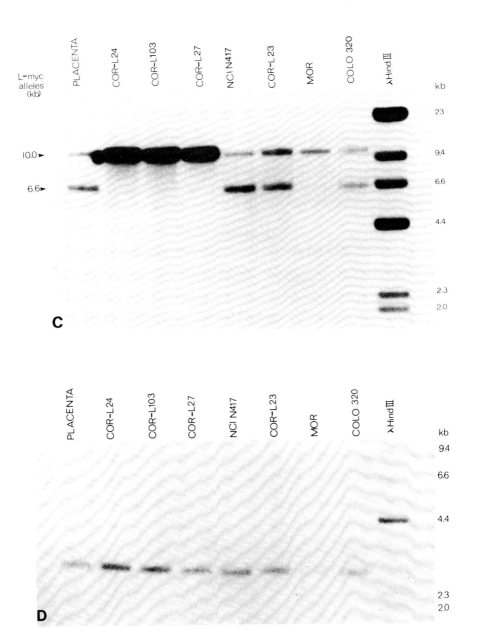

Figure 3 Continued

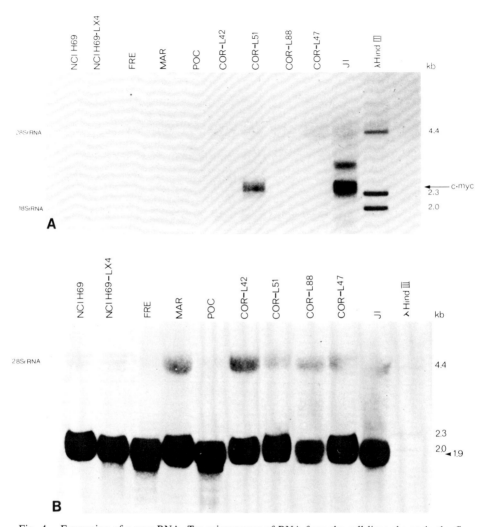

Fig. 4.   Expression of c-myc RNA. Ten micrograms of RNA from the cell lines shown in the figure was denatured and separated in 1.4% agarose gels. The RNA was total cellular RNA except for FRE, POC, COR-L88, and COR-L103, which were cytoplasmic preparations. The RNA was transferred to nylon, and the filter was hybridised to the c-myc exon 1 probe as described in "Materials and Methods" (**A,C**). The c-myc mRNA runs at ~2.4 kb using coelectrophoresed glyoxylated bacteriophage lambda DNA digested with HindIII as size markers. This c-myc probe hybridises nonspecifically to ribosomal RNA (A,C). Variations in loading and transfer were normalised by reprobing the washed filters with an actin probe pRT3, as shown in **B** and **D**. Actin RNA is 1.9 kb and the pRT3 probe also detects 28S ribosomal RNA. (Continued on following page)

rangement of an L-myc or L-myc-related allele. When digested with EcoRI, HindIII, XbaI, SacI, or KpnI, COR-L47 DNA showed novel hybridising species in comparison with other L-myc amplifed or single-copy cell lines (Fig. 3A and data not shown). The novel fragments were of single-copy intensity and may be an unamplified L-myc allele, perhaps present on a third copy of chromosome 1 (cells of COR-L47 are diploid or tetra/quatraploid). Alternatively, the novel fragments may represent a myc-related gene, which, when amplified, is detectable by some homology with the L-

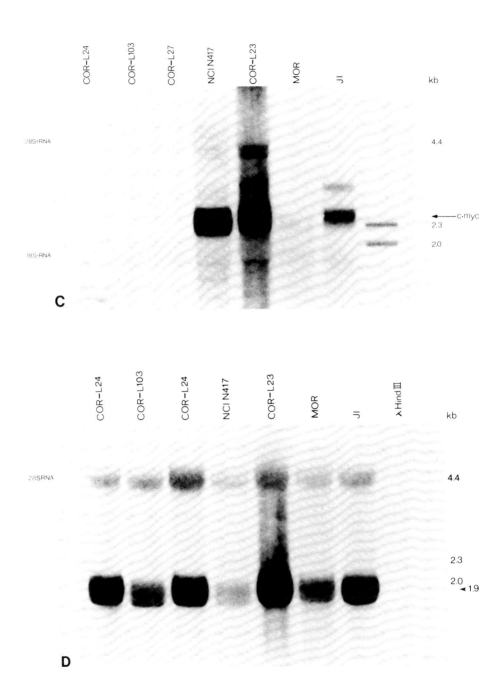

Figure 4 Continued

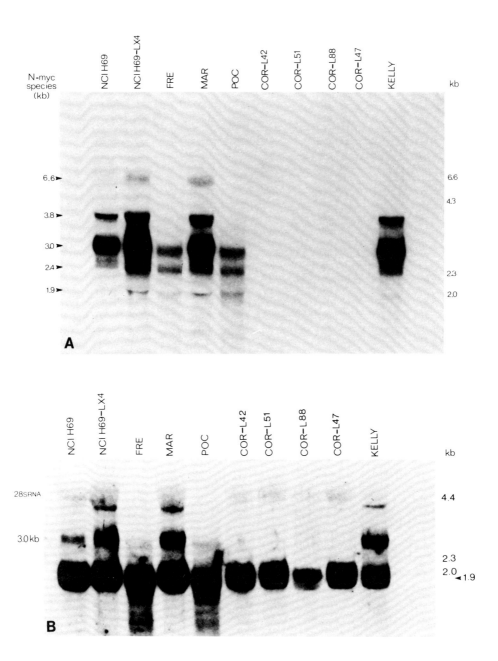

Fig. 5.   Expression of N-myc mRNA. Ten micrograms of RNA (samples were total or cytoplasmic just as in Fig. 4) from the cell lines shown in the figure was treated as for Figure 4. After probing the two filters with the Nb-1 probe and detection of a major 3-kb N-myc transcript (**A,C**), they were washed and reprobed with the actin probe (**B,D**). Note that the Nb-1 signal has not been fully removed prior to probing for actin mRNA. (Continued on following page)

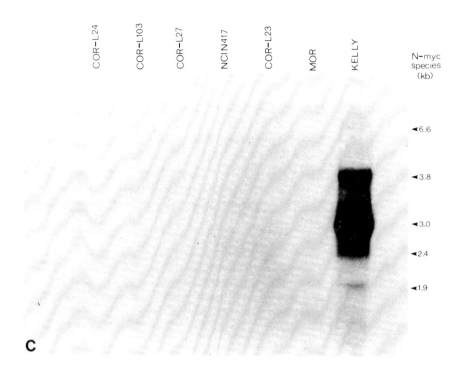

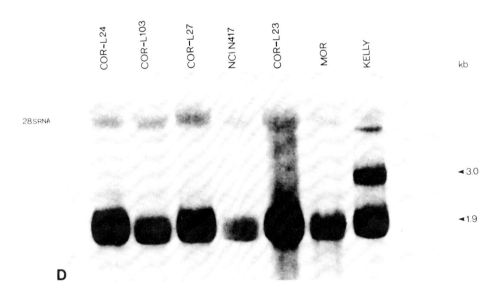

Figure 5 Continued

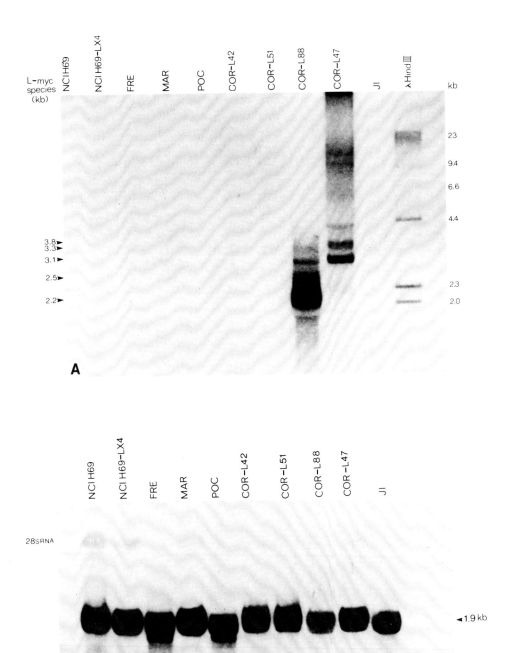

Fig. 6.   Expression of L-myc mRNA. Ten micrograms of RNA (samples total or cytoplasmic as in Fig. 4) from the cell lines shown in the figure was treated as for Figure 4. After probing with the L-myc transcript (**A,C**), the figures were reprobed with the actin probe (**B,D**). The major L-myc transcript is 2.2 kb; sizes of other hybridising species are shown. (Continued on following page)

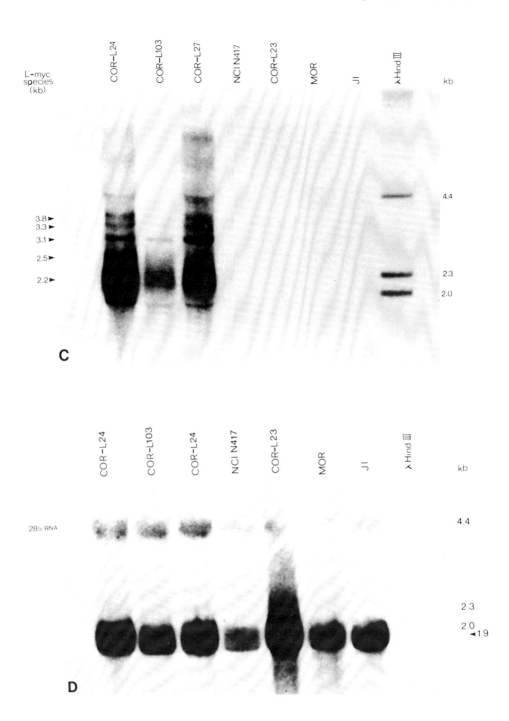

Figure 6 Continued

myc probe. Although there are no reports of more than one member of the characterised myc gene family being amplified in a single SCLC cell line, this apparent exclusion may not be universal and may not extend to more distantly related genes. Interestingly, in COR-L47 the major RNA species hybridising to the L-myc probe was a 3.1-kb species, present in the other L-myc expressing lines at a lower molar ratio than the normal 2.2-kb transcript (Figs. 6A,C).

myc Gene Expression in SCLC Cell Lines

RNA was prepared from cells growing in log phase and was analysed by Northern filter hybridisation. Expression of a particular myc RNA was detected only in cell lines shown to have amplified that myc gene (Figs. 4–6), with the exception of COR-L51 (Fig. 4A), which has single-copy c-myc. For this line, some other mechanism of activation leading to c-myc expression may be involved. For all three myc genes, the level of expression correlated well with the level of gene amplification (determined using the immunoglobulin and actin gene controls in sections band D of Figs. 1–6 for loading and transfer variation). As myc gene amplification seemed exclusive (see above), so the cell lines were found to express only one myc gene (as far as could be detected by Northern filter hybridisation).

All c-myc amplified lines expressed the normal 2.2- and 2.4-kb transcripts (only resolved as two discrete bands on short exposures), as did COR-L51 (Fig. 4A,C), even where novel restriction fragments were present (COR-L23). The N-myc probe detected two nuclear precursor species of 3.8 and 6.6 kb (in Fig. 5A FRE and POC are cytoplasmic RNA preparations) and the major 3-kb translated transcript [40] (Fig. 5A,C). The nature of the remaining hybridising species is being further investigated. The L-myc probe detected a major 2.2-kb transcript and several larger species (Fig. 6A,C), one of which is that (3.1 kb) in higher molar ratio in COR-L47 (see above), and two of which are nuclear (3.3 and 3.8 kb; COR-L103 in Fig. 6C was a cytoplasmic preparation).

Chromosome 3 Abnormalities in SCLC Cell Lines

Although a deletion in the short arm of chromosome 3 has often been observed in SCLC cell lines and in biopsy samples, the extent to which this is a diagnostic feature of SCLC is not clear [10, 13–18, 43]. Using the cell lines listed in Table II, metaphase spreads were prepared, and at least 20 metaphases were examined for each cell line. A number of abnormalities of chromosomes 1, 5, 6, 10, 11, 12, 16, 17, 19, and 20 were observed, but the most common abnormality was a deletion in the short arm of chromosome 3 ([44]; only chromosome 3 abnormalities are described here). Both interstitial and terminal deletions were observed. The extent of the deletion was constant for a given cell line but varied between cell lines (Fig. 7). The minimum common region of overlap mapped to the 3p23–3p24 band border, with breakpoint clusters at 3p12, 3p14, and 3p24. In this set of cell lines the SCLC of "classic" phenotype had a 3p$^-$ chromosome, with the single exception of the c-myc expressing line COR-L51 (this cell line has a translocation t(3;11)(p14;p15.2)). The three "biochemical variant" SCLC cell lines had a 3q$^-$ chromosome, with no minimal region of overlap, while the "morphological variant" NCI N417 had no 3p$^-$ or 3q$^-$ but showed extra material on 3q.

Although the cells of every cell line examined in this study had an abnormal chromosome 3, they possessed at least one normal chromosome 3. In triploid cells,

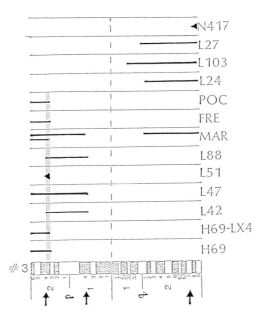

Fig. 7. Abnormalities of chromosome 3 seen in the majority of cells examined from each cell line. Abnormalities of each line are shown in relation to the idiogram of a G-banded chromosome 3. Solid bar, deleted regions of chromosome 3; triangle, translocations; arrow, known constitutive fragile sites on chromosome 3 (3p24.2; 3p14.2; 3q27); shaded area, common region of deletion overlap.

there were always two normal and one abnormal chromosome 3s rather than two abnormal 3s. Tetraploid cells had two normal and two abnormal chromosome 3s.

DISCUSSION
Oncogene Amplification

In order to assess the significance of the myc gene family in SCLC we have studied a set of SCLC cell lines established in Britain for copy number and expression of these genes. Ten of 12 SCLC cell lines showed myc gene amplification and expression, including 5 of 7 lines established from untreated patients. In comparison, Dr. J. Minna has reported at this meeting a finding of c-, N-, or L-myc amplification in 23 of 38 SCLC cell lines. Gene amplification is an adaptive mechanism allowing increased expression of genes conferring a selective advantage on cells [44,45]. Growing the SCLC cells in culture is likely to allow for such selection to occur. Eight of our 12 SCLC cell lines have been in culture for over a year. If, as the high occurrence of myc gene amplification in SCLC cell lines strongly suggests, myc amplification confers some selective advantage on SCLC cells, the time in culture may explain the higher proportion of lines with myc gene amplification. Until something is known of the function of the myc gene products, we cannot explain this selective advantage nor the apparent exclusion of the myc gene family; as found by other workers [8,9,12], no cell line showed amplification or expression of more than one of the three myc genes.

Amplification would certainly appear to be the most common mechanism of myc gene activation in SCLC. All except one of our amplified lines had cytogenetic markers of gene amplification, and hence translocation of the amplified genes may also have been involved in most cases. Rearrangement of the myc genes was uncommon, perhaps owing to flanking DNA protecting the myc genes from aberrations of translocation. Of the two unamplified lines, COR-L42 may have amplification of a myc-related gene detected by the c-myc exon 1 probe. The other line, COR-L51, expressed c-myc from a single-copy gene. As c-myc is expressed in many normal tissues [46–48], it is perhaps unnecessary to invoke aberrations of the c-myc gene as having activated its expression.

Several reports suggest an association of c-myc amplification with the "morphological variant" subclass of amplified cell lines [7,9,10], believed to represent a more aggressive form of SCLC in patients [9]. These reports document c-myc amplification in a higher proportion of "morphological variant" cell lines than of "biochemical variant" or "classic" cell lines. The present study is in agreement with such observations, c-myc expression being detected in only one "classic" SCLC cell line and in none of the "biochemical variant" cell lines. With only one "morphological variant" line we cannot comment on the importance of c-myc amplification in this phenotype. We note, however, that while it is more common for c-myc to be amplified in this subclass, other myc genes can be amplified and expressed while maintaining the "morphological variant" phenotype [12]. We also found c-myc amplification and expression in a LCLC and an adenocarcinoma cell line; c-myc amplification and expression is thus not exclusive to SCLC among lung cancers. Until more is known about the nature of the contribution of myc gene expression to the cellular phenotype we cannot interpret the apparently more restricted expression of c-myc, as opposed to N- and L-myc among SCLC subclasses.

Chromosome 3

This study included eight "classic" and four "variant" SCLC cell lines, mainly from untreated patients and from different sites. The "classic" cell lines all showed abnormalities in 3p (7 deletions and 1 translocation), whereas the "variant" cell lines had normal 3ps but deletions in 3q. More SCLC cell lines will need to be studied to determine if this distribution of 3p and 3q abnormalities among SCLC subtypes is significant. Published data on 3p deletions in SCLC often do not involve a distinction between "classic" and "variant" lines [16,43,52]. However, Whang-Peng et al [13] reported 3p deletions in both SCLC subtypes. Saksela et al [10] found 3q abnormalities in two "variant" SCLC cell lines, while de Leij et al [17] found 3p deletions in three "variant" lines. Hence, although our "classic" and "variant" lines were distinct in terms of 3p/3q abnormalities, not all pubished data would agree with this.

Chromosome 3 abnormalities are not confined to SCLC; Zech et al [15] reported 3p deletions in a squamous, a LCLC, and an adenocarcinoma cell line. In fact, abnormalities of chromosome 3 are common in both solid and haematopoietic tumours [50], and 3p is the single most consistent site of chromosome change in rhabdomyosarcoma cells [51]. The presence of three constitutive fragile sites on chromosome 3 (Fig. 7) may predispose to such abnormalities [52]. The 3p deletion is therefore not an abnormality specific to lung cancer, but as a consistent feature of at least "classic" SCLC the possible significance of the DNA of this region 3p14–3p24 should be considered. The presence of three copies of chromosome 3 in the majority of the "classic" SCLC cell lines, one copy of which has the 3p$^-$, raises the possibility that the deletion may contribute to tumorigenesis or tumour progression by uncovering a recessive mutant allele, analogous to the retinoblastoma system [6]. It will be of interest to determine which genes map to the 3p deletion region. As the c-raf proto-oncogene maps to 3p25 [53], it may be affected by some 3p deletions (Fig. 7). Molecular probes will also allow more accurate deletion mapping than conventional cytogenetics has been able to achieve.

ACKNOWLEDGMENTS

We thank F. Gilbert for the cell line Kelly, Dr. J. Minna for the line NCI N417 and the L-myc probe, Drs. D. Carney and A. Gazdar for the line NCI H69, Dr. M. Ellison for the lines MAR, FRE, POC, and MOR, Dr. G. Lenoir for the line JI, Dr. J.M. Bishop for the line COLO 320 HSR, and DR. J. Rogers for the actin clone pRT3.

REFERENCES

1. Rowley JD: Nature 301:290, 1983.
2. Dalla-Favera R, Martinotti S, Gallo RC: Science 219:963, 1983.
3. Heisterkamp N, Stephenson JR, Groffen J, Hansen PF, de Klein A, Bartram CR, Grosveld G: Nature 306:239, 1983.
4. Weinberg RA: Science 230:770, 1985.
5. Slater RM: Cancer Genet Cytogenet 19:37, 1986.
6. Cavenee WK, Dryja TP, Phillips RA, Benedict WF, Godbout R, Gallie BL, Murphree AL, Strong LC, White RL: Nature 305:779, 1983.
7. Little CD, Nau MM, Carney DN, Gazdar AF, Minna JD: Nature 306:194, 1983.
8. Nau MM, Brooks BJ, Battey J, Sausville E, Gazdar AF, Kirsch IR, McBride OW, Bertness V, Hollis GF, Minna JD: Nature 318:69, 1985.
9. Carney DN: Semin Surg Oncology XII:289, 1985.
10. Saksela K, Bergh J, Lehto V, Nilsson K, Alitalo K: Cancer Res 45:1823, 1985.
11. Gazdar AF, Carney DN, Nau MM, Minna JD: Cancer Res 45:2924, 1985.
12. Nau MM, Brooks BJ, Carney DN, Gazdar AF, Battey JF, Sausville EA, Minna JD: Proc Natl Acad Sci USA 83:1092, 1986.
13. Whang-Peng J, Bunn Jr PA, Kao-Shan CS, Lee EC, Carney DN, Gazdar AF, Minna JD: Cancer Genet Cytogenet 6:119, 1982.
14. Wurster-Hill DH, Cannizzaro LA, Pettengill OS, Sorenson GD, Cate CC, Maurer LH: Cancer Genet Cytogenet 13:303, 1984.
15. Zech L, Bergh J, Nilsson K: Cancer Genet Cytogenet 15:335, 1985.
16. Falor WH, Ward-Skinner R, Wegryn S: Cancer Genet Cytogenet 16:175, 1985.
17. de Leij L, Postmus PE, Buys CHCM, Elema JD, Ramaekers F, Poppema S, Brouwer M, van der Veen AY, Mesander G, The TH: Cancer Res 45:6024, 1985.
18. De Fusco P, Frytak S, Dahl R, Dewald G: Proc ASCO 5:20, 1986.
19. Carney DN, Gazdar AF, Bepler G, Guccion JG, Marangos PJ, Moody TW, Zweig MH, Minna JD: Cancer Res 45:2913, 1985.
20. Gazdar AF, Carney DN, Guccion JG, Baylin SB: In Greco FA, Oldham RK, Bunn PA (eds): "Small Cell Carcinoma of the Lung." New York: Grune and Stratton, 1981, p 145.
21. Gazdar AF, Zweig MH, Carney DN, Van Stierteghen AC, Baylin SB, Minna JD: Cancer Res 41:2773, 1981.
22. Carney DN, Mitchell JB, Kinsella TJ: Cancer Res 43:2806, 1983.
23. Abeloff MD, Eggleston JC, Mendelsohn G, Ettinger DS, Baylin SB: Am J Med 66:757, 1979.
24. Radice PA, Matthews MJ, Ihde DC, Gazdar AF, Carney DN, Bunn PA, Cohen MH, Fossieck BE, Makuch RW, Minna JD: Cancer 50:2894, 1982.
25. Nau MM, Carney DJ, Battey J, Johnston B, Little C, Gazdar AF, Minna JD: Curr Top Microbiol Immunol 113:172, 1984.
26. Brodeur GM, Seeger RC, Schwab M, Varmus HE, Bishop JM: Science 224:1121, 1984.

27. Schwab M, Ellison J, Busch M, Rosenau W, Varmus HE, Bishop JM: Proc Natl Acad Sci USA 81:4940, 1984.
28. Seeger RC, Brodeur GM, Sather H, Dalton A, Siegel SE, Wong KY, Hammond D: N Eng J Med 313:1111, 1985.
29. Bernheim A, Berger R, Lenoir G: Cancer Genet Cytogenet 3:307, 1981.
30. Alitalo K, Schwab M, Lin CC, Varmus HE, Bishop JM: Proc Natl Acad Sci USA 80:1707, 1983.
31. Schwab M, Alitalo K, Klempnauer K-H, Varmus H, Bishop JM, Gilbert F, Brodeur G, Goldstein M, Trent J: Nature 305:245, 1983.
32. Twentyman PR, Fox NE, Wright KA, Bleehen NM: Br J Cancer 53:529–537, 1986.
33. Baillie-Johnson H, Twentyman PR, Fox NE, Walls GA, Workman P, Watson JV, Johnson N, Reeve JG, Bleehen NM: Br J Cancer 52:495, 1985.
34. Southern E: J Mol Biol 98:503, 1975.
35. Thomas PS: Proc Natl Acad Sci USA 77:5201, 1980.
36. Rigby PWJ, Dieckmann M, Rhodes D, Berg P: J Mol Biol 113:237, 1977.
37. Seabright M: Lancet 2:971, 1971.
38. Rabbitts TH, Baer R, Davis M, Forster A, Hamlyn PH, Malcolm S: Curr Top Microbiol Immunol 113:166, 1984.
39. Watt R, Stanton LW, Marcu KB, Gallo RC, Croce CM, Rovera G: Nature 303:725, 1983.
40. Kohl NE, Legouy E, DePinho RA, Nisen PD, Smith RK, Gee CE, Alt FW: Nature 319:73, 1986.
41. Taub R, Kirsch I, Morton C, Lenoir G, Swan D, Tronick S, Aaronson S, Leder P: Proc Natl Acad Sci USA 79:7837, 1982.
42. Dalla-Favera R, Martinotti S, Gallo R: Science 219:963, 1983.
43. Buys CHCM, van der Veen AY, de Leij L: In 8th International Chromosome Conference, Lubeck FRG, 1983.
44. Schimke RT: Cell 37:705, 1984.
45. Schimke RT: Cancer Res 44:1735, 1984.
46. Gonda TJ, Sheiness DK, Bishop JM: Mol Cell Biol 2:617, 1982.
47. Pfeifer-Ohlsson S, Goustin AS, Rydnert J, Wahlstrom T, Bjersing L, Stehelin D, Ohlsson R: Cell 38:585, 1984.
48. Erikson J, ar-Rushdi A, Drwinga HL, Nowell PC, Croce CM: Proc Natl Acad Sci USA 80:820, 1983.
49. Reeve JG, Stewart J, Watson JV, Wulfrank D, Twentyman PR, Bleehen NM: Br J Cancer 53:519, 1986.
50. Mark J: Adv Cancer Res 24:165, 1977.
51. Trent JM, Casper J, Meltzer P, Thompson F, Fogh J: Cancer Genet Cytogenet 16:189, 1985.
52. Yunis JJ, Soreng AL: Science 226:1199, 1984.
53. Bonner T, O'Brien SJ, Nash WG, Rapp UR, Morton CC, Leder P: Science 223:71, 1984.
54. Waters JJ, Ibson JM, Twentyman PR, Bleehen NM, Rabbitts PM: Cancer Genet Cytogenet, 1987 (submitted).

Journal of Cellular Biochemistry 34:39–46 (1987)
Cellular and Molecular Biology of Tumors and
Potential Clinical Applications 129–136

Autostimulatory Mechanisms in Myeloid Leukemogenesis

J.W. Schrader, K.B. Leslie, H.J. Ziltener, and S. Schrader

The Walter and Eliza Hall Institute of Medical Research, P.O. Royal Melbourne Hospital, Victoria 3050, Australia

WEHI-274 is a monocytic leukemia that arose in a BALB/c mouse infected with Abelson murine leukemia virus. A series of subclones were derived from early passages of this tumor. Three subsets of these leukemogenic subclones were identified. Two subsets demonstrated autostimulatory patterns of growth. This was due to the ectopic production of the T-cell lymphokine the panspecific hemopoietin IL-3 in one case and of the T-cell lymphokine granulocyte-macro-phage colony-stimulating factor (GM-CSF) in the other. The third type of subclone did not secrete any autostimulatory growth factor. In the subclone producing IL-3, one copy of IL-3 gene was rearranged and abnormal IL-3 RNA transcripts were present in the nucleus. Subclones producing GM-CSF also contained abnormal GM-CSF RNA transcripts, although no rearrangement of the GM-CSF gene was detected. All three sets of subclones shared a common rearrangement of one c-*myb* oncogene, suggesting that they share a common ancestor. These results suggest that initiation or progression of leukemogenic behavior in this abnormal clone occurred in three different ways, two of which involved autostimulation by the ectopic activation of T-cell lymphokine genes.

Key words: c-*myb* rearrangement, granulocyte-macrophage colony-stimulating factor, panspecific hemopoietin, interleukin-3, autostimulation, myeloid leukemia

There are now many examples of soluble polypeptides that stimulate the growth of specific types of cell. It is also well-established that the growth of tumor cells is usually much less dependent on such soluble growth factors than is that of their normal counterparts. In 1961 Hsu [1] proposed that one way in which a cell could become independent of exogenous sources of a growth factor would involve infection by a virus that carried the gene coding for that growth factor. Based on observations that tumor cells released "transforming growth factors" that caused nontransformed cells to assume some of the growth characteristics of transformed cells, Sporn and Todaro [2] elaborated upon the autocrine hypothesis and pointed to its implications

The present address for all authors is The Biomedical Research Centre, The University of British Columbia, Vancouver, British Columbia, Canada V6T 1W5.

Received March 25, 1986; revised and accepted December 18, 1986.

for new therapeutic strategies. Evidence that the initiation of the production of an autostimulatory factor could actually cause a change to an oncogenic growth pattern came from experiments showing that the initiation of the ectopic production of a hemopoietic growth factor normally released from activated T cells, coincided with leukemogenesis [3]. Shortly thereafter two groups noted that the *v-sis* oncogene of the simian sarcoma virus encoded a product that closely resembled platelet-derived growth factor [4,5]. These experiments validated Hsu's earlier speculation and strongly supported the link between pathological production of an autostimulatory growth factor and oncogenesis.

Because the physiological source of several of the hemopoietic growth factors is well established, the hemopoietic system has provided several clear instances of tumors exhibiting ectopic production of hemopoietic growth factors [3,6,7]. In the case of the myelomonocytic leukemia WEHI-3B it is now clear that the ectopic production of a T-cell lymphokine panspecific hemopoietin (IL-3) or interleukin-3 (IL-3) results from pathological disruption of the growth factor gene [8]. Another monocytic leukemia, WEHI-274.14, also constitutively produces IL-3 and moreover appears to require this factor for its growth [7].

The myelomonocytic leukemia WEHI-3B provides an instructive example of how the behavior of tumor cells can change with continued passage. When initially isolated, WEHI-3B required an exogenous source of hemopoietic growth factors for optimal growth in agar. However, with one possible exception [9], the clones of WEHI-3B that are in use today no longer respond to IL-3. This loss of responsiveness to IL-3 probably reflects strong selective pressure during its long passage history against cells that depended on an autostimulatory mechanism and responded to IL-3 and selection for variants that no longer depended on IL-3 and thus had a growth advantage over the autostimulatory parental cell, especially at low cell densities.

The monocytic leukemia WEHI-274 arose in a BALB/c mouse that had been infected with the Abelson murine leukemia virus. Based on the history of WEHI-3B, we reasoned that cell lines that had been selected for the capacity to grow from single cells in vitro in the absence of exogenous sources of growth factors could differ substantially from the major population of leukemic cells in vivo. Therefore, we thawed an early frozen sample of WEHI-274 and plated out the cells in vitro in the presence or absence of a source of IL-3, namely, medium that had been conditioned by WEHI-3B. In parallel, cells were also cultured in vitro at high cell density in medium alone. Cells from both populations were then plated in agar, either in the presence or absence of WEHI-3–conditioned medium. Much higher numbers of colonies grew in the cultures in which WEHI-3–conditioned medium was present, suggesting that the bulk of cells in the original tumor responded to IL-3 in vitro. A number of these clones were plucked from the agar cultures and studied further. Subsequent experiments with fractionated WEHI-3B–conditioned medium and with purified or synthetic IL-3 demonstrated that the active factor in the WEHI-3B–conditioned medium was IL-3.

Previously we had shown that one such clone, WEHI-274.14, showed an autostimulatory pattern of growth when plated in agar at varying cell densities. Thus, whereas in the presence of WEHI-3–conditioned medium, WEIII-274.14 formed colonies in agar at cell densities ranging from 10^2 to 10^4/ml, in the absence of WEHI-3B–conditioned medium, colony growth occurred only at the highest cell density of 10^4/ml [7]. This pattern of dependence on an exogenous source of growth factor at low cell densities but not higher cell densities is a characteristic sign of an autostimulatory mechanism. The presence of this mechanism was confirmed when conditioned medium was harvested from high density cultures of WEHI-274 (10^5/ml) grown in the absence of exogenous sources of IL-3 and was shown to enhance in a dose-dependent fashion the growth of WEHI-274.14 cells at low cell densities [7].

The nature of this autostimulatory factor was further investigated by biochemical techniques and shown to be indistinguishable from T cell-derived IL-3 in terms of its apparent molecular weight on gel filtration and behavior on reverse-phase HPLC [7]. Here we describe further the molecular nature of the factor produced by WEHI-274 and present evidence that one IL-3 gene in WEHI-274.14 has undergone a pathological rearrangement. We report that other clones of WEHI-274 isolated in parallel with WEHI-274.14 also show evidence of an autostimulatory mechanism but one that involves not IL-3 but a second T-cell lymphokine, GM-CSF. These subclones of WEHI-274 together with a third class of clone, which appears to produce neither IL-3 nor GM-CSF, share a common rearrangement of a c-*myb* gene, indicating that they arose from a common progenitor.

MATERIALS AND METHODS

Frozen stocks of WEHI-274 cells that had been passaged several times from the animal to high density in vitro cultures and back were obtained through the kindness of Dr. A. Harris at the Hall Institute. Conditioned medium was produced from WEHI-3B cells as described elsewhere [6]. The medium used was RPMI 1640 supplemented with 10% fetal calf serum, 2-mercaptoethanol 5×10^{-5} M, and glutamine 2.8×10^{-3} M supplemented with WEHI-3B–conditioned medium (3% of 10-fold concentrate) as indicated. In some experiments the medium was gelled by the inclusion of 0.3% Bacto-agar (Difco Laboratories, Detroit, MI).

Total cellular RNA was extracted by standard methods, and polyadenylated RNA was isolated using an oligo-dT cellulose column. Southern and Northern blot analyses were peformed by standard methods. The IL-3 probe was the 400 bp HindIII-XbaI cDNA fragment containing most of the coding region of the mature protein. The GM-CSF probe was a PstI-EcoRI cDNA fragment containing the entire coding region of the mature protein. The c-*myb* probe consisted of the 1.3 kb HindIII-EcoRI genomic DNA fragment, which comprises the second exon of the murine c-*myb* gene. All probes were labeled by random priming with random hexamers after the method of Feinberg [10].

Antipeptide antibodies were raised against synthetic peptides corresponding to defined regions of the IL-3 sequence and were affinity-purified and coupled to Sepharose beads as detailed elsewhere [11].

IL-3 was assayed as described elsewhere using a PSH-dependent line, R6X. GM-CSF was assayed using a colony assay as described elsewhere [6].

RESULTS
Evidence of Pathology of IL-3 Gene in WEHI-274.14

Southern blot analysis of DNA from the WEHI-274.14 subclone using a IL-3-specific probe indicated that one copy of the IL-3 gene was rearranged (see Table I). Digestion of normal mouse liver DNA with EcoRI resulted in hybridization with a

TABLE I. Organization of the IL-3 and c-*myb* Genes by Southern Blot Analysis of an EcoRI Genomic Digest

	IL-3 cDNA probe		c-myb genomic probe	
DNA source	No. of bands	Fragment size (kb)	No. of bands	Fragment size (kb)
Germline	1	8.5	1	6.5
274.14	2	8.5 and 9.1	2	6.5 and 2.8
274.28	1	8.5	2	6.5 and 2.8
274.3	1	8.5	2	6.5 and 2.8

single 8.5 kb fragment corresponding to that reported for the germline IL-3 gene [8]. However, in the case of DNA from WEHI-274.14, the IL-3 probe hybridized with two bands, one corresponding to a single germline copy of the IL-3 gene and the other to a larger, 9.1 kb fragment (Table I). Digestion of DNA from WEHI-274.14 with Bam-HI and hybridization with a IL-3 probe revealed a band of 3.1 kb in addition to the germline bands of 2.8 kb and 8.5 kb. Information from restriction maps of a IL-3 gene and data from other experiments in which DNA from WEHI-274.14 was digested with various restriction enzymes localized the rearrangement of the IL-3 gene in WEHI-274.14 to a region betwen 0.5 and 1.5 kb 5' to the transcription-initiation site of the normal IL-3 gene.

Abnormal IL-3 Transcripts in WEHI-274.14

Northern blot analysis of whole-cell, polyadenylated RNA extracted from WEHI-274.14 cells revealed a surprising result (Fig.1). The IL-3-specific probe hybridized with three major transcripts of 8.0 kb, 4.5 kb, and 1.5 kb, contrasting with the 1.3 kb primary transcript seen in activated T cells. As shown in Table II, the 8.0 kb species was the major transcript and was present at high levels, which were markedly disproportionate to the relatively small amounts of biologically active IL-3 released by this cell line. Fractionation experiments indicated that the large, 8.0 kb and 4.5 kb transcripts occur predominantly in the nucleus and that, in accord with the low levels of IL-3 activity produced, only low levels of the smaller 1.5 kb cytoplasmic species could be detected. It is interesting to contrast this with the situation in the myelomonocytic leukemia WEHI-3B where the IL-3 RNA transcripts are indistinguishable from those in activated T cells.

Nature of the IL-3 Molecule Released by WEHI-274.14

Data showing that the IL-3 gene was rearranged in WEHI-274.14 (Table I) and that there were abnormal IL-3 transcripts present (Table II) strongly supported biochemical and biological evidence suggesting that WEHI-274.14 released a molecule related to IL-3 [7]. Experiments using antibodies specific for defined peptides corresponding to regions of the IL-3 amino acid sequence have further clarified the nature of the molecules with IL-3 bioactivity secreted by WEHI-274.14 cells. Thus antibodies specific for epitopes determined by the six N-terminal amino acids of IL-3 bound up to 70% of bioactivity released by WEHI-274.14 [12]. This observation indicated that these six amino acids, which are present on the primary products secreted by activated T cells but which had been cleaved from the subpopulation of molecules analyzed as IL-3 by Ihle et al [13], are also present on the bulk of IL-3 secreted by WEHI-274.14.

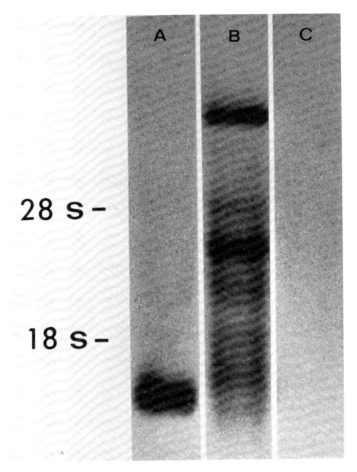

Fig. 1.   Northern blot analysis using a IL-3-cDNA probe of whole cell polyadenylated RNA from A) WEHI-3B, showing a normal-sized 1.3 kb transcript; B) WEHI-274.14, showing the abnormal transcripts; and C) a control line, the IL-3-dependent R6-X, showing no IL-3 transcripts.

TABLE II. Detection of Specific IL-3 and GM-CSF Gene Transcripts by Northern Blot Analysis of Whole Cell Polyadenylated RNA

Source of RNA	IL-3 cDNA probe		GM-CSF cDNA probe	
	Presence of transcript	Dominant transcript (kb)	Presence of transcript	Dominant transcript (kb)
Activated T cell	+	1.3	+	1.1
274.14	+	8	−	—
274.28	−	—	+	10
274.3	−	—	−	—

Similar experiments showed that antibodies to peptides corresponding to the N-terminal 29 amino acids predicted by the nucleotide sequence of the IL-3 cDNA clones and also to peptides corresponding to the middle of the molecule (residues 91–112) also bound IL-3 bioactivity from WEHI-274.14 (Ziltener et al, in preparation). Together with data on the apparent Mr. and hydrophobicity of the IL-3 from WEHI-274.14 [7], these experiments indicate that the IL-3 from this leukemia is very similar, if not identical, to the T-cell product.

IL-3 and GM-CSF Genes in Other Subclones of WEHI-274

When other subclones of WEHI-274 that were derived at the same time as WEHI-274.14 were examined for abnormalities of IL-3 genes, different results were obtained. Although in two cases, ie WEHI-274.28 and WEHI-274.25, the cells released an autostimulatory factor, in neither case could IL-3 bioactivity be detected in supernatants of high density cultures. Moreover, there was no evidence for rearrangement of the IL-3 gene (Table I). Analysis of the factor in conditioned medium form WEHI-274.25 or WEHI-274.28 suggested that these lines produced a second T-cell lymphokine, GM-CSF. Southern blot analysis revealed a rearrangement of the GM-CSF gene in these subclones (Leslie et al, in preparation).

GM-CSF RNA in Subclones of WEHI-274

Northern blot analysis showed no evidence of RNA transcripts that hybridized with a GM-CSF probe in either WEHI-274.14 or WEHI-274.3 (or WEHI-3b). However, in WEHI-274.28 and WEHI-274.25 the GM-CSF probe hybridized with a strikingly abnormal pattern of transcripts, somewhat reminiscent of that seen in WEHI-274.14 with IL-3 probes. Thus there was a large (10 kb), abnormal transcript, together with one smaller transcript (about 1 kb) present at lower levels. In contrast, in activated T cells the GM-CSF transcript was about 1 kb in size. Fractionation experiments indicated that the dominant 10 kb transcript was present in the nucleus and was not detectable in the cytoplasm. None of the transcripts in leukemic cells hybridized with a probe specific for the LTR of Moloney murine leukemia virus.

Rearrangement of the c-myb Gene

The results detailed above suggested that there were at least three types of subclones in the mouse carrying the original WEHI-274 leukemia, those producing IL-3 transcripts, eg, WEHI-274.14, those producing abnormal GM-CSF transcripts, eg, WEHI-274.28 or WEHI-274.25, and those producing neither, eg, WEHI-274.3. The relationship between these clones was clarified by experiments that examined the c-*myb* gene in these clones (Table I), and indicated that in all three classes of subclones there was a common abnormality of one c-*myb* gene. This observation strongly suggested that all three subclones were derived from a common progenitor cell.

DISCUSSION

Our experiments show that autostimulatory mechanisms are operating in WEHI-274, a myeloid leukemia that arose in vivo. In this instance there is good biological evidence that factors that are secreted by leukemic cells, ie, IL-3 in the case of WEHI-274.14 and GM-CSF in the cases of WEHI-274.25 and WEHI-274.28, act as auto-stimulatory factors. At present it is not possible to say whether the production of these factors is critical for the leukemogenic behavior of these clones or merely enhances their growth; experiments attempting to stop the growth of the leukemic cells with antibodies specific for IL-3 or GM-CSF should shed light on this point. Certainly it is striking that in this one tumor, progression of different subclones has occurred through autostimulatory mechanisms that involve two distinct T-cell lymphokines. If the activation of the IL-3 and GM-CSF genes represent completely independent events, and the rearrangements of the respective genes strongly suggest that this is the case, their occurrence in subclones of a single tumor suggests that the aberrant activation of lymphokine genes might be a relatively common mechanism of oncogenic progression in the appropriate target cells.

The common origin of the three classes of subclones, which was demonstrated by their sharing of a common c-*myb* rearrangement, provides an intriguing insight into the history of this tumor. It seems reasonable to postulate that the initiating event was aberrant activation of one c-*myb* gene in a macrophage precursor. Activation of this c-*myb* gene probably resulted in immortalization of this clone.

Although there is no direct evidence, it may well be that this immortalized clone remained dependent on the growth factors to which monocytic progenitors respond, ie, IL-3, GM-CSF, or CSF-1. If this were the case this clone, although immortal, would not have behaved as a transplantable leukemia. Progression to the leukemic state (or enhanced leukemogenicity) appears to have involved at least three discrete mechanisms. Thus leukemogenic subclones represented by WEHI-274.14 resulted from aberrant activation of the IL-3 gene, whereas leukemogenic subclones represented by WEHI-274.28 or WEHI-274.25 resulted from an activation of a second T-cell lymphokine gene, GM-CSF. In the third group of leukemic clones exemplified by WEHI-274.3, the leukemogenic mechanism has yet to be identified. It should be noted that v-abl sequences were not detected in any of these clones. These experiments point to the power of recombinant DNA techniques in establishing the aberrant production of autostimulatory growth fractor by tumors cells and set the scene for experiments investigating the therapeutic potential of antibodies and other measures designed to interrupt autostimulation.

ACKNOWLEDGMENTS

We thank Ms. Joanne Ringham, Denise Galatis, Angela Milligan, and Mr. Gary Coe for excellent technical assistance. This work was supported by the N.H. & M.R.C., Canberra; PHS grant 5R01 CA386484-02 awarded by the National Cancer Institute, DHHS; The Bushell Trust; and The Windermere Hospital Foundation. K.B.L. was a Wenkart Scholar, and H.J.Z. was supported by a Fellowship from the Swiss Academy of Medical Sciences.

REFERENCES

1. Hsu TC: Int Rev Cytol 12:69, 1961.
2. Sporn MB, Todaro GJ: N Engl J Med 303:878, 1980.
3. Schrader JW, Crapper RM: Proc Natl Acad Sci USA 80:6892, 1983.
4. Doolittle RF, Hunkapiller MW, Hood LE, Devare SG, Robbins KC, Aaronson SA, Antoniades HN: Science 221:275, 1983.
5. Waterfield MD, Scrace GT, Whittle N, Stroobant P, Johnson A, Wateson A, Westermart B, Heldin GH, Huang JS, Duel TF: Nature 304:35, 1983.

6. Clark-Lewis I, Kent SBH, Schrader JW: J Biol Chem 259:7488, 1984.

7. Schrader JW, Schrader S, Leslie K, Dunn A: In Gale RP, Golde DW (eds):"Leukemia: Recent Advances in Biology and Treatment." New York: Alan R. Liss, Inc., 1985, pp 293–302.

8. Ymer S, Tucker QJ, Sanderson CJ, Hapel AJ, Campbell HD, Young IG: Nature 317:255, 1985.

9. Whetton AD, Bazill GW, Dexter TM: J Cell Physiol 123:73, 1985.

10. Feinberg AP, Vogelstein B: Anal Biochem 132:6, 1983.

11. Ziltener HJ, Clark-Lewis I, Hood LE, Kent SBH, Schrader JW: J Immunol 138:1099, 1987.

12. Ziltener HJ, Clark-Lewis I, Fazekas de St. Groth B, Hood LE, Kent SBH, Schrader JW: J Immunol 138:1105, 1987.

13. Ihle JN, Keller J, Oroszlan S, Henderson LE, Copeland TD, Fitch F, Prystowsky MB, Goldwasser E, Schrader JW, Palasynski E, Dy M, Lebel B: J Immunol 131:282, 1983.

Journal of Cellular Biochemistry 34:71–79 (1987)
Cellular and Molecular Biology of Tumors and
Potential Clinical Applications 137–145

Differential Induction of Transcription of c-*myc* and c-*fos* Proto-Oncogenes by 12-O-tetradecanoylphorbol-13-acetate in Mortal and Immortal Human Urothelial Cells

Jan Skouv, Britta Christensen, and Herman Autrup

Laboratory of Environmental Carcinogenesis, The Fibiger Institute, DK-2100 Copenhagen Ø, Denmark

The effect of the skin tumor-promoter TPA (12-O-tetradecanoylphorbol-13-acetate) on expression of cellular proto-oncogenes has been examined in cell lines derived from human urothelium. A single treatment with TPA (1 μg/ml) increased the transcription of c-*fos* and c-*myc* proto-oncogenes at least 20-fold in the mortal cell line HU 1752. The induction was transient and was accompanied by a rapid but transient change in cell morphology. When immortalized cell lines were treated with TPA a similar rapid and transient morphological response was observed, but the TPA treatment only increased the level of c-*fos* mRNA, suggesting that the normal regulation of c-*myc* transcription is altered in immortalized cells irrespective of their tumorigenic properties. The levels of c-Ha-*ras* and c-Ki-*ras* mRNAs were unaffected by TPA treatment in all cell lines.

Key words: TPA, oncogene expression, human epithelial cells, phorbol ester, immortalization, c-*myc*, c-*fos*

It is generally accepted that the development of cancer in man and experimental animals is a multistage process [1,2]. Evidence supporting this view has been obtained from the experimental induction of skin cancer in mice and bladder cancer in rats [3–5]. In these models the carcinogenic process has been separated into at least three different stages: initiation, promotion, and malignant conversion [6–8]. In our laboratory, a series of human urothelial cell lines has been developed that have been classified into three catagories: 1) mortal and nontumorigenic, 2) immortal but nontumorigenic, and 3) immortal, tumorigenic cell lines [19,20]. It has been suggested that these cell lines provide an in vitro model representing successive stages in multistage carcinogenesis [19].

Received April 8, 1986; revised and accepted November 12, 1986.

One of the most potent tumor-promoter substances in experimental animal models is the phorbolester 12-O-tetradecanoylphorbol-13-acetate (TPA) [9]. TPA as well as the naturally occurring mitogens platelet-derived growth factor (PDGF) and epidermal growth factor (EGF) have been found to elicit transient transcription of two cellular oncogenes, c-*myc* and c-*fos*, in serum-starved rodent cells [10–12]. In contrast to these observations, we have previously reported that TPA increased c-*fos* expression but did not increase expression of c-*myc* in the immortalized, nontumorigenic human bladder epithelial cell line HCV 29 [13]. Since altered regulation of c-*myc* has been implicated in the genesis of tumors [17,18] we questioned whether the apparent resistance of c-*myc* to induction by TPA was correlated to the growth and tumorigenic properties of the cells. Accordingly, we have examined the effect of TPA on oncogene expression in human cell lines representing the mortal, the immortal, and the tumorigenic classes.

MATERIALS AND METHODS
Cell Lines and Growth Conditions

The cell lines used in this study are described briefly in Table I. The cells were serially propagated as previously described [19]. The mortal line HU 1752 was cultured in FIB41B medium [21] supplemented with seven nonessential amino acids (7NEA) and 20% fetal bovine serum (FBS). The immortalized cell lines were cultured in FIB41B medium supplemented with 7NEA and 5% FBS.

Oncogene Probes

By nick translation [22] ^{32}P-labelled DNA probes with a specific activity of approximately 10^8 cpm/μg were prepared. The probes were the 1.3-kb *ClaI-EcoRI* fragment of the human c-*myc*, the 2.4-kb *EcoRI* fragment of the human c-Ki-*ras*-2, the 2.8-kb *SacI* fragment of the human c-Ha-*ras*-1, and the 1,050-bp *PstI* fragment of the v-*fos* gene of FBJ murine osteosarcoma virus [23].

TPA Exposure

Cultures, approximately 80% confluent, were treated with a single dose of TPA dissolved in dimethyl sulfoxide (DMSO). The final concentrations of TPA and DMSO were 1 μg/ml and 0.1%, respectively. The cells were incubated with TPA at 37°C for various periods of time as indicated in Figures 2, 3, and 5.

RNA Isolation and Filter Hybridization

Total cellular RNA was prepared by a variation of the guanidine thiocyanate method by using a ten-times-higher amount of beta-mercaptoethanol than originally

TABLE I. Properties of Cell Lines

Cell line	Life span in vitro[a]	Tumorigenicity in nude mice[b]
HU 1752	Mortal	Nontumorigenic
HCV 29	Immortal	Nontumorigenic
HU 609	Immortal	Nontumorigenic
HCV 29T	Immortal	Tumorigenic
HU 609T	Immortal	Tumorigenic

[a]We define immortal as survival for more than 75 passages in vitro (equivalent to more than 200 population doublings).
[b]The tumorigenic properties were tested by subcutaneous inoculation of 10^7-10^8 trypan-blue-negative cells into 6–8 wk-old inbred BALB/c athymic nude mice as previously reported [19].

described [24]. The integrity of each RNA sample was confirmed by gel electrophoresis of glyoxylated RNA [25]. Only RNA samples showing intact 28S and 18S ribosomal bands with a 28S:18S ratio bigger than 2:1 were analysed further. The relative levels of oncogene-related RNA were determined by a modification of the dot blot technique [26,27] with a Minifold II apparatus and BA 85-3B nitrocellulose filter (Schleicher and Schuell, Dassel, West Germany). Hybridization of serial dilutions (10, 5, 2.5 μg) of RNA was performed at high stringency (50% formamide at 45°C) as described elsewhere [28,29]. The hybridization was followed by stringent washing 3× for 20 min in 2× SSC (1 × SSC-buffer is 0.15 M NaCl + 0.015 Na citrate), 0.1% sodium dodecylsulfate (SDS) at 50°C and 3× for 20 min in 0.1 × SSC, 0.1% SDS at 50°C. Autoradiograms were prepared by using Agfa Structurix D7 film (Agfa, Leverkusen, West Germany). This film shows a linear response to ^{32}P without preflashing.

RESULTS

When human urothelial cells cultured in vitro were treated with a single dose of TPA (1 μg/ml), a rapid change in morphology was observed (Fig. 1). This change was seen in all cell lines regardless of their life span in vitro. The effect of TPA on the cell morphology was transient. The change in cell appearance was seen within 20 min of exposure and seemed most apparent after approximately 1 hr of TPA exposure. Cells treated with TPA for extended periods of time (10 hr or more) had an almost normal appearance.

The transient change in cell morphology was correlated with changes in the levels of oncogene-related RNAs. A single dose of TPA (1 μg/ml) enhanced the level of c-*fos* RNA in all cell lines, irrespective of their life span in vitro. After 50 min of exposure the level of c-*fos* RNA was enhanced at least 20-fold in the mortal, nontumorigenic cell line HU 1752 (Fig. 2). The level of c-*fos* returned to the pretreatment level during the following 2 hr of continued exposure to TPA. A similar transient increase in the c-*fos* level was seen in the immortalized, nontumorigenic cell lines HU 609 and HCV 29. The immortalized, tumorigenic cell lines HCV 29T (Fig. 5) and HU 609T also responded to the TPA treatment by a transient increase (approximately tenfold) in the c-*fos* level. The time course of this induction followed the kinetics observed in the case of the two immortal but nontumorigenic cell lines HU 609 and HCV 29.

The level of c-*myc* increased (at least 20-fold) in the mortal cell line HU 1752 in response to a single dose to TPA (Fig. 2). The increase in the c-*myc* RNA level in this cell line appeared to be transient, like the increase of c-*fos* RNA. However, as has been reported by others [10–12], the decay of the elevated c-*myc* level was slower than the decay in the c-*fos* level (Fig. 2). In contrast to the result obtained in the HU 1752 cell line, we did not observe any increase in the c-*myc* level in the immortalized cell lines. The levels of c-Ha-*ras* and c-Ki-*ras* RNA were unaffected by the TPA treatment in all cell lines studied.

To investigate if the apparent resistance of immortalized cell lines to TPA-enhanced c-*myc* levels was due to the relatively high concentration of TPA used, a dose-response experiment was performed (Fig. 3). The immortalized HCV 29 cell line was exposed to various concentrations of TPA ranging from 5 to 1,000 ng/ml. The exposure time was 45 min. Whereas the level of c-*fos* RNA was positively related

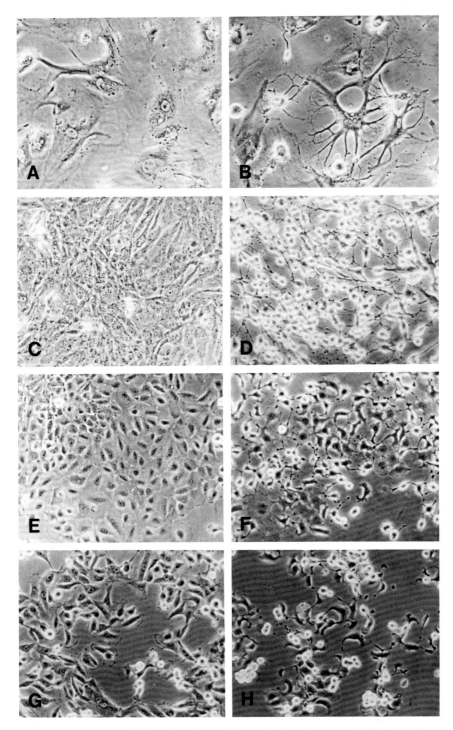

Fig. 1.   Effect of TPA (1 μg/ml) on the cell morphology of various human urothelial cells. The mortal HU 1752 cell line before (**A**) and after (**B**) 40 min of exposure. The immortalized HU 609 cell line before (**C**) and after (**D**) 110 min of exposure. The tumorigenic cell lines HCV 29T before (**E**) and after (**F**) exposure for 40 min and HU 609T before (**G**) and after (**H**) 90 min exposure to TPA. ×100.

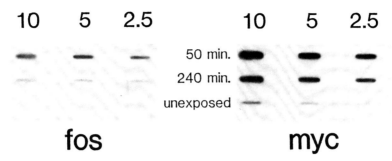

Fig. 2. Slot blot analysis of oncogene expression in the mortal cell line HU 1752 treated with a single dose of TPA (1 μg/ml) in vitro. Cells were lysed and total cellular RNA was extracted after 0, 50, and 240 min exposure, spotted in twofold dilutions (10, 5, and 2.5 μg per slot), and hybridized with radiolabelled DNA probes specific for the *fos* and c-*myc* oncogenes, respectively.

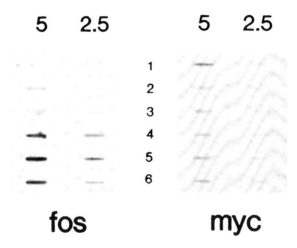

Fig. 3. Slot blot analysis of oncogene expression in the immortalized but nontumorigenic cell line HCV 29. The cells were treated for 45 min with a single dose of TPA: **1**) 5 ng/ml, **2**) 20 ng/ml, **3**) 80 ng/ml, **4**) 200 ng/ml, **5**) 700 ng/ml, and **6**) 1,000 ng/ml. See also legend to Figure 2.

to the TPA concentration, we did not observe any enhancement of the c-*myc*, c-Ha-*ras*, or c-Ki-*ras* RNA levels. The "typical" TPA-induced change in the cell morphology was observed at all concentrations (data not shown).

The basal level of c-*fos* and c-*myc* RNA was measured in all cell lines. The basal level of c-*fos* was essentially the same in all cell lines examined. In contrast, the basal level of c-*myc* RNA varied substantially between cell lines (Fig. 4). The tumorigenic cell lines HCV 29T and HU 609T both showed an enhanced level of c-*myc*. Also the immortalized HU 609 cell line showed an increased basal level of c-*myc* compared to the immortalized HCV 29 and the mortal HU 1752 cell lines.

In order to be able to compare the basal level of oncogene expression in HU 1752 cultured in 20% FBS to the level observed in the other cell lines cultured in 5% FBS, the effect of different serum concentration was examined in HCV 29 (Fig. 4). Neither the basal level of c-*fos* nor c-*myc* was found to be significantly influenced by the serum concentration in the media.

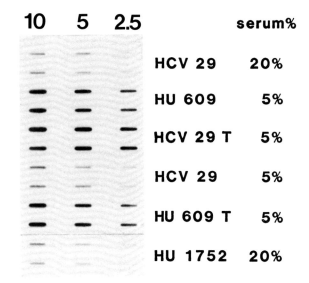

Fig. 4.   Basal level of c-*myc* RNA in various human urothelial cell lines. Total cellular RNA was extracted from the indicated cell lines cultured in media containing 5 or 20% fetal bovine serum, respectively. For each cell line RNA was extracted from two independent culture flasks and spotted onto a nitrocellulose filter in twofold dilutions (10, 5, and 2.5 μg). The filter was hybridized with ^{32}P-labelled DNA specific for the human c-*myc*.

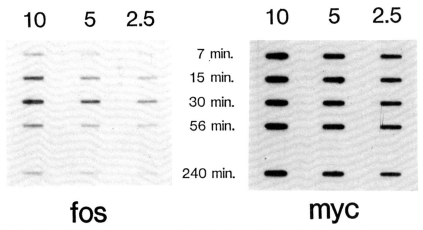

Fig. 5. Slot blot analysis of oncogene expression in the immortal, tumorigenic cell line HCV 29T treated with a single dose of TPA (1 μg/ml) for various times. See also legend to Figure 2.

DISCUSSION

The c-*myc* oncogene has been implicated both in the acquisition of cell immortality and in the ability of cells to form tumors [14–18]. Some information pertaining to this point can be derived by examining the basal level of c-*myc* expression in the cell lines used in this study. The cell lines HU 609, HU 609T, and HCV 29T all show increased levels of c-*myc* RNA, which is consistent with the view that immortalization is related to c-*myc* overexpression. However, the low level of c-*myc* basal expression observed in the immortal line HCV 29 suggests that elevated c-*myc* expression is not always required for immortalization.

Previous work in our laboratory has demonstrated that a single dose of TPA induced expression of the c-*fos* proto-oncogene of HCV 29 cells transiently [13]. This transient induction of c-*fos* correlated with a rapid change in HCV 29 cell morphology. Evidence presented here indicates that TPA transiently induces c-*fos* expression in human urothelial cells irrespective of their life span in vitro and their tumorigenic properties in nude mice. TPA also induced a marked change in cell morphology of all cells investigated. Thus human urothelial cells seem to be susceptible to the action of TPA. Morphological changes have also been observed in other human epithelial cells after TPA treatment—eg, cells of the colon, endometrium, and lung [30–32]. It is interesting to note that the TPA-induced changes in morphology of lung, endometrial, and urothelial cells were transient.

TPA binds to and mediates its cellular effects through the activation of the phospholipid and Ca^{++}-dependent enzyme protein kinase C (pkC) [33–35]; pkC plays a central role in the intracellular signal transduction of a variety of biologically active substances affecting cellular functions and proliferation [34–36]. The enzyme has been found in all tissues so far tested [35], including human urothelial cells [37]. There is ample evidence that substances which activate pkC either directly, like TPA, or indirectly via an enhanced phosphoinositide turnover, like PDGF, transiently activate the transcription of a group of genes named "competence" genes that includes the c-*myc* and c-*fos* proto-oncogenes [10–12,38–43]. Since all urothelial cells judged by the morphology were susceptible to the TPA treatment and since TPA induced at least one of the "competence" genes—namely, c-*fos*—it could be expected that c-*myc* would also be activated by the TPA treatment. Such a coupled induction of both c-*myc* and c-*fos* was, however, observed only in the mortal cell line HU 1752, suggesting a difference in the c-*myc* regulation between immortalized and nonimmortalized human urothelial cells. TPA induces both c-*fos* and c-*myc* expression in the immortalized BALB/c-3T3 [10,43] and immortalized A431 human carcinoma cells [41], thus showing that the immortalization process per se does not cause a decoupling between c-*fos* and c-*myc* in all cell types.

Since the experiments were performed at a high concentration of TPA it was considered possible that the decoupling between c-*fos* and c-*myc* in the immortalized cells was caused by a toxic effect specifically abolishing the activation of c-*myc*. We consider this explanation unlikely because no activation of c-*myc* was observed at low doses of TPA in a dose-response experiment with the immortalized HCV 29 cell line. In this context it is interesting that TPA induced the "characteristic" change in cell morphology at all concentrations investigated. Since c-*fos* only was activated at TPA concentrations higher than 80 ng/ml, the dose-response experiment thus indicates that the morphological change and the c-*fos* activation are two separate responses.

It is probably reasonable to anticipate that cells have a limited capacity for c-*myc* transcription. Thus it is conceivable that activation of pkC may not be able to induce any further c-*myc* expression in cells already expressing maximal levels of this proto-oncogene. Three out of four of the immortalized urothelial cell lines we examined showed an enhanced basal level of c-*myc* which was comparable to the level of c-*myc* expression induced by TPA in HU 1752. It cannot be excluded that c-*myc* expression was maximally expressed in these three cell lines before the TPA treatment. This explanation cannot, however, account for the response of HCV 29 to TPA treatment. This cell line expressed a basal level of c-*myc* RNA that was indistinguishable from the level in the mortal HU 1752, thus illustrating that the activation of c-*fos* and c-*myc* can also become decoupled in cells expressing low levels of c-*myc*.

Continuous labelling of the urothelial cells with ^{3}H-thymidine showed that 99–100% of the immortalized cells were in the growth fraction, whereas no more than 63% of the mortal HU 1752 cells were in the growth fraction [44]. This indicates that a relative large fraction of the mortal cells (approximately 40%) were at rest at the time of TPA treatment, in contrast to less than 1% of the immortalized cells. We therefore propose that the difference in c-*myc* inducibility between mortal and immortal cell lines reported here is a consequence of the distribution of quiescent vs actively dividing cells. This hypothesis is currently being investigated.

ACKNOWLEDGMENTS

We thank Dr. J. Kieler and S.N. Stacey for valuable discussions and for their attentive help during the preparation of this manuscript. Furthermore, we thank Inge Skibshøj and Helle Jensen for excellent and indispensable technical help. Oncogene probes were kindly provided by Dr. G. Yoakum, Laboratory of Human Carcinogenesis, National Cancer Institute, Bethesda, MD (c-Ha-*ras*-1), Dr. S.A. Aronsen, Laboratory of Cellular and Molecular Biology, National Cancer Institute, Bethesda, MD (c-*myc* and c-Ki-*ras*-2), and Dr. R. Müller, European Molecular Biology Laboratory, Heidelberg, FRG (v-*fos*). This work was supported by a grant from the Danish Cancer Society. B.C. and J.S. are recipients of fellowships from the Danish Cancer Society.

REFERENCES

1. Doll R: Cancer Res 38:3573, 1978.
2. Moolgravkar SH, Knudson AG Jr: J Natl Cancer Inst 66:1037, 1981.
3. Slaga TJ, Fischer SM, Weeks CE, Klein-Szanto AJP, Reiners J: J Cell Biochem 18:99, 1982.
4. Hicks RM: Br Med Bull 36:39, 1980.
5. Cohen SM, Greenfield RE, Ellwein LB: Environ Health Perspect 49:209, 1983.
6. Hennings H, Shores R, Wenk ML, Spangler EF, Tarone R, Yuspa SH: Nature 304:67, 1983.
7. Hicks RM: Carcinogenesis 4:1209, 1983.
8. Hennings H, Yuspa SH: J Natl Cancer Inst 74:735, 1985.
9. Slaga TJ, Nelson KG: In Weinstein IB, Vogel HJ (eds): "Genes and Proteins in Oncogenesis." New York: Academic Press, 1983, pp 125–142.
10. Greenberg ME, Ziff EB: Nature 311:43, 1984.
11. Müller R, Bravo R, Burckhardt J, Curran T: Nature 312:716, 1984.
12. Kruijer W, Cooper JA, Hunter T, Verma I: Nature 312:711, 1984.
13. Skouv J, Christensen B, Skibshøj I, Autrup H: Carcinogenesis 7:331, 1986.
14. Land H, Parada LF, Weinberg RA: Nature 304:596, 1984.
15. Mogneau E, Lemieux L, Rassoulzadegan M, Cuzin F: Proc Natl Acad Sci USA 81:5758, 1984.
16. Connan G, Rassoulzadegan M, Cuzin F: Nature 314:277, 1985.
17. Klein G, Klein E: Nature 315:190, 1985.
18. Adams JM, Harris AW, Pinkert CA, Corcoran LM, Alexander WS, Cory S, Palmiter RD, Brinster RL: Nature 318:533, 1985.
19. Christensen B, Kieler JVF, Vilien M, Don P, Wang CY, Wolf H: Anticancer Res 4:319, 1984.
20. Kieler JVF: Cancer Metastasis Rev 3:265, 1984.
21. Kieler J, Moore J, Biczowa B, Radikowski C: Acta Pathol Microbiol Scand [A] 79:529, 1971.
22. Rigby PWJ, Dieckmann M, Rhodes C, Berg P: J Mol Biol 113:237, 1977.
23. Curran T, Peters G, Van Beveren C, Teich NM, Verma IM: J Virol 44:674, 1982.
24. Chirgwin JM, Przybyla AE, MacDonald RJ, Rutter WJ: Biochemistry 18:5294, 1979.

25. McMaster GK, Carmichael GC: Proc Natl Acad Sci USA 74:4835, 1977.
26. Kafatos FC, Jones CW, Efstratiadis A: Nucleic Acids Res 7:1541, 1979.
27. Müller R, Slamon DJ, Trembly JM, Cline MJ, Verma IM: Nature 299:640, 1982.
28. Wahl G: "Schleicher and Schuell Technical Literature No. 371." Schleicher and Schuell Inc., Keene, USA.
29. Barinaga M, Franco R, Meinkoth J, Ong E, Wahl GM: "Schleicher and Schuell Technical Literature Nos. 352–354." Schleicher and Schuell Inc., Keene, USA.
30. Friedman EA: In Harris CC, Autrup NH (eds): "Human Carcinogenesis." New York: Academic Press, 1983, pp 325–368.
31. Kaufman DG, Siegfried JM, Dorman BH, Nielson KG, Walton LA: In Harris CC, Autrup NH (eds): "Human Carcinogenesis." New York: Academic Press, 1983, pp 469–508.
32. Gescher A, Reed DJ: Cancer Res 45:4315, 1985.
33. Blumberg PM, Köenig B, Sharkey NA, Leach KL, Jaken S, Jeng AY, Börzsönyi M, Lapis K, Day NE, Yamasaki H (eds): "Models, Mechanisms and Etiology of Tumour Promotion." Lyon: IARC, 1984, pp 139–156.
34. Nishizuka Y: Nature 308:693, 1984.
35. Takai Y, Kaibuchi K, Tsuda T, Hoshijima M: J Cell Biochem 29:143, 1985.
36. Berridge MJ: Sci Am 253:124, 1985.
37. Verma AK, Bryan GT, Reznikoff CA: Carcinogenesis 6:427, 1985.
38. Cochran BH, Reffel AC, Stiles CD: Cell 33:939, 1983.
39. Kelly K, Cochran BH, Stiles CD, Leder P: Cell 35:603, 1983.
40. Cochran BH, Zullo J, Verma IM, Stiles CD: Science 226:1080, 1984.
41. Bravo R, Burckhardt J, Curran T, Müller R: EMBO J 4:1193, 1985.
42. Coughlin SR, Lee WMF, Williams PW, Giels GM, Williams LT: Cell 43:243, 1985.
43. Zullo JN, Cochran BH, Huang AS, Stiles CD: Cell 43:793, 1985.
44. Christensen B, Kieler J, Bem W: Submitted for publication.

Journal of Cellular Biochemistry 34:247–258 (1987)
Cellular and Molecular Biology of Tumors and
Potential Clinical Applications 147–158

Structure of Amplified DNA, Analyzed by Pulsed Field Gradient Gel Electrophoresis

P. Borst, A.M. Van Der Bliek, T. Van Der Velde-Koerts, and E. Hes

Division of Molecular Biology, The Netherlands Cancer Institute, Plesmanlaan 121, 1066 CX Amsterdam, The Netherlands

Pulsed field gradient electrophoresis allows the separation of large DNA molecules up to 2,000 kilobases (kb) in length and has the potential to close the resolution gap between standard electrophoresis of DNA molecules (smaller than 50 kb) and standard cytogenetics (larger than 2,000 kb). We have analysed the amplified DNA in four cell lines containing double minute chromosomes (DMs) and two lines containing homogeneously staining regions. The cells were immobilized in agarose blocks, lysed, deproteinized, and the liberated DNA was digested in situ with various restriction endonucleases. Following electrophoretic separation by pulsed field gel electrophoresis, the DNA in the gel was analysed by Southern blotting with appropriate probes for the amplified DNA. We find that the DNA in intact DMs is larger than 1,500 kb. Our results are also compatible with the notion that the DNA in DMs is circular, but this remains to be proven. The amplified segment of wild-type DNA covers more than 550 kb in all lines and possibly up to 2,500 kb in some. We confirm that the repeat unit is heterogeneous in some of the amplicons. In two cell lines, however, with low degrees of gene amplification, we find no evidence for heterogeneity of the repeats up to 750 (Y1-DM) and 800 kb (3T6-R50), respectively. We propose that amplicons start out long and homogeneous and that the heterogeneity in the repeat arises through truncation during further amplification events in which cells with shorter repeats have a selective advantage. Even if the repeats are heterogeneous, however, pulsed field gradient gels can be useful to establish linkage of genes over relatively short chromosomal distances (up to 1,000 kb). We discuss some of the promises and pitfalls of pulsed field gel electrophoresis in the analysis of amplified DNA.

Key words: dihydrofolate reductase, gene amplification, double minute chromosomes, multi-drug resistance, Kirsten-ras, homogeneously staining regions

Many tumour cells contain amplified DNA in the form of double minute (DM) chromosomes or chromosomes with homogeneously staining regions (HSR) or abnor-

Abbreviations used: ABR, abnormal banding region; CHO, chinese hamster ovary; DHFR, dihydrofolate reductase; DM, double minute (chromosomes); HSR, homogeneously staining region; MTX, methotrexate.

Received March 7, 1986; accepted May 1, 1986.

mal banding regions (ABR). In some cells amplification is induced and maintained by drug selection and the products of amplified genes are involved in drug metabolism. In other cells amplification of oncogenes is found, probably maintained by the selective advantage of oncogene overexpression in the tumour or tissue culture [see refs. 1–12 for recent reviews].

The analysis of amplified DNA by standard gel electrophoretic techniques is complicated by the large size of the amplified units, which exceeds by far the limit of resolution of this technique (about 50 kilobases [kb]). We have therefore turned to pulsed field gradient (PFG) gel electrophoresis, a novel technique for the size-fractionation of large DNA molecules, developed by Schwartz and Cantor [13]. This technique allows the sizing of DNA molecules up to 1,500 kb and probably even larger. We have used this to study two questions:

1. What is the size and size heterogeneity of the amplicon?
2. What is the size and structure of DMs?

We summarize here the results obtained in the past 2 years with this approach in our lab. Some of the results have been briefly reported elsewhere [14,15].

MATERIALS AND METHODS

Cell Lines

The MTX-resistant EL4/8 and EL4/12 mouse lymphoma cell lines [16,17] were obtained from Dr. C.J. Bostock, MRC Mammalian Genome Unit, Dept. of Zoology, University of Edinburgh (Edinburgh, Scotland).

The MTX-resistant 3T6-R50 mouse cell line [16,17] was obtained from Dr. R.T. Schimke, Dept. of Biological Sciences, Stanford University, (Stanford, CA).

The Y1-DM and Y1-HSR sub-lines of the mouse adrenocortical tumour [18–20] were obtained from Dr. D.L. George, University of Pennsylvania, Dept. of Human Genetics, The School of Medicine/G3 (Philadelphia, PA).

The multi-drug resistant Chinese hamster ovary cell line CH^RC5 [8,21] was obtained from Dr. V. Ling, The Ontario Cancer Institute (Toronto, Canada).

All cell lines were grown in the medium and with the drug concentrations specified by the suppliers.

Lysis and Deproteinization of Cells in Agarose

The procedure developed by Schwartz and Cantor [13] for yeast, was adapted to mammalian cells as described by Van der Bliek et al [15].

PGF Gel Analysis In-Gel Digestion, and DNA Blotting and Hybridization Procedures

This was done essentially as described by Schwartz and Cantor [13] with small modifications [15]. In some experiments long pulse times (60, 70, 90, or 150 sec) were used as described by Johnson and Borst [22]. In-gel digestion with restriction endonucleases was done as described by Bernards et al [23]. Blotting and hybridization was done as described by Van der Bliek et al [15].

Source of DNA Probes

The DHFR gene was detected with a mouse cDNA probe-pR400-12 obtained from Dr. A.D. Levinson, Dept. of Molecular Biology, Genentech Incorporated (South

San Francisco, CA). In the hybridization we used the gel-purified insert containing the complete DHFR encoding sequence with a single point mutation [24].

The c-Ki-ras gene was detected with a probe derived from the Ki-MusV clone HiHi-3 obtained from Dr. R.W. Ellis, Lab Tumor Virus Genetics, NCI (Bethesda, MD), via Dr. R. Nusse of this institute. A 380 base-pair (bp) SacII/XbaI fragment, devoid of repetitive sequences [25], was gel-purified and used in the hybridizations.

RESULTS

General Features of PFG Gel Analysis of Mammalian (Amplified) DNA

To study the structure of amplified DNA, we have lysed and deproteinized cultured cells in agarose blocks, which allows handling of pure DNA without degradation by shear. The DNA in the blocks was then digested with a restriction endonuclease, the blocks were inserted into the slots of a 1% agarose gel, and the digests subjected to PFG gel electrophoresis. For most experiments we used the modified Schwartz-Cantor [13] box depicted in the left half of Figure 1. In this setup the DNA runs approximately in the diagonal, but with occasional twists owing to the field gradient. In some experiments the modified Carle-Olson [26] box depicted in the right half of Figure 1 was used.

To size the DNA, we have primarily used oligomers of phage lambda DNA [23,26]. Under optimal conditions this provides size marking up to 1,000 kb and, with some luck, up to 1,500 kb. With a pulse time of 35 sec good separation is obtained up till 650 kb; larger DNA migrates in a compression zone. Very large linear DNA (and circular DNA > 10 kb) is trapped in the slot. By increasing the

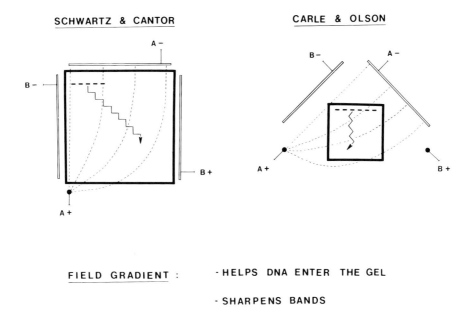

Fig. 1. Gel boxes used for PFG gel electrophoresis. The Schwartz-Cantor box has a field gradient only in the N-S direction (A$^-$-A$^+$), the Carle-Olson box in both directions. See text for further explanation.

pulse time, the compression zone can be shifted to higher DNA molecular weights. As reliable markers > 1,500 kb are not available, it is not known what the upper limit of the technique is. It could possibly be up to 3,000 kb at pulse times of 150 sec and longer [see ref. 22].

Undigested mammalian DNA of the cell lines studied was completely retained in the slot at all pulse frequencies. This is illustrated in Figure 2 for Y1-DM DNA. Treatment of the DNA in agarose with pancreatic DNAse I in the presence of Mn^{2+}, which introduces duplex breaks at semirandom positions [27], initially results in the appearance of DNA in the compression zone, even at long pulse times when the compression zone is well separated from the 1,000-kb area (Fig. 2). The same result is obtained when the fate of the DM DNA is analysed by blotting the gel onto nitrocellulose and hybridizing the blot with a probe for the amplified c-Ki-ras gene, located in the DMs [18–20]. At longer DNase incubations all DNA is removed from slot and compression zone and appears as smear lower in the gel.

The same result was obtained for all DM-containing cell lines, whether DNase I was used or a restriction endonuclease. We conclude that all DMs studied by us must contain DNA > 1,500 kb and possibly > 3,000 kb. The fact that undigested DNA does not enter the gel at all suggests but does not prove that intact DMs contain circular DNA, as also indicated by the lack of free ends in DM nucleoprotein spread and visualized by EM [28].

To test the size and homogeneity of the repeats contained in these DMs, we have digested the DNA in agarose blocks with restriction endonucleases that cut mammalian DNA infrequently. In our hands MluI (ACGCGT), NaeI (GCCGGC), NotI (GCCCCGC), SacII (CCGCGG), and SfiI (GGCCNNNNNGGCC) were most useful. This may be related to the long recognition site (NotI and SfiI) and/or the presence of CpG doublets, which are underrepresented in mammalian DNA [29] and

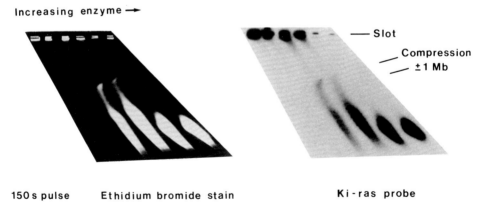

Fig. 2. DNA fragments generated by digestion of Y1-DM DNA with pancreatic DNase I in the presence of Mn^{2+}. Cells of Y1-DM were embedded in agarose, lysed, and deproteinized. The blocks were pre-incubated for 1 hr at room temperature with various DNase I concentrations in 0.05 M Tris-HCl, pH 8.0; 0,1 % gelatine; 0.1 mM phenylmethylsulfonylfluoride (PMSF). After the addition of 0.6 mM MnCl$_2$ the blocks were incubated for 1 hr at 37°C. The DNaseI reaction was stopped by extensive washing with 0.1 M EDTA, pH 8.0, at 4°C. The fragments were size-fractionated by PFG gel electrophoresis using a pulse of 150 sec. The gel was blotted onto nitrocellulose and hybridized with a probe for the c-Ki-ras gene. From left to right the DNaseI concentrations were 0.5-1-5-10-50-100 pg/ml. See Materials and Methods for further details of procedures.

often methylated [30]. The results obtained with this approach are summarized in Table I and briefly discussed in the following sections.

The Mouse EL4/8, EL4/12 and 3T6-R50 Lines (DHFR Gene)

The MTX-resistant lines EL4/8 and EL4/12 were isolated by Bostock and coworkers from mouse EL4 lymphoma cells by stepwise MTX selection. EL4/8 has 750–1,120 times the wild-type DHFR gene copy number; EL4/12 650–1,360 times. In EcoR I digests, EL4/12 only shows the parental DHFR DNA fragments; EL4/8 has additional bands associated with rearrangements close to the 3′ end of the DHFR gene in a subportion of the amplified DNA [1]. Cytogenetically EL4/8 and /12 have "variable numbers of DMs, which vary in size up to forms that appear as rings" [1]. Whether extra DHFR genes are also present in chromosomes is not known, but this is not impossible [cf. ref. 1]. We have verified by cytogenetics (Diamidinophenylin-dole [DAPI] and Giemsa staining) that EL4/12, as used in our experiments, still contains numerous DMs.

The 3T6-R50 was obtained from a clonal line 3T6-S5 by stepwise selection with MTX. It contains DMs and a 50× elevation of the number of DHFR genes without rearrangements detectable in Southern blots [16,17].

Figure 3A compares the fragments obtained when DNA from EL4/8, EL4/12, and 3T6-R50 is digested in agarose with NotI. 3T6-R50 yields a single band of 300 kb and no other DNA; EL4/12 yields approximately equal bands of 250, 350, and 550 kb, but in addition some DNA in the compression zone and in the slot that does not completely disappear even with large excess of enzyme; EL4/8 gives a complex pattern of nonstoichiometric bands with a majority of the hybridization over compression zone and slot.

The interpretation of these patterns is aided by the analysis of two mouse cell lines without DHFR gene amplification, L1210 and Y1-DM, shown in Figure 3B. L1210 only yields a single band at about 1,000 kb, well separated from the compression zone in this 150-sec PFG gel. The same band is also present in the Y1-DM line, but in addition this line yields a 300-kb band which comigrates with the 300-kb band in 3T6-R50. The two bands in the Y1-DM DNA are not equally intense, but this could easily be due to some trapping of the larger DNA in the slot. This is often seen with long pulse times [22]. These results suggest that the two bands in Y1-DM are allelic and that L1210 is homozygous for the long fragment. The 3T6-R50 cell line

TABLE I. Structure of Amplified DNA

| Cell line | Selected gene | Estimated size in kb of | | |
		Intact DMs	Subrepeats	Repeats
DM lines				
Mouse EL4/12	DHFR	>1,500	250, 350, 550	>1,150
Mouse EL4/8	DHFR	>1,500	Complex	?
Mouse 3T6 R5O	DHFR	>1,500	None ?	>800
Mouse Y1 DM	c-Ki-ras	>1,500	None ?	2,500 ?
HSR lines				
Mouse Y1 HSR	c-Ki-ras		Complex	>2,000 ?
Hamster CH^{R}C5	P-glycoprotein		>800	>1,100
Hamster CHOC 400.5	DHFR			>800

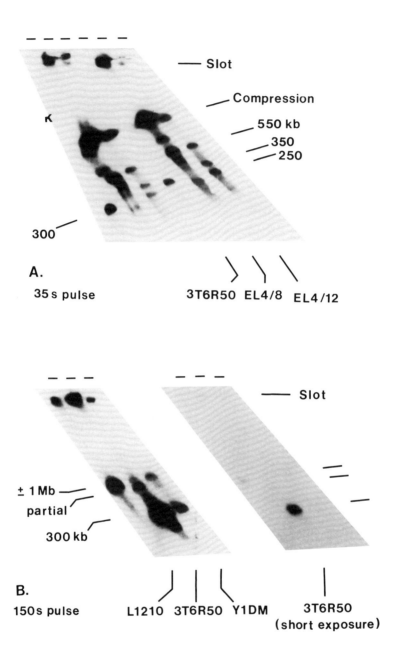

Fig. 3. PFG gel analysis of restriction fragments containing amplified and wild-type DHFR genes. Cells from the lines indicated were embedded in agarose, lysed, and deproteinized and the DNA was cleaved in-gel with endonuclease NotI. The fragments were size-fractionated by PFG gel electrophoresis using pulse times of 35 sec (A) or 150 sec (B). The gels were blotted onto nitrocellulose and hybridized with a probe for the DHFR gene. The figure shows the autoradiograms of this hybridization. In L1210 and Y1-DM the DHFR gene is not amplified; in the other lines it is. The molecular weights indicated were deduced from ladders of lambda DNA oligomers, run in adjacent slots (not shown). **A:** The left three lanes were digested with 10 U NotI for 3 hr at 37°C. The right three lanes were digested with 50 U NotI for 6 hr at 37°C. **B:** The blocks were digested with 50 U NotI for 6 hr at 37°C. The left part was exposed for 5 days at −70°C, the right part was exposed for 1 hr at −70°C.

would then contain an amplicon derived from the allele with the short NotI DHFR fragment. Homogeneity of the amplicons is suggested by the amplification of the intact 300-kb NotI fragment and by the partial digestion product of about 800 kb, visible in Figure 3B. This is the only partial seen in NotI digests of 3T6-R50 DNA. Note that the weak band at 1,000 kb in 3T6-R50 comigrates with the WT allele found in Y1-DM and L1210 DNA. In EL4/8 and EL4/12 DNA the amplified DHFR gene resides on very large NotI fragments (Fig. 3A), which could easily have arisen from the WT long NotI fragment.

We cannot link the polymorphism in the NotI fragments to the observation by Federspiel et al [17] of two alleles of the mouse DHFR gene, which diverge about 50 kb downstream of the gene, because the 3T6 line only contains one of these alleles [17].

We have done many experiments to get more information on the repeats of EL4/12 DNA with only limited success. All enzymes tested, including SfiI, gave fragments < 300 kb that were useless for long-range mapping. Only NaeI gave large fragments, which comigrate with the major fragments obtained with NotI, as shown in Figure 4A,B. It is known from previous work that a GC-rich area with one NotI and two NaeI sites lies directly upstream of the mouse DHFR gene [31]. The simplest interpretation of our results is therefore that the 550-, 350-, and 250-kb fragments actually run from this upstream cluster to the upstream cluster of the DHFR gene in the next repeat. There are various ways in which multiple repeats may have arisen. The simplest model is that the initial amplicon was 550 kb or larger and that shorter repeats were formed during additional rounds of amplification, either by recombination, or deletion.

We have attempted to define the relation between the three major repeats in the amplified DNA by partial digestion analysis. Figure 4 shows examples. At low incubation time the 550-kb band is most prominent. This suggests that the 250- and 350-kb fragments are linked in the amplified DNA and that the expected 600-kb band comigrates with the 550-kb band. This is certainly within the error limits of our size determinations. The larger fragments appearing at shorter digestion times are compatible with a tandem arrangement of 550/350/250-kb fragments in the intact DNA, but the predicted size distribution for the partials expected from other arrangements, eg, runs of 250s, 350s, and 550s, is not sufficiently different from the one observed to exclude these alternatives.

Figure 4 also illustrates two peculiarities in this type of analysis: crooked lanes caused by the field gradient and unusual partials. The partial digests are unusual in that final digestion products appear at the earliest time points and that the relative concentration of partials is never high at any digestion condition. We return to this probelem below.

The Y1 Mouse Adrenocortical Tumour Cell Lines

The Y1 clonal cell line was established in culture in 1966 and two sublines with amplified c-Ki-ras gene are available, the Y1-DM and the Y1-HSR line [see 18–20]. Our results with the Y1-DM line can be summarized in two points: 1) Each restriction endonuclease that cleaves the Y1-DM DNA into large fragments yields a single homogeneous fragment that hybrizidizes with the Ki-ras cDNA probe. The largest fragments are obtained with MluI and NotI, which both give a 750-kb band, showing that the repeat is homogeneous over a large region. The homogeneity over an even

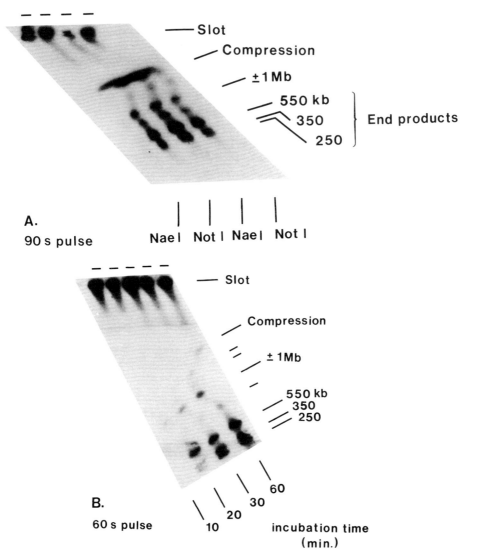

Fig. 4. PFG gel analysis of partial digestion products of EL4/12 DNA cleaved with NaeI or NotI. The experiment was carried out as in Figure 3, but using variable enzyme concentrations or incubation times to generate partial products. In A the pulse time was 90 sec, in B 60 sec. A: From left to right: EL4/12 blocks were digested with 12 U NaeI for 30 min at 0°C; 12 U NotI for 2 hr at 37°C; 12 U NaeI for 60 min at 0°C; 12 U NotI for 4 hr at 37°C. B: EL4/12 blocks were digested with 12 U NaeI at 15°C with an incubation time as indicated.

larger segment is indicated by the appearance of defined, partial digestion products, too large to size, at short incubation times. 2) In the ethidium-stained gel of Y1-DM DNA cut with MluI or NotI, DNA bands are visible superimposed on the heterogeneous DNA background. The relative intensity of these bands is proportional to their size; they are specific for Y1-DM DNA; and only one of these bands (the 750-kb band) hybridizes with the Ki-ras probe. We infer that each of these bands is derived from the DM and that the repeat size of the amplified DNA is at least equal to the sum of these bands, ie, > 2,500 kb.

The amplified DNA in the Y1-HSR is more complex and yields multiple nonstoichiometric bands with NotI and MluI. A full account of our work on the Y1-DM and Y1-HSR lines will be published elsewhere.

The CH^{R}C5 Chinese Hamster Ovary Line

The CH^{R}C5 line was selected for colchicine resistance by Ling and coworkers and is cross-resistant to a wide variety of other, unrelated drugs. We have isolated DNA probes for five genes that are overexpressed and amplified in the resistant line relative to the sensitive parent and used these probes to construct a map of the amplicon, which is complex and covers at least 1,100 kb in wild-type DNA [15]. Three other multi-drug-resistant hamster lines amplify subsets of these genes that are adjacent in the map [32]. Although we have been unable to construct a precise restriction map of the amplicon, PFG gel analysis has been very useful in this case to establish linkage of genes [15]. In fact, short-range linkage studies may become one of the most useful applications of PFG gel analysis.

Practical Problems in the PFG Analysis of (Amplified) Mammalian DNA

1) PFG analysis is still somewhat of an art. Although improved classical PFG boxes [22] and the orthogonal field alternation gel system [26] give less crooked lanes and more reproducible results than the original PFG system, good results still require more fiddling, feeling, and repeated experiments than standard electrophoresis. In fact, uninterpretable results are easy to get with this method. It is possible that the new system developed by Carle et al [33], will solve these problems.

A major source of problems in PFG gels is the field gradient, which makes adjacent lanes nonequivalent and therefore difficult to compare. According to Schwartz and Cantor [13] the field gradient is essential for stretching large DNA, ie, > 500 kb. Without gradient this DNA tends to stick in the slot. This is also our experience.

2) The number of enzymes available that cleave mammalian DNA into large fragments is still limited. The enzymes that do, have GC-rich recognition sites. These sites are often clustered, because of the presence of GC-rich areas in mammalian DNA. Potentially the usefulness of such enzymes could be further limited by methylation of C residues in recognition sites. This may be less of a problem in the study of amplified DNA, as active genes are usually undermethylated and amplified genes are selected for activity. Shimada and Nienhuis [34] have verified that in the case of DHFR gene amplification all amplified copies are equally undermethylated.

Ingenious methods have been devised to cut DNA into large fragments by combining the use of specific DNA methylases with a restriction enzyme that only cuts methylated DNA [35]. This approach, however, has been applied with only limited success to DNA embedded in agarose [23].

3) An appealing feature of PFG gel electrophoresis is the high resolution over a large range, because mobility is a linear function of the DNA size (rather than of the logarithm of size as in standard electrophoresis). This is why under optimal conditions lambda DNA 20-mers and 21-mers can be completely separated [23]. Remaining drawbacks are the following: a) The occurrence of compression zones at unexpected positions in the gel; these depend on the exact conditions of the run [23]. b) The fact that mobility is not exclusively dependent on size but that DNA sequence makes a minor contribution [23]. The reasons for sequence dependence remain unknown. c) The uncertainty of sizing above 1,500 kb because of the lack of suitable markers.

The problems in size calibration complicate the interpretation of partial digestion products and the construction of restriction maps.

4) We have had difficulties in getting good series of partial digestion products in our PFG analysis. Usually we get only minor amounts of partials and complete digestion products at the earliest time points, or the lowest enzyme concentrations. It is possible that the enzyme does not readily diffuse into the agarose blocks and hence tends to completely digest whatever DNA it encounters on its slow influx. We have tried to promote partial digestion by digesting at 0°C for long periods, or by partially preventing digestion with drugs that bind to DNA, like actinomycin D. The results have been unsatisfactory. It should be added, however, that we have had no problems in getting partial digestion in agarose blocks of lambda DNA with MluI, of adeno 12 DNA with NotI and of adeno 5 DNA with SfiI. In view of this we cannot rule out that the problems seen with infrequently cutting enzymes are due to site clusters, making the generation of detectable partials unlikely.

DISCUSSION

Our initial results with PFG gels, summarized in Table I, lead to three tentative conclusions:

1) In several cell lines (EL4/8, EL4/12 and Y1-HSR) we find gross heterogeneity in the size of the amplified unit. This is most pronounced when the copy number of amplified genes is high, but it is also seen in the multi-drug-resistant CHO cell line CH^{R}C5 in which amplification is 30-fold. This confirms the results of standard gel analysis of highly amplified DNA, which has shown multiple joints and increasing heterogeneity of flanking sequences as one moves away from the gene that has been selected for [see 1,2,17,36].

2) The size of the wild-type segment found amplified in some of the cell lines studied is large, up to 2,500 kb in Y1-DM. Although this also confirms previous estimates [see 1,2,37], we note that these estimates were based on data with a considerably larger margin of uncertainty than our results.

3) Some amplified units are homogeneous over distances of at least 750 kb (Y1-DM) or 800 kb (3T6-R50) and they may well be homogeneous over all of the amplicon. This is unexpected in view of the pronounced heterogeneity reported for all amplicons studied in depth [see 2,17,36] with the possible exception of the short DHFR amplicon in Chinese hamster cell line CHOC 400 [38]. Why this discrepancy? We do not think that lack of resolution of the PFG gel system is responsible, because some amplicons yield bands that are nearly as sharp as bands visualized after standard gel electrophoresis. We also do not think that heterogeneity is a side effect of drug selection. It might be argued that selection with MTX or N-(phosphonacetyl)-L-aspartate inhibits DNA synthesis by substrate limitation and would therefore promote formation of short amplicons, if amplification is mainly due to rereplication of partially replicated DNA segments. The results with the 3T6-R50 line show, however, that drug selection does not necessarily lead to heterogeneous amplicons.

We therefore favour the interpretation that the homogeneity or heterogeneity of the amplicon is mainly determined by the degree of amplification, heterogeneity being the result of multiple rounds of amplification imposed by stringent selection. We propose that amplicons start out long and homogeneous and that heterogeneity arises later. If the initial amplicon were 3,000 kb, a 1,000-fold amplification would double the haploid DNA content of the cell. This would be such an extra load that any deletion that would shorten the amplified unit by removing co-amplified DNA would confer a selective advantage on the cell containing it. The multiple rounds of selection required for high degrees of amplification would obviously provide ample opportunity for deletions to occur. This proposal is compatible with published data and testable.

ACKNOWLEDGMENTS

We thank Dr. V. Ling, The Ontario Cancer Institute, Toronto, Canada; Dr. C.J. Bostock, MRC Mammalian Genome Unit, University of Edinburgh, Scotland; Dr. R.T. Schimke, Dept. of Biological Sciences, Stanford University, California; and Dr. D.L. George, Dept. of Human Genetics, University of Pennsylvania, Philadelphia, Pennsylvania for supplying us with cell lines; and Dr. A.D. Levinson, Dept. of Molecular Biology, Genentech Incorporated, South San Francisco, California, and Dr. R.W. Ellis, Lab. Tumor Virus Genetics, NCI, Bethesda, Maryland, for DNA probes. We are indebted to our colleagues Dr. M. de Bruijn and Dr. F. Baas for advice and critical comments. This work was supported in part by grant NKI 84-20 of the Queen Wilhelmina Fund.

REFERENCES

1. Bostock CJ, Tyler-Smith C: Genome Evolution 20:69, 1982.
2. Stark GR, Wahl GM: Annu Rev Biochem 53:447, 1984.
3. Schimke RT: Cell 37:705, 1984.
4. Schmike RT: Cancer Res 44:1735, 1984.
5. Curt GA, Cowan KH, Chabner BA: J Clin Oncol 2:62, 1984.
6. Borst P: Nature 309:580, 1984.
7. Hamlin JL, Milbrandt JD, Heintz NH, Azizkhan JC: Int Rev Cytol 90:31, 1984.
8. Riordan JR, Ling V: Pharmacol Ther 28:51, 1985.
9. Alitalo K: TIBS 10:194, 1985.
10. Schwab M: TIG 1:271, 1985.
11. Sager R, Gadi IK, Stephens L, Grabowy CT: Proc Natl Acad Sci USA 82:7015, 1985.
12. Glanville N: Mol Cell Biol 5:1456, 1985.
13. Schwartz DC, Cantor CH: Cell 37:67, 1984.
14. Van Der Bliek AM, Bernards A, Borst P: J Cell Biochem [Suppl] 9C:32, 1985.
15. Van Der Bliek AM, Van Der Velde-Koerts T, Ling V, Borst P: Mol Cell Biol 6:1671, 1986.
16. Brown PC, Beverley SM, Schimke RT: Mol Cell Biol 1:1077, 1981.
17. Federspiel NA, Beverley SM, Schilling JW, Schimke RT: J Biol Chem 259:9127, 1984.
18. George DL, Francke U: Cytogenet Cell Genet 28:217, 1980.
19. George DL, Scott AF, De Martinville B, Francke U: Nucl Acids Res 12:2731, 1984.
20. George DL, Scott AF, Trusko S, Glick B, Ford E, Dorney DJ: EMBO J 4:1199, 1985.
21. Ling V, Kartner N, Sudo T, Siminovitch L, Riordan JR: Cancer Treat Rep 67:869, 1983.
22. Johnson PJ, Borst P: Gene 43:213, 1986.
23. Bernards A, Kooter JM, Michels PAM, Moberts RMP, Borst P: Gene 42:313, 1986.
24. Simonson CC, Levinson AD: Proc Natl Acad Sci USA 80:2495, 1983.
25. Ellis RW, DeFeo D, Shih TY, Gonda MA, Young HA, Tsuchida N, Lowy DR, Scolnick EM: Nature 292:506, 1981.
26. Carle GF, Olson MV: Nucl Acids Res 12:5647, 1984.
27. Melgar E, Goldthwait DA: J Biol Chem 213:4409, 1968.
28. Hamkalo BA, Farnham PJ, Johnston R, Schimke RT: Proc Natl Acad Sci USA 82:1126, 1985.
29. Setlow P: In Fasman GD (ed): "Handbook of Biochemisty and Molecular Biology." Cleveland, Ohio: CRC Press, 1976, pp 312–318.
30. Razin A, Cedar H: Int Rev Cytol 92:159, 1984.

31. Crouse GF, Simonson CC, McEwan RN, Schimke RT: J Biol Chem 257:7887, 1982.
32. De Bruyn MHL, Van Der Bliek AM, Biedler JL, Borst P: Mol Cell Biol 6:4717, 1986.
33. Carle GF, Frank M, Olson MV: Science 232:65, 1986.
34. Shimada T, Nienhuis AW: J Biol Chem 260:2468, 1986.
35. McClelland M, Kessler LG, Bittner M: Proc Natl Acad Sci USA 81:983, 1984.
36. Roberts JM, Buck LB, Axel R: Cell 33:53, 1983.
37. Cowell JK: Annu Rev Genet 16:21, 1982.
38. Montoya-Zavala M, Hamlin JL: Mol Cell Biol 5:619, 1985.

Cellular and Molecular Biology of Tumors and Potential Clinical Applications 159–166 (1988)

Mechanisms of Chromosome Translocations in B- and T-Cell Neoplasms

Frank G. Haluska, Lawrence R. Finger, Yoshihide Tsujimoto, and Carlo M. Croce

The Wistar Institute, Philadelphia, Pennsylvania 19104

Most leukemias and lymphomas exhibit characteristic, nonrandom chromosome translocations (Yunis, 1983). This feature of hematopoietic malignancy underlies many of the recent exciting advances in our understanding of the molecular genetic basis of human oncogenesis. It has become clear over the past several years that in the hematologic neoplasias carrying specific chromosome translocations, the loss of genetic control consequent to the chromosome translocation is the primary oncogenic event in the pathogenesis of the malignancy. In particular, the chromosome translocations juxtapose cellular oncogenes with genetic loci capable of altering the expression of the oncogenes. Importantly, these loci may exert their effects in cis over relatively large genetic distances [Croce et al, 1984]. Thus, a fruitful avenue of investigation has been to construct molecular clones of the chromosome regions directly involved in the translocations, to isolate these clones using defined probes from the genetic segments surrounding the translocation breakpoints, and to examine their structure. Using this approach, we have studied and characterized several translocations involving the immunoglobulin loci [Croce et al, 1984; Croce and Nowell, 1985]. These include the t(11;14) translocation characteristic of chronic lymphocytic leukemia [Tsujimoto et al, 1984a], the t(14;18) translocation seen in follicular lymphoma (Tsujimoto et al, 1984b], and the t(8;14) translocation of Burkitt lymphoma and acute lymphoblastic leukemia [Haluska et al, 1986]. Recently this approach has been extended to translocations involving the T-cell alpha locus [Finger et al, 1986]. These investigations have demonstrated that the enzymatic machinery which physiologically functions in immunoglobulin gene V-D-J recombination [Tonegawa, 1983], as well as in T-cell receptor gene recombination [Yancopoulos et al, 1986], aberrantly joins segments of DNA from the translocated chromosomes, and thus is directly responsible for the non-random translocations.

The immunoglobulin heavy chain locus maps to chromosome region 14q32 [Croce et al, 1979], which is prone to involvement in translocations characterizing a number of lymphoid tumors. One such malignancy is chronic lymphocytic leukemia (CLL) of

Received September 3, 1986.

the B-cell type, which exhibits a t(11;14) (q13;q32) translocation [Nowell et al, 1981]. We cloned the translocation breakpoint from a case of CLL, CLL 271 [Tsujimoto et al, 1984a] in order to study the involved segments of both of these chromosomes. A genomic library was constructed in the phage vector EMBL 3A from CLL 271 cells. This library was screened with genomic probes corresponding to the immunoglobulin heavy chain mu constant region ($C\mu$) and the joining region (J_H). Two classes of recombinant clones were obtained. One of these represented the productively rearranged mu allele. The second class of clones represented the joining of chromosomes 11 and 14; this was demonstrated by Southern blotting of subcloned probes against DNAs from somatic cell hybrids containing only human chromosome 11 or only human chromosome 14. We designated this region of chromosome 11, which is involved in the t(11;14) translocations of CLL 271, as bcl-1 (B-cell leukemia/lymphoma-1).

Subsequently we were able to demonstrate that specific genomic probes from the bcl-1 region of chromosome 11 recognize rearranged restriction fragments in several other cases of CLL, as well as in a case of diffuse large cell lymphoma, all of which carry the t(11;14) translocation [Tsujimoto et al, 1985a]. Utilizing the chromosome 11-specific probes derived from the CLL 271 breakpoint clone, we screened a genomic library constructed from a second case of CLL, CLL 1386, and obtained two clones which hybridized with both the bcl-1 and J_H probes. This indicated that these clones contained the translocation breakpoint from this leukemia. Detailed restriction mapping showed that the breakpoints on chromosome 11 from CLL 271 and CLL 1386 were quite close to one another, and thus we obtained the nucleotide sequences surrounding these breakpoints. Analysis of the sequences revealed several features. First, the breakpoints of these two CLLs are within eight nucleotides of each other on chromosome 11. Second, both breakpoints occur immediately 5' to the IgH J4 segment on chromosome 14. Third, at the breakpoints, short stretches of nucleotides having homology to neither chromosome 11 nor 14 were observed. Finally, the normal region of chromosome 11 has a sequence homologous to the heptamer-nonamer recognized by the immunoglobulin recombinase [Sakano et al, 1979]. These features strongly suggested that these translocations occurred through the action of the immunoglobulin V-D-J recombinase, which functions during physiologic rearrangement of the immunoglobulin locus during B-cell maturation [Tonegawa, 1983]. This putative enzyme is hypothesized to recognize heptamer-nonamer signal sequences apposed to the recombining segments. Recombination takes place when a signal sequence having a 12-base pair spacer is paired with one having a 23-base pair spacer [Sakano et al, 1981]. Furthermore, V-D-J joining results in deletions, substitutions, or in the addition of extra nucleotides (N regions), presumably by the action of terminal deoxynucleotide transferase [Desiderio et al, 1984], at the joining sites. The characteristics of the translocation breakpoint sequences, including breakage 5' of J_H at the site where a D segment is normally joined, the presence of heterogeneous N nucleotides, and correctly spaced heptamer-nonamer signal sequences on chromosome 11, all strongly implicate the V-D-J recombinase in the mechanism of the t(11;14) translocation in malignant B-cells [Tsujimoto et al, 1985a].

A second lymphoid malignancy commonly exhibiting a translocation involving the 14q32 region is follicular lymphoma, one of the most common B-cell malignancies [Fukuhara et al, 1979].The observed translocation in these cases is usually t(14;18)(q32;q21). Employing an approach analogous to that described above for bcl-

1, we have cloned the region on chromosome 18 involved in these translocations [Tsujimoto et al, 1984b]. We took advantage of the cell line 380, which was established from a patient with acute lymphoblastic leukemia, and which carries both the t(8;14)(q24;q32) and the t(14;18)(q32;q21) translocations [Pegoraro et al, 1984]. Using DNA from this cell line, we constructed a genomic library and screened it with the J_H probe [Tsujimoto et al, 1984b]. Two classes of recombinant clones were obtained. Using subcloned probes from these phages to probe Southern-blotted DNAs from somatic cell hybrids containing only chromosomes 8, 14, or 18, we showed that one of these classes contained the t(8;14) breakpoint, while the second class contained the t(14;18) breakpoint. The region of chromosome 18 involved in these translocations was designated bcl-2 (B-cell leukemia/lymphoma-2). Genomic probes derived from the bcl-2 region immediately surrounding the t(14;18) breakpoints were shown to detect rearrangements in greater than 60% of follicular lymphoma DNAs [Tsujimoto et al, 1985b]. Additionally, these probes detect three RNA transcripts of 8.5, 5.5, and 3.5 kilobases (kb) on Northern blots [Tsujimoto and Croce, 1986]. Together these data indicate that the points of chromosome breakage are clustered in the majority of follicular lymphomas having t(14;18) translocations, and that in these cases the bcl-2 gene is directly involved in tumorigenesis.

A genomic bcl-2 probe was used to screen genomic libraries constructed from the DNA from four cases of follicular lymphoma [Tsujimoto et al, 1985c]. From each of these libraries, recombinant clones were obtained which hybridized to both the bcl-2 probes and to the immunoglobulin J_H probe, demonstrating that, as was the case for bcl-1, the heavy chain joining segment was the site of chromosome translocation. Nucleotide sequence analysis of the 380 breakpoint clone and the four additional follicular lymphoma clones revealed features reminiscent of the t(11;14) breakpoints, and again suggestive of recombinase involvement. In each case, the site of joining on chromosome 14 is at the 5' end of a J_H segment, where a D segment physiologically recombines. N regions are found at the joining sites in each case. And in the three cases where the normal region of chromosome 18 was compared, heptamer-nonamer signal sequences occur. Thus, the mechanism of chromosome translocation in follicular lymphomas having the t(14;18) is the same as for CLLs having the t(11;14): these translocations result from mistakes in V-D-J joining.

Given that in these two types of common B-cell malignancies the characteristic translocations occur through the operation of the recombinase, it seemed reasonable to suppose that the same might be true of Burkitt lymphoma. The most common translocation observed in Burkitt lymphoma is the t(8;14)(q24;q32) [Manolov and Manolova, 1972; Zech et al, 1976]; a similar translocation occurs in pre-B-cell acute lymphoblastic leukemia [Williams et al, 1984]. This juxtaposes the IgH locus with the cellular oncogene c-*myc* [Dalla Favera et al, 1982]. As noted above, the cell line 380 carried both the t(14;18) translocation and the t(8;14) translocation [Pegoraro et al., 1984], and screening a 380 genomic library with a J_H probe yielded recombinant clones corresponding to both translocations [Tsujimoto et al, 1984b]. We demonstrated that one of these clones contained sequences from chromsome 8 by probing a panel of DNAs from somatic cell hybrids containing only human chromosome 8 or 14 [Haluska et al, 1986]. This chromosome 8-specific probe was then used to detect rearrangements in restriction endonuclease digested genomic DNAs from the African Burkitt lymphomas P3HR-1 and Daudi [Haluska et al, 1986] as well as the undifferentiated lymphoma EW 36 (unpublished observations).These data indicated that the t(8;14) translocation breakpoints in these lymphoma are clustered near one another.

We thus attempted to clone these breakpoints by constructing genomic libraries from P3HR-1 and Daudi; in addition, we employed the 380 library previously utilized [Tsujimoto et al, 1984b]. We initially screened the P3HR-1 library with the J_H probe, and secondarily screened the recombinant clones obtained with the chromosome 8-specific probe, whereas the Daudi and 380 libraries were screened directly with the chromosome 8 probe [Haluska et al, 1986]. The resulting phage clones were subjected to analysis by restriction endonuclease digestion and Southern blotting, allowing us to categorize the clones as containing only chromosome 8 sequences, or the joining between chromosome 8 and 14. From P3HR-1 we obtained the breakpoint clone, and from 380 the breakpoint was obtained previously. We also obtained clones spanning the normal region of chromosome 8 from 380, and only normal clones from Daudi.

Figure 1 illustrates the nucleotide sequence of the (8;14) breakpoints from 380 and P3HR-1 as well as the corresponding segment of chromosome 8. The analysis of these sequences strongly implicates the V-D-J recombinase in the mechanism of translocation. The 380 breakpoint on chromosome 8 occurs at a sequence homologous to the canonical heptamer (bracketed in Fig. 1). This heptamer is perfectly palindromic; however, a nonamer is lacking. Yet the alignment of the J6 segment with the 380 sequence clearly demonstrates that chromosome 14 would be correctly positioned for the utilization of the J6 heptamer-nonamer during recombination. Furthermore, an N region is observed, including a stretch of GCs, as often occurs [Tonegawa, 1983]. At the P3HR-1 breakpoint, a heptamer is found. Twelve bases downstream is a nonamer. On chromosome 14, although the break is greater than 100 bases 5' of J5, an almost-perfect heptamer-nonamer is observed, with 23-basepair spacing. Recombination according to the 12/23 rule could occur. The 50 nucleotides 3' of this chromosome 14 nonamer comprise 16 possible codons (including a stop) and a GT splice signal, as in a J segment, and thus might constitute an additional signal recognized by the recombinase. Imprecision is also observed at the breakpoint. Finally, single base changes which may occur as a consequence of somatic mutation following F-D-J recombination are exhibited in both breakpoints. In both of these translocations, then, sequence analysis strongly suggests that the translocation occurred through the action of the recombinase in a sequence-specific manner.

It is noteworthy that Burkitt lymphoma is a heterogeneous disease. It occurs as a sporadic form, in Europe and North America, or as an endemic, African form. The phenotype of the sporadic Burkitt lymphoma cell is that of a relatively differentiated B-cell, which secretes IgM [Benjamin et al, 1982]. That of the endemic form suggest a less differentiated cell, one which is positive for cytoplasmic or surface Ig, but which does not secrete Ig. Additionally, most African Burkitt lymphomas are associated with EBNA (Epstein-Barr virus nuclear antigen). We have previously shown that sporadic Burkitt lymphomas with a rearranged c-myc gene are at a more advanced stage of differentiation than African Burkitt lymphomas [Croce and Nowell, 1986], and that in these cases translocation occurs into the IgH switch region [Showe et al, 1985]. In African Burkitt lymphomas, however, and in pre-B-cell ALL, our analysis of the mechanism of translocation indicates the involvement of the V-D-J recombinase. This enzyme functions at the pre-B-cell stage of differentiation [Korsmeyer et al, 1983], as does terminal transferase [Desiderio et al, 1984]. Thus, when examined at the immunophenotypic level or at the molecular genetic level, the cell of origin of the African Burkitt lymphoma or the pre-B-cell ALL differs from that of the sporadic lymphoma. African Burkitt lymphoma cases originate in a cell which is at an early stage of ontogeny, and is subject to mistakes in V-D-J joining, whereas the sporadic Burkitt cases originate from more differentiated cells, in which switching mistakes occur.

T-cell malignancies, like those of B-cells, are characterized by nonrandom chromosome abnormalities. Frequently translocations are observed which involve the 14q11-q13 region [Hecht et al, 1984; Williams et al, 1984]. By analogy with the 14q32 region involved in B-cell neoplasia, one might have predicted that this region would prove to comprise genes expressed in a T-cell specific manner, and indeed, this is precisely the case. The alpha chain of the T-cell receptor maps to 14q11-q12 [Croce et al, 1985]. Furthermore, the direct involvement of the Tα locus in these translocations has been demonstrated at the molecular level: analysis of somatic cell hybrids derived from T-ALLs revealed that the Tα locus was split by t(11;14) (p13;q11) translocation (Erikson et al, 1985). In addition, we showed that a translocation placing the Tα locus in proximity to c-*myc* resulted in deregulation of the c-*myc* gene [Erikson et al, 1986]. In this case, we studied two T-cell leukemias carrying the t(8;14)(q24;q11) translocation. Southern blot experiments on one of these leukemias, DeF, demonstrated no DNA rearrangements with characterized probes. But analysis of somatic cell hybrids between human tumor cells and mouse leukemic cells demonstrated that Cα was translocated 3′ to c-*myc* on the 8q+ chromosome, while the 14q- retained Vα. Moreover, based on the known restruction map 3′ of c-*myc*, it was determined that the breakpoint on chromosome 8 was at least 38 kb from c-*myc*. Southern blot experiments of the second leukemia, SKW-3, did reveal rearranged restriction fragments. The breakpoint was shown to lie within approximately three kb of the third exon of c-*myc*. These breakpoints are consistent with those of the variant Burkitt lymphomas, which juxtapose c-*myc* and the kappa Ig locus on chromosome 2, or the lambda Ig locus on chromosome 22 [Croce and Nowell, 1985]. There appears to be heterogeneity of chromosome breakpoints on chromosome 8 in both the variant Burkitt lymphomas as well as in T-cell leukemias carrying the t(8;14).

The availability of a DNA probe detecting a rearrangement in SKW-3 DNA allowed us to clone and sequence the breakpoint of this leukemic cell line [Finger et al, 1986]. We constructed a genomic library in the lambda phage EMBL 3A, and screened it with the probe, derived from the 3′ flanking sequences of c-*myc* on chromosome 8, which detected the rearrangement. Two groups of recombinant clones were obtained, one corresponding to the germline configuration of c-*myc*, and the second containing chromosome 14 sequences. This was demonstrated by employing subclones to probe DNAs from rodent x human somatic cell hybrids containing only human chromosomes 8 or 14. Comparison of the phage restriction maps with that of the Tα locus (Showe and Harvey, unpublished data) revealed that the chromosome 14 portion of the breakpoint clones corresponded to a region of the Jα locus approximately 36-kb 5′ to the Cα segment. Thus, the juxtaposition of Tα and c-*myc* reflects the same head-to-tail orientation previously demonstrated for the t(2;8) and t(8;22) variant Burkitt lymphoma translocations (Croce and Nowell, 1985).

The nucleotide sequence of the SKW-3 breakpoint is illustrated in Figure 2, as are those of the normal chromosomes 8 and 14. Nucleotides 78–131 on chromosome 14 compose a Jα segment, so designated on the basis of the conserved phe-gly-x-gly motif, conserved in T-cell receptor J segments [Yoshikai et al, 1985; Winoto et al, 1985; Arden et al, 1985]. Donor splice signals are present at the 3′ boundary of the Jα. Immediately 5′ of the J segment are situated heptamer-nonamer recombination

Fig. 1.

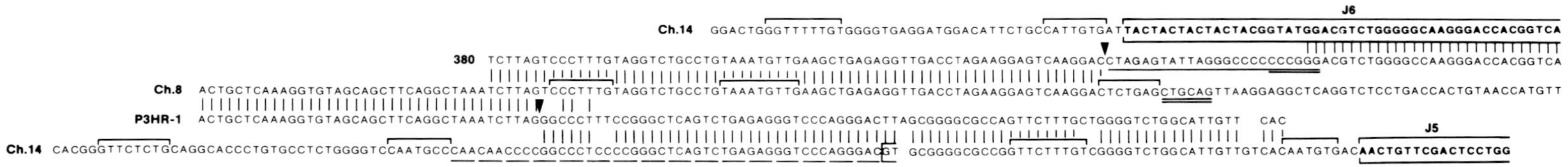

Ch.14   GGACTGGGTTTTTGTGGGTGAGGATGGACATTCTGCCATTGTGATT**TACTACTACTACGGTATGGACGTCTGGGGCAAGGGACCACGGTCA**

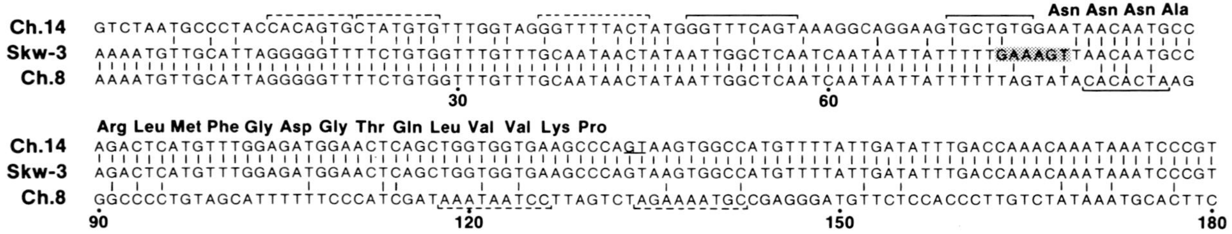

                                                                                                    J6

            380 TCTTAGTCCCTTTGTAGGTCTGCCTGTAAATGTTGAAGCTAGAAGGAGTCAAGGACTAGAGTATTAGGGCCCCGGGAGTGCTGGGGCAAGGGACCACGGTCA
                 ||||||||||||||||||||||||||||||||||||||||||||||||||||||||||||||||||||||||||
Ch.8   ACTGCTCAAAGGTGTAGCAGCTTCAGGGTAA TCTTAGTCCCTTTGTAGGTCTGCCTGTAAATGTTGAAGCTAGAAGGAGTCAAGGACTCTGAGCTCGAGTTAAGGAGGCTCAGGTCTCCTGACCACTGTAACCATGTT

P3HR-1 ACTGCTCAAAGGTGTAGCAGCTTCAGGGTAAATCTTAGGGCCCTTTCCGGGCTCAGTCTGAGAGGGTCCCAGGGACCGGCCAGTTCTTTGCTGGGGTCTGGCATTGTT   CAC
                 ||||||||||||||||||||||||||||||||||||||||||||||||||||||||
Ch.14   CACGGGTTCTCTGCGAGGCACCCTGCCTCTGGGGTCCAATCCCGGCCTCCCGGGCTCAGTCTGAGAGGGTCCCAGGGACCGG GCCGGGCGGCCCGGTTCTTTGTCGGGTCTGCATTGTTGTCAAATGTGTCAAGTCACAATGTGACAGTGA **AACTGTTCGACTCCTGG**

                                                                                                    J5

Fig. 2.

Ch.14   GTCTAAATGCCCTACCACCAGTGCTATGTGTTTGGGTAGGGTTTCAGTAAAGGCAGGAAGTGCTGGAATAACAATGCC
Skw-3   AAAATGTTGCATTAGGGGGGTTTTCTGTGGTTTGTTTGCAATAACTA—TAATTGGCTCAATCAATAATTATTTT-**GAAAG**-TAACAATGCC
Ch.8   AAAATGTTGCATTAGGGGGGTTTTCTGTGGTTTGTTTGCAATAACTA—TAATTGGCTCAATCAATAATTATTTT-----TAACAATGCC

                                                                                    60   **Asn Asn Asn Ala**

        Arg Leu Met Phe Gly Asp Gly Thr Gln Leu Val Val Lys Pro
Ch.14   AGACTCATGTTTGGAGGATGGAACTCAGCTGGTGGTGAAGCCCAG AAGTGGCCATGTTTTATTGATATTTGACCAAAACAAATAAATCCCGT
Skw-3   AGACTCATGTTTGGAGATGGAACTCAGCTGGTGGTGAAGCCCAGTAAGTGGCCATGTT-TATT-GATATTTGACCAAAACAAATAAATCCCGT
                                                                                    120
Ch.8   GGCCCCTGTAGCATTTTTCCCATCGATAAATAATCCTTAGTCTAGAAAATGCGAGGGATGTTCTCCACCCTTGTCTATAAATGCACTTC
                                                    90   150   180

signals. At the breakpoint, six nucleotides having homology to neither chromosome 8 nor 14 are found. Finally, on chromosome 8 a heptamer is situated at the breakpoint, although a suitable nonamer does not occur until a point 30 base pairs downstream is reached. Thus, as has been shown in B-cells, the mechanism of translocation in T-cells seems to involve the recombinase. The translocation breakpoint occurs 5' to a Jα segment; it includes a region of N nucleotides, which have been directly demonstrated in rearranged T gamma genes [Quertermous et al, 1986]; and it occurs in proximity to heptamer-nonamer sequences, which apparently are recognized by the same enzymatic apparatus as that which functions in B-cells [Yancopoulos et al, 1986].

Thus a productive approach to defining the cellular elements which underlie hematologic oncogenesis has been to employ defined molecular probes to study the structure of nonrandom chromosome translocations. These probers are derived from genetic loci which might serve to activate abnormally juxtaposed genes in restricted cell populations. In particular, we have utilized DNA probes from the immunoglobulin heavy chain locus to demonstrate activation in B-cells of aberrantly situated c-*myc* and bcl-2 genes. Furthermore, we have shown that the mechanism of translocation involves the operation of the recombinase, which is expressed in lymphoid progenitors. A similar situation is becoming evident in T-cells. Activation of c-*myc* is implicated in T-cell oncogenesis, and the mechanism of translocation also involves the recombination enzymes. The progress that has been made in broadening this approach allows us to predict that by extensioin of these techniques it will in the future be possible to identify most of the genes involved in B-and T-cell neoplasia, and to gain insight into their mechanisms of action as an eventual basis for rational diagnosis and therapy.

REFERENCES

1. Arden B, Klotz JL, Siu G, Hood LE: Nature 316:783–787, 1985.
2. Croce CM, Isobe M, Palumbo A, Puck J, Ming J, Tweardy D, Erikson J, Davis M, Rovera G: Science 227:1044–1047, 1985.
3. Croce CM, Nowell PC: Blood 65:1–7, 1985.
4. Croce CM, Nowell PC: Adv Immunol 38:245–274, 1986.
5. Croce CM, Shander M, Martinis J, Cicurel L, D'Ancona GG, Dolby TW, Koprowski H: Proc Natl Acad Sci USA 76:3416–3420, 1979.
6. Croce CM, Tsujimoto Y, Erikson J, Nowell PC: Lab Invest 51:258–267, 1984.
7. Dalla-Favera R, Bregni M, Erikson J, Patterson D, Gallo R, Croce CM: Proc Natl Acad Sci USA 79:7824–7827, 1982.

Fig. 1. Nucleotide sequence of the joining site between chromosome 8 and 14 in P3HR-1 and 380, and the corresponding normal chromosome 8 region. The triangles designate points at which the P3HR-1 and 380 sequences diverge from the chromosome 8 sequence; vertical lines indicate identical nucleotides. Bold sequences indicate the J5 and J6 heavy chain joining segments. The bracketed regions are conserved heptamer-nonamer signal sequences, and a putative N region is underlined at the 380 joining site. The underlined region of chromosome 14 comprises 16 potential codons and a splice signal (see text).

Fig. 2. Sequence of SKW-3 t(8;14) breakpoint, and corresponding regions of chromosomes 8 and 14. Brackets indicate the conserved heptamer and nonamer regions adjacent to the breakpoint. Other homologous heptamer and nonamer segments are indicated by dashed lines. The possible N-region nucleotides are shown as a gray box. The 3' splice donor site is underlined.

8. Desiderio SV, Yancopoulos GD, Paskind M, Thomas E, Boss MA, Landau N, Alt FW, Baltimore D: Nature 311:752–755, 1984.
9. Erikson J, Finger L, Sun L, Ar-Rushdi A, Nishikura K, Minowada J, Finan J, Emanuel BS, Nowell PC, Croce CM: Science 232:884–886, 1986.
10. Erikson J, Williams DL, Finan J, Nowell PC, Croce CM: Science 229:784–786, 1985.
11. Finger LR, Harvey RC, Moore RCA, Showe LC, Croce CM: Science (in press), 1986.
12. Fukuhara S, Rowley JD, Variakojis D, Golomb HM: Cancer Res 39:3119–3128, 1979.
13. Haluska FG, Finver S, Tsujimoto Y, Croce CM: Nature 324:158–161, 1986.
14. Hecht F, Morgan R, Hecht BK, Smith SD: Science 226:1445–1447, 1984.
15. Korsmeyer SJ, Arnold A, Bakhshi A, Ravetch JV, Siebenlist U, Hieter PA, Sharrow SO, Lebien TW, Kersey JH, Poplack DG, Leder P, Waldman TA: J Clin Invest 71:301–313, 1983.
16. Manolov G, Manolova Y: Nature 237:33–34, 1972.
17. Nowell P, Shankey TV, Finan J, Guerry D, Besa A: Blood 57:444–451, 1981.
18. Pegoraro L, Palumba A, Erikson J, Fauda M, Giovanazzo B, Emanuel BS, Rovera G, Nowell PC, Croce CM: Proc Natl Acad Sci USA 81:7166–7170, 1984.
19. Quertermous T, Strauss W, Murre C, Dialynas DP, Strominger JL, Seidman JG: Nature 322:184–187, 1986.
20. Sakano H, Huppi K, Heinrich G, Tonegawa S: Nature 280:280–294, 1979.
21. Sakano H, Kurosawa Y, Weigert M, Tonegawa S: Nature 290:562–565, 1981.
22. Showe LC, Ballantine M, Nishikura K, Erikson J, Kaji H, Croce CM: Mol Leuk Biol 5:501–509, 1985.
23. Tonegawa S: Nature 302:575–581, 1983.
24. Tsujimoto Y, Cossman J, Jaffe E, Croce CM:Science 228:1440–1443, 1985b.
25. Tsujimoto Y, Croce CM: Proc Natl Acad Sci USA 83:5214–5218, 1986.
26. Tsujimoto Y, Finger LR, Yunis J, Nowell PC, Croce CM: Science 226:1079–1099, 1984b.
27. Tsujimoto Y, Gorham J, Cossman J, Jaffe E, Croce CM: Science 229:1390–1393, 1985c.
28. Tsujimoto Y, Jaffe E, Cossman J, Gorham J, Nowell PC, Croce CM: Nature 315:340–343, 1985A.
29. Tsujimoto Y, Yunis J, Onorato-Showe L, Erikson J, Nowell PC, Croce CM: Science 224:1403–1406, 1984a.
30. Williams DL, Wok AT, Melvin SL, Roberson PK, Dahl G, Flake T, Stass S: Cell 36:101–109, 1984.
31. Winoto A, Mjolsness S, Hood L: Nature 316:832–836, 1985.
32. Yancopoulos GD, Blackwell TK, Suh H, Hood L, Alt FW: Cell 44:251–259, 1986.
33. Yoshikai Y, Clark SP, Taylor S, Sohn U, Wilson BI, Minden, Mak TW: Nature 316:837–840, 1985.
34. Yunis JJ: Science 221:227–236, 1983.
35. Zech L, Haglund U, Nilsson K, Klein G: Int J Cancer 17:47–56, 1976.

Cellular and Molecular Biology of Tumors and Potential
Clinical Applications 167–177 (1988)

DNA Rearrangement, Relocation, and Amplification in Neuroblastoma Cell Lines and Primary Tumors

Samuel Latt, Yosef Shiloh, Kazuo Sakai, Elise Rose, Garrett Brodeur, Tim Donlon, Bruce Korf, Naotoshi Kanda, Michael Heartlein, John Kang, Helene Stroh, Peter Harris, Gail Bruns, and Robert Seeger

Departments of Pediatrics (S.L., Y.S., K.S., E.R., T.D., B.K., N.K., M.H., J.K., H.S., P.H., G.B.) and Genetics (S.L.), Harvard Medical School, Boston, Massachusetts 02114; Howard Hughes Medical Institute (S.L., H.S., P.H.), Washington University School of Medicine, St. Louis, Missouri 63110 (G.B.); Department of Pediatrics, UCLA School of Medicine and the Children's Cancer Study Group, Los Angeles, California 90024 (R.S.)

DNA amplification in neuroblastoma and some retinoblastoma lines, as manifested by either homogeneously staining regions (HSRs) or double minute bodies (DMs), is accompanied by DNA relocation and, in some cases, interesting DNA rearrangement. Extensive amplification of the oncogene N-myc and, to a systematically lesser extent, other DNA fragments highly amplified in neuroblastoma cell lines is found in advanced stage neuroblastomas. The hierarchy with which DNA fragments are amplified in primary neuroblastomas and neuroblastoma cell lines may contain information about the relative ordering of DNA fragments around N-myc in differently sized amplification units in these cells. Experiments utilizing somatic hybrid DNA panels, DNA dosage blotting, and in situ hybridization map those DNA fragments which are extensively amplified in neuroblastoma cells to the top of the human chromosome 2 short arm, near band 2p24. In contrast, some DNA fragments amplified in the neuroblastoma line IMR-32, but not in primary tumors, map either to the middle or the proximal part of this chromosome arm. Evidence thus far is compatible with a splicing of DNA from these three widely spaced regions of human 2p into amplification units contained in the HSRs of IMR-32. In other neuroblastoma cell lines and primary tumors, DNA amplification is associated with extensive rearrangement. For one particular amplified DNA fragment, this rearrangement occurs at a specific point, bordered by DNA rich in A-T base pairs. In at least one neuroblastoma cell line, NB-9, this rearrangement does not reflect a simple DNA recombination. Instead, a complex, at least three-component, splice event has occurred. The mechanisms underlying the unusual DNA recruitment, rearrangement, and amplification in these neuroectodermal tumors and cell lines should prove of basic interest in understanding the dynamics with which the human genome changes.

Received February 13, 1986.

Key words: NB-9 cells, IMR-32 cells, primary neuroblastoma, DNA splicing, in-situ renaturation
gels

Analysis of DNA amplification in primary neuroblastomas, neuroblastoma cell lines, and in embryologically related tissues such as retinoblastoma has provided clinically useful information and insight about some totally unexpected complexities of DNA amplification in human malignancy. While the full significance of the unusual DNA sequence fluidity in neuroectodermal tissue is not yet clear, information already obtained has detected some novel DNA relocation, splicing, and rearrangement phenomena. A reasonable intermediate conclusion is that these phenomena reflect basic processes operative in other disease conditions and in general provide hints at the molecular level of changes in chromosome structure apparent at a cytological level. The present communication will outline salient features of the DNA amplification process described in detail elsewhere [1–7], present data using some new methods that will facilitate more detailed studies, and consider some broader implications of the information thus far obtained.

Our studies of DNA amplification in neuroblastoma began with flow sorting and cloning of a homogeneously staining region (HSR)-containing No. 1 chromosome in the neuroblastoma cell line IMR-32 [8–10]. Through a subsequent series of experiments [11], evidence for a new oncogene, often termed "N-myc," was obtained. Independent studies directed more specifically at oncogene detection led to similar conclusions [12–14]. As expected from the initial studies on IMR-32 [10], N-myc mapped to the short arm of human chromosome 2, independent of the site(s) of its ultimate amplification [11,15,16], which could be multiple [10,17]. Studies of N-myc in primary neuroblastomas indicated that extensive ($\geqslant \times 10$) amplification was restricted to grade III or IV tumors [16,18] and associated with a poor clinical prognosis [19]. Additional studies of N-myc and related sequence amplification in neuroblastomas, retinoblastomas, (neuroectodermal) [16,20,21], and a few small cell lung tumors (which express some neuron-specific markers) [22] continue to refine conclusions about the clinical significance of such DNA amplification. DNA transfection studies [23,24] have corroborated the potential of the intact N-myc sequence to transform cells if used in conjunction with DNA from "Ras" type oncogenes.

Our generalized approach to amplified sequence analysis of the HSR of IMR-32 cells [10,11] led to additional observations, beyond the oncogene component of the amplicon, which promise to reveal general aspects of DNA amplification in malignancy. An early observation [16,25] was the existence of a nested hierarchy of DNA amplification in different primary neuroblastomas (Fig. 1). This observation has since been extended to neuroblastoma cell lines (Fig. 2) [25]. DNA segments included in these diagrams have been independently shown to hybridize with DNA in or adjacent to human chromosome 2 band p24 [15,16]. Yet, within this region, the tumor and cell line amplification data indicate a relative ordering of the DNA segments that defines central and peripheral regions of 2p24 that constitute a variably sized amplicon (Fig. 3). Given the approximate size of band 2p24, ie, 5,000–10,000 kilobases (kb), the lack of molecular proximity, detectable by DNA blots, among the DNA fragments described in Figures 1–3 is not surprising.

Isolation of many more amplified sequences, as well as a more global view of the amplicons to be characterized in IMR-32 and other neuroblastoma material, is clearly needed. Two relatively new approaches can provide some of the desired DNA

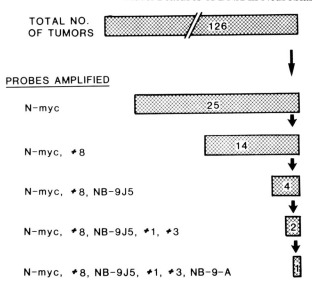

Fig. 1. Hierarchy of DNA amplification in primary neuroblastomas (updated and patterned after Figure 1 of Shiloh et al, [16].

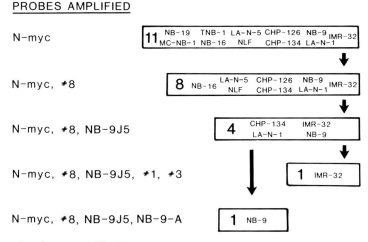

Fig. 2. Hierarchy of DNA amplification in neuroblastoma cell lines. The source of the cell lines used is given in Shiloh et al (1986) [25].

sequences. One employs the phenol-enhanced DNA reassociation technique (PERT) of Kunkel et al (1985) [27], initially used to detect DNA in chromosome deletions, to enrich for amplified DNA. Essentially, one carries out reassociation of MboI-digested DNA (eg, from IMR-32) containing amplified sequences, in the presence of sheared, normal DNA, to a point at which the amplified segments dominate the MboI-terminated duplexes, which are then cloned into pBR322. Results to date suggest that at least a fivefold enrichment can be achieved for amplified sequences in IMR-32, with more general analysis of this approach (Shiloh et al, 1987) yielding consistent results.

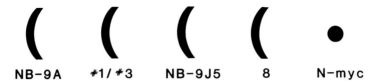

NB-9A   #1/#3   NB-9J5   8   N-myc

Fig. 3.   Mapping of DNA probes in the neuroblastoma amplicons relative to N-myc. Proposed spatial organization of the DNA fragments used in this study in normal DNA. The relative distance from N-myc (without any knowledge of lateral orientation) is determined according to the frequency with which the probe is amplified in tumors and cell lines. It can be deduced that, relative to the other probes, N-myc is the closest to the core of the amplified domain. An additional probe, pG21 [26] maps just proximal to probe 8 by this methodology.

A second approach for isolating sequences amplified in neuroblastoma tissue utilizes the in situ agarose gel renaturation technique of I. Roninson (1983) [28]. Self-reannealing of IMR-32 DNA indicates a heterogeneity in amplification extent (Fig. 4) for different Hind III-cut DNA segments, with a simple inspection suggesting that the more extensively amplified segments either obscure each other or fail to account for most of the 2,000–3,000-kb amplified unit (referred to here as amplicon) in this neuroblastoma cell line (30–40 bands $\times$ 5-kb average size; 50 fold repeat $\leqslant$ 1,000 kb). Cross-annealing studies, using DNA from IMR-32 as probe and DNA from either IMR-32 or the neuroblastoma cell line NB-19 as driver, indicate that only a fraction of the amplified DNA is common to both cell lines, a finding consistent with recent, independent observations [30]. Isolation of amplified DNA segments is in principle possible directly from such gels [32]. Alternatively, one can utilize a candidate segment as driver DNA, the tumor DNA as probe, and identify an amplified segment with minimal obscuration from nonspecific sequence repeats (Fig. 5). Both of these approaches, augmented by chromosome 1 and 2-specific recombinant DNA libraries produced from flow-sorted metaphase chromosomes, should soon permit isolation of many more amplified DNA sequences from IMR-32 and other neuroectodermal tumor cell lines or tumors. Ordering of the small DNA segments within the amplicon could then conceivably be accomplished using pulse gel electrophoresis [eg, 33] to isolate very large, overlapping DNA fragments in agarose gels for probing with the many smaller DNA fragments.

Even at the current stage of amplified DNA segment isolation from IMR-32 cells and related neuroectodermal tissue, two interesting new phenomena have been discovered. The first is a long-range DNA splicing, into the amplified segment of IMR-32, of DNA segments widely separated on the short arm of human chromosome 2 (Fig. 6). Evidence for the separation of the DNA on 2p includes in situ hybridization, hybrid cell mapping, and quantitative DNA blotting [16]. DNA linkage data, using restriction-fragment-length polymorphisms for the segments involved [eg, 34], should complement and refine these studies, positioning DNA segments along the short arm of chromosome 2. The generality of this DNA splicing, associated with DNA amplification and relocation, remains to be established.

Another interesting preliminary finding is the likely retention of an unamplified DNA segment on chromosome 2. This conclusion has thus far been based on indirect observations, via in situ hybridization (unpublished data) on IMR-32 or by DNA dosage blotting of the unrearranged and unamplified DNA comlementary to IMR-32 probe 8 in NB-9 DNA (Harris et al, unpublished data). Experiments to cross-check

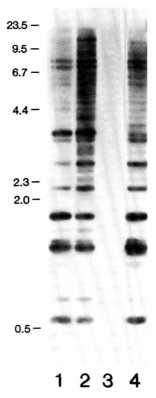

Fig. 4. Use of Roninson (1983) [28] in situ reassociation gels to demonstrate the spectrum and variability of DNA amplification in neuroblastoma cell lines IMR-32 and NB-19. The probe in all cases was ^{32}p end-labeled Hind III-cleaved IMR-32 DNA, 2×10^6 cpm (4.7×10^7 cpm/μg). The driver DNA was 15 μg of Hind III-digested nuclear DNA per lane: **(1)** 46,XY; **(2)** IMR-32; **(3)** nothing; **(4)** NB-19. Constant bands in lanes 1, 2, and 4 are at 9.5, 5.5, and 1 kb (probably traces of mitochondrial DNA) and a 1.9 kb Hind III satellite DNA [29]. One can resolve some 30–40 bands of average size near 10 kb in lane 2 and somewhat fewer in lane 4. Some are common to both lanes; some are unique. Even without densitometry, the unequal intensity (and hence differential amplification) of various bands is clearly apparent.

this finding by metaphase chromosome sorting using material from a cell line in which the HSR-containing chromosomes, can be separated from the apparently normal No. 2 chromosome and DNA from each checked DNA sequence content by Southern (1975) [29] blotting are possible. In view of additional constraints—eg, that the amplified DNA sequences, when relocated, are not always changed in size and are not always transcribed—simple mechanisms may not be sufficient to account for the DNA amplification-relocation process. One alternative, involving mobile extra-chromosomal elements [eg, 35], is theoretically possible but potentially difficult to establish definitively, especially if it occurred in the past and is no longer active.

An equally interesting observation is the complexity involved in some of the DNA rearrangement events. One of particular interest is that associated with ampli-fication of one unusual DNA segment, probe 8 (the eighth-largest segment initially isolated from the HSR of IMR-32 [10]). Early studies [11] indicated that DNA homologous to probe 8 was rearranged prior to amplification in neuroblastoma NB-9 DNA (Fig. 7). DNA restriction mapping had suggested that this rearrangement was

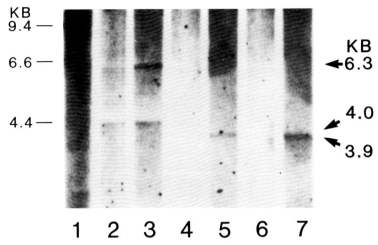

Fig. 5. Identification of additional DNA sequences amplified in IMR-32 using Roninson (1983) [28] in situ DNA reassociation gels. Tracer DNA was end-labeled with ^{32}P (approximately 5 × 10^7 cpm/μg) after Hind III digestion. In **lanes 1, 3, 5,** and **7** this was IMR-32 DNA; in lanes **2, 4, 6** this was 46,XY DNA. 10^6 cpm per lane was used. Driver DNA was 50-ng insert in plasmid pBR322 (lanes 2,3) or in Charon 21A phage (lanes 4-7) digested with Hind III. Lane 1 contained no driver DNA. Probe IMR-32 [10] was used as a control in lanes 2 and 3; on standard Southern (1975) [31] blots this gives a very high background. The 6.3-kb band is more intense in lane 3 than lane 2, indicating its amplification. Bands of equal intensity are also seen in lanes 2 and 3 at the site expected for pBR322. Background at higher MW (lanes 4-7) is probably due to phage arms. Two new amplified inserts (#14, 4.0 kb) and (#15, 3.9 kb) are evident in lanes 4, 5 and 6, 7, respectively. Unlike previous studies of Kanda et al [10], no effort was made to preselect against phage containing AluI sequences that would have obscured a Southern blot.

a simple recombinational event (Fig. 8), not unlike that envisioned for sister chromatid exchange [36–41]. However, isolation and use of DNA probes close to the presumed rearrangement point with restriction endonuclease digests of 46,XY DNA indicated an unexpected complexity in the hybridization pattern (Fig. 9). By multiple use of the same blots with different probes, it could be excluded that incomplete DNA digestion was responsible for this complexity. These observations prompted a DNA sequence analysis (Sakai et al, preliminary data) using M13-dideoxynucleotide methodology [42,43] across this region in NB-9, which revealed the interposition of a 155-base pair (bp) fragment, by a mechanism yet to be determined, which is not adjacent to the flanking moieties of the 3.2-kb Hind III fragment homologous to probe 8 in normal DNA (Fig. 10). Immediately evident is the complex nature of DNA rearrangement involved in this NB-9 amplification process. A plausible speculation is that DNA segments like the 155-bp fragment interposed between the larger, rearranged moieties in NB-9 DNA may play a more general role in DNA sequence rearrangements in tumors and tumor cell lines.

A further indication of the lability of DNA sequences in specific segments amplified in neuroblastomas, and perhaps other tumors, becomes evident upon examining both the detailed sequence near the probe 8 interchange point, as well as the probe 8-homologous DNA interchange point in another neuroblastoma cell line (Fig. 11). The interchange point in tumor line TNB-1 (Kanda et al, submitted), is based here on restriction fragment analysis of amplified segments, and can be considered only an approximate indication of a common DNA interchange point.

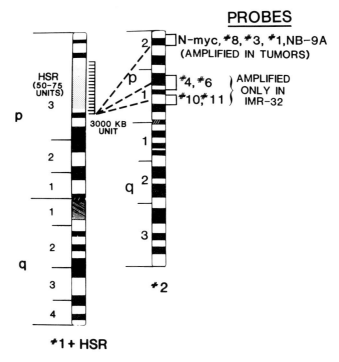

Fig. 6. A schematic showing the three different domains on human chromosome 2p, defined by different DNA probes, and the proposed assembly of sequences from these domains into one amplification unit in the HSR of IMR-32 cells [16].

Particularly interesting is the A-T-rich segment in probe 8 just adjacent to the interchange point in NB-9 DNA and quite likely in the other neuroblastoma tissues, reminiscent of sequences 5′ to some known genes (eg, globin) and sequences 3′ to the KpnI repeat family [45]. The DNA adjacent to the 155-bp insert in NB-9 is also very A-T rich. One testable hypothesis suggested by these observations is that the A-T-rich sequences somehow facilitate recombinational processes in human neuroblastomas. Substantiation of these preliminary observations should reveal general features of DNA rearrangement that may well prove to be of general relevance for DNA amplification and chromosome reorganization in malignancy [46]. Recent observations [eg, 47] of increased rates of chromosomal evolution in malignant versus nonmalignant cells could somehow relate to these observations. Fundamental in all of these questions, of course, is whether the tumorigenicity predisposes to chromosomal fluidity, whether chromosomal evolution triggers neoplastic behavior, or whether both are correct and either event triggers an accelerating cascade of events resulting in increased malignant behavior. Identification of putative signal sequences and rearrangement splice sequences, which in turn can be used to assay for proteins, eg, topoisomerase II, [48,49] mediating DNA interchange and chromosome structural change constitute one set of observables by which this complex chain of events might be dissected.

ACKNOWLEDGMENTS

The advice of Dr. Igor Roninson in adapting in situ gel renaturation technology, Dr. Ulrich Mueller and Dr. Phillipe Gros in using this technology for identifying

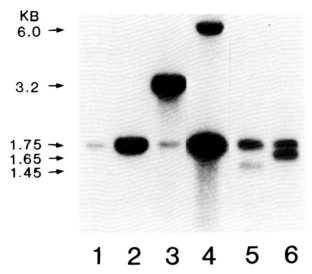

Fig. 7. Blot showing rearrangements detected by IMR-32 probe 8 in Hind III-digested DNA from different neuroblastoma cell lines and in a primary neuroblastoma. Two micrograms of Hind III-digested DNA from 46,XY (lane 1), IMR-32 (lane 2), NB-9 (lane 3), neuroblastoma 86 (lane 4),CHP-126 (lane 5), and TNB-1 (lane 6) were electrophoresed in 0.8% agarose gels. The Southern [29] blot was probed with IMR-32 probe 8 [10]. In addition to the single copy (lanes 1,3) or amplified (other lanes) 1.75-kb bands, the 3.2-kb amplified band in NB-9 (lane 3), 6-kb in neuroblastoma 86 (lane 4), 1.45-kb (lane 5), and 1.65-kb (lane 6) bands are evident.

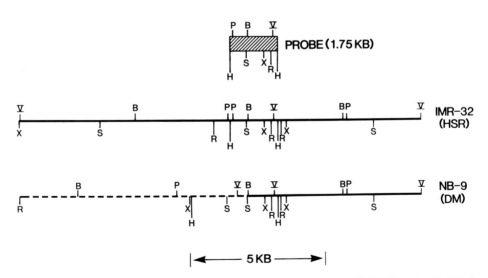

Fig. 8. Resolution at restriction map level of rearrangement involving part of IMR-32 probe 8 in NB-9 DNA. Comparison of DNA restriction maps of the region amplified in IMR-32 and NB-9 cells and exhibiting sequence homology to probe 8 isolated by Kanda et al [10] from the HSR of IMR-32 cells. Restriction enzyme abbreviations: H3, Hind III; B, BamHI; RI, EcoRI; RV, EcoRV; S, SacI. The heavy line in the IMR-32 and NB-9 maps indicates the extent of homology between the amplified sequences in the corresponding genomic DNA apparent by the restriction mapping utilized. The thin lines to the left represent DNA regions outside of this domain of apparent homology [11].

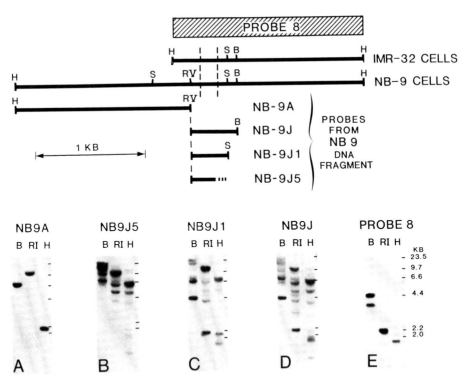

Fig. 9. Complexity of NB-9 rearrangement of IMR-32 probe 8 revealed by DNA blots using probes progressively closer to the putative DNA rearrangement point. Three micrograms of 46,XY genomic DNA digested with BamHI **(B)**, EcoRI **(RI)** or Hind III **(H)** were electrophoresed in 0.8% agarose gels and blotted onto nitrocellulose. Probes NB-9A **(A)** and IMR-32 8 **(E)** define opposite ends of the 3.2-kb probe 8 homologous fragment amplified in NB-9 cells. Probes NB9J, NB9J1, and NB9J5, covering progressively smaller segments of the junctional region adjacent to probe 8 homology, show first **(lanes D,C)** increasing complexity and then **(lane E)**, once probe 8 homology is gone, a new pattern.

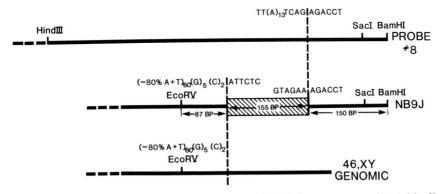

Fig. 10. Partial DNA sequence revealing 155-bp insert making NB-9 rearrangement detected by IMR-32 probe 8 at least a three-way splice [44]. Identification of a 155-base pair insert at the junction between DNA homologous to probe 8 which is amplified in NB-9 DNA and flanking DNA amplified in NB-9 cells but not IMR-32 cells. A description is also given of the DNA sequence bordering the sites at which the DNA segments flanking this insert are spliced, as well as the first few base pairs inside of the inserted segment (Sakai et al. preliminary data).

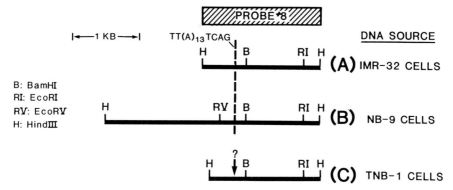

Fig. 11. Current low-resolution DNA restriction map diagram suggestive of a common point on IMR-32 probe 8 or DNA rearrangement in different human neuroblastoma cell lines. Results were obtained from amplified DNA digested with BamHI (B), EcoRI (E), or Hind III (H). Current experiments, on cloned variant-sized fragments, continue to be performed in greater detail. As evidenced by the arrows, and consistent (for TNB-1) with unpublished data of Kanda et al (to be submitted), the interchange point may be at or near the same location on probe 8 in all DNA sources shown.

amplified DNA segments, and Dr. Louis Kunkel in adapting phenol-accelerated DNA reassociation is greatly appreciated, as is the continuing interaction with Drs. Fred Alt and Nancy Kohl. This study was supported by grant CD-36 from the American Cancer Society (S.A.L.), and grants HD18526 (S.A.L.), GM21121/33579 (S.A.L.), CA22794 (R.C.S.), and CA39771 (G.M.B.), CA01027 (G.M.B.), CA27678 (R.C.S.) from the N.I.H. Yosef Shiloh was a Chaim Weizmann postdoctoral fellow.

REFERENCES

1. Biedler JL, Spengler BA: Science 191:185, 1976.
2. Balaban-Malenbaum G, Gilbert F: Science 198:739, 1977.
3. Alt FW, Kellems RE, Bertino JR, Schimke RT: J Biol Chem 253:1357, 1978.
4. Barker PE, Hsu TC: J Natl Cancer Inst 62:257, 1979.
5. Schimke RT (ed): "Gene Amplification." Cold Spring Harbor: Cold Spring Harbor Laboratory, 1982, p 339.
6. Hamlin JL, Milbrandt JD, Heintz NH, Azizkhan JC: Int Rev Cytol 90:31, 1984.
7. Stark GR, Wahl GM: Annu Rev Biochem 53:447, 1984.
8. Tumilowicz JJ, Nichols WW, Cholon JJ, Greene AE: Cancer Res 30:2110, 1970.
9. Latt SA, Alt FA, Schreck RR, Kanda N, Baltimore D: In Schimke RT (ed): "Gene Amplification." Cold Spring Harbor: Cold Spring Harbor Laboratory, 1982, pp 283–289.
10. Kanda N, Schreck R, Alt F, Bruns G, Baltimore D, Latt S: Proc Natl Acad Sci USA 80:4069, 1983.
11. Kohl NE, Kanda N, Schreck RR, Bruns G, Latt SA, Gilbert F, Alt FW: Cell 35:359, 1983.
12. Schwab M, Alitalo K, Klempanuer K-H, Varmus H, Bishop JM, Gilbert F, Brodeur G, Goldstein M, Trent J: Nature 305:245, 1983.
13. Montgomery KT, Biedler JL, Spengler BA, Melera PW: Proc Natl Acad Sci USA 80:5724, 1983.
14. Michitsch RW, Montgomery KT, Melera PW: Mol Cell Biol 4:2370, 1984.
15. Schwab M, Varmus HE, Bishop JM, Greschik K-H, Naylor SL, Sakaguchi AY, Brodeur G, Trent J: Nature 308: 288, 1984a.
16. Shiloh Y, Shipley J, Brodeur GM, Bruns G, Korf B, Donlon T, Schreck RR, Seeger R, Sakai K, Latt SA: Proc Natl Acad Sci USA 82:3761, 1985.
17. Emanuel BS, Balaban G, Boyd JP, Grossman A, Negishi M, Parmiter A, Glick MC: Proc Natl Acad Sci USA 82:3736, 1985.
18. Brodeur GM, Seeger RC, Schwab M, Varmus HE, Bishop JM: Science 224:1121, 1984.
19. Seeger RC, Brodeur GM, Sather H, Dalton A, Siegel SE, Wong KY, Hammond D: N Engl J Med 313:1111, 1985.

20. Lee W-H, Murphree AL, Benedict WF: Nature 309:458, 1984.
21. Sakai K, Kanda N, Shiloh Y, Donlon T, Schreck R, Shipley J, Dryja T, Chaum E, Chaganti RSK, Latt S: Cancer Genet Cytogenet 17:95, 1985.
22. Nau NM, Carney DW, Johnson JB, Little C, Gozdan A, Minna JD: Curr Top Microbiol Immunol 113:172, 1984.
23. Schwab M, Ellison J, Busch M, Rosenau W, Varmus HE, Bishop JM: Proc Natl Acad Sci USA 81:4940, 1984b.
24. Yancopoulos GD, Nisen PD, Tesfaye A, Kohl NE, Goldfarb MP, Alt FW: Proc Natl Acad Sci USA 83:1827, 1986.
25. Shiloh Y, Korf B, Kohl NE, Sakai K, Brodeur GM, Harris P, Kanda N, Seeger RC, Alt F, Latt SA: Cancer Res 46:5297, 1986.
26. Kohl NE, Gee CE, Alt FWT: Science 226:1335, 1984.
27. Kunkel LM, Monaco AP, Middlesworth W, Ochs H, Francke U, Latt SA: Proc Natl Acad Sci USA 82:4778, 1985.
27a. Shiloh Y, Rose E, Colletti-Feener C, Korf B, Kunkel LM, Latt SA: Gene 51:53, 1986.
28. Roninson IB: Nucleic Acids Res 11:5413, 1983.
29. Manuelidis L, Bird PA: Nucleic Acids Res 10:3221, 1982.
30. Nakatani H, Tahara E, Sakamoto H, Terada M, Sugimura T: Biochem Biophys Res Commun 130:508, 1985.
31. Southern EM: J Mol Biol 98:503, 1975.
32. Roninson IB, Abelson HT, Housman DE, Howell N, Varshavsky A: Nature 309:636, 1984.
33. Schwartz DC, Cantor CR: Cell 37:67, 1984.
34. Shiloh Y, Kanda N, Kunkel LM, Bruns G, Sakai K, Latt SA: Nucleic Acids Res 13:5403, 1985.
35. Shapiro J (ed): "Mobile Genetic Elements." New York: Academic Press, 1983, 688 p.
36. Taylor JH, Woods PS, Hughes WL: Proc Natl Acad Sci USA 43:1, 1957.
37. Latt SA: Proc Natl Acad Sci USA 70:3395, 1973.
38. Latt SA: Proc Natl Acad Sci USA 71:3162, 1974a.
39. Latt SA: Science 185:74, 1974b.
40. Latt SA: Annu Rev Genet 15:11, 1981.
41. Latt SA, Schreck RR, D'Andrea A, Kaiser TN, Schlesinger F, Lester S, Sakai K: In Tice RR, Hollaender A (eds): "Sister Chromatid Exchanges: 25 Years of Experimental Research." New York: Plenum Press, 1984, p 11.
42. Messing J, Gronenborn B, Muller-Hill B, Hofschneider PH: Proc Natl Acad Sci USA 74:3642, 1977.
43. Sanger F, Nicklen S, Coulson AR: Proc Natl Acad Sci USA 74:5463, 1977.
44. Latt SA, Shiloh Y, Sakai K, Brodeur G, Donlon T, Korf B, Shipley J, Bruns G, Heartlein M, Kanda N, Kohl N, Alt F, Seeger R: In Ramel C, Lambert B, Magnusson J (eds): "Genetic Toxicology of Environmental Chemicals, Part A: Basic Principles and Mechanisms of Action." New York: Alan R. Liss, Inc., 1986, p 601.
45. Grimaldi G, Skowronski J, Singer MF: EMBOJ 3:1753, 1984.
46. Klein G, Klein E: Nature 315:190, 1985.
47. Sager R, Gadi IK, Stephens L, Grabowy CT: Proc Natl Acad Sci USA 82:7015, 1985.
48. Wang JC: Annu Rev Biochem 54:665, 1985.
49. Pommier Y, Zwelling LA, Chien-Song K-S, Whang-Peng J, Bradley MO: Cancer Res 45:3143, 1985.

Cellular and Molecular Biology of Tumors and Potential
Clinical Applications 179–183 (1988)

Augmented Expression of Epidermal Growth Factor Receptor in Human Pancreatic Carcinoma Cells Exhibiting Alterations of Chromosome 7

Paul S. Meltzer, Jeffrey M. Trent, and Murray Korc

*Departments of Pediatrics (P.S.M.), Radiation Oncology (J.M.T.) and Internal Medicine,
(M.K.), University of Arizona, Tucson, Arizona 85724*

The gene encoding the epidermal growth factor (EGFR) is located on the short arm of human chromosome 7. We have examined the relationship of alterations of chromosome 7 to EGFR levels in four human pancreatic carcinoma cell lines. Saturation binding studies with ^{125}I-EGF demonstrated enhanced numbers of EGFR in all four cell lines. Numerical or structural abnormalities of chromosome 7 were found in each cell line. No EGFR gene amplification was observed. Our results suggest a possible relationship between alterations of chromosome 7 and EGFR levels in pancreatic carcinoma.

Key words: oncogenes, cytogenetics, tyrosine kinase

As the relationship of growth factors to the control of normal cellular proliferation has been elucidated, it has become of increasing interest to investigate these cellular regulatory systems in cancer cells [1]. The observation of structural homologies among growth factors, growth factor receptors, and retroviral oncogenes has lent considerable impetus to these investigations. Epidermal growth factor (EGF) and its receptor (EGFR) have been well characterized and provide a particularly suitable system for study [2]. EGFR signal transduction is most likely related to its intrinsic tyrosine kinase activity, and it is of interest that the EGFR kinase domain is highly homologous to the v-*erb* B oncogene [3]. High levels of EGFR expression have been reported in several tumor types, including breast cancer [4], melanoma [5], squamous cell lung cancer [6], brain tumors [7], and epidermoid carcinoma [8]. However, levels of EGFR have varied widely both within and between tumor types studied. In order to clarify the role of EGFR in cancer it will be important to determine the factors which account for this variability.

In this report, we examine the relationship of chromosomal alterations to EGFR levels in four human pancreatic carcinoma cell lines. Studies using the cloned EGFR

Received April 17, 1986.

cDNA have localized the EGFR gene to the short arm of human chromosome 7 [8]. Structural anomalies of chromosome 7 and EGFR gene amplification have been related to EGFR overexpression in the epidermoid carcinoma cell line A-431 [8]. Recently, it has also been suggested that augmented EGFR expression in melanoma is the consequence of numeric changes in chromosome 7 [5]. Although underlying mechanisms controlling the growth of pancreatic cancer are poorly understood, it is recognized that EGF exerts a trophic effect on normal pancreatic cells, and these cells are known to display EGFR [9]. We therefore sought to establish whether a relationship exists between aberrations of chromosome 7 and levels of EGFR expression in pancreatic carcinoma.

MATERIALS AND METHODS
Cell Culture

Cells were propogated as previously described [10].

Chromosomal Analysis

G- and Q- banded karyotypes of PANC-1, T_3M_4, and UACC-462 were performed as previously described [11].

EGF Binding Studies

EGF binding at 4° C was carried out using iodinated purified mouse EGF [10]. Scatchard analysis [12] of saturation data was used to determine the number of binding sites per cell.

Blot Hybridization

DNA was extracted from UACC 462, T_3M_4, PANC-1, and A-431 cells, digested with Eco RI; size fractionated on agarose gels; and blotted onto nylon membranes [10]. Blots were probed with pHEB [13] a human genomic clone isolated on the basis of homology to v-erbB.

RESULTS

All four pancreatic carcinoma cell lines demonstrated abnormalities of chromosome 7. These included both numeric and structural alterations. UACC 462 had a modal chromosome number of 54 and contained five copies of a normal chromosome 7. PANC-1 had a modal number of 58 and contained a deleted chromosome 7 (del(7)(p 15)) and four unaltered copies of chromosome 7 (Fig. 1) T_3M_4 had a modal number of 56 and carried two copies of a normal chromosome 7 and two abnormal derivatives of chromosome 7 [rcpt(7:7)(p11;q11.2)]. COLO 357 has been previously reported [14] to have a modal number of 53 and carry one normal chromosome 7 and two abnormal derivatives of chromosome 7 [iso(7p) and t(7;10)(p15;q11)].

Scatchard analysis of EGF binding data demonstrated a single order of binding sites and the following number of binding sites per cell: UACC 462, 8.5×10^4; PANC-1, 4.0×10^5; T_3M_4, 1.2×10^6; and COLO 357, 2.5×10^5.

Determination of EGFR gene copy number by Southern blot hybridization did not demonstrate EGFR gene amplification in any of the pancreatic carcinoma cell lines studied (Fig. 2).

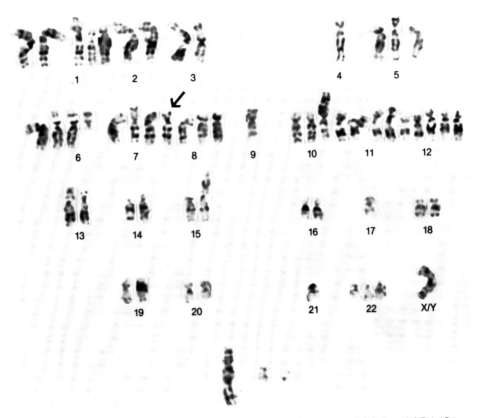

Fig. 1.   G-banded karyotype of PANC-1. Arrow denotes chromosome 7 deletion (del(7)(p15)).

DISCUSSION

Normal rat pancreatic cells display 20,000 EGF receptors on their surface [9]. All four pancreatic carcinoma cell lines studied exhibited considerably higher than normal numbers of EGFR, and it is important to determine the cellular mechanisms which result in EGFR overexpression. In A-431 cells, gene amplification has been implicated as a mechanism of increased EGFR gene expression [8]. However, none of the four pancreatic carcinoma cell lines studied demonstrated significant EGFR gene amplification. EGFR biosynthesis and turnover are complex processes, and high levels of EGFR would be expected from alterations at several points in this process. Nonetheless, the presence of abnormalities of chromosome 7 in all four pancreatic carcinoma cell lines studied raises the possibility of a relation between these altera-tions and increased EGFR gene expression. Our interest in this hypothesis has been heightened by RNA dot blot analysis, which has shown that EGFR mRNA levels correlate with EGFR number in these cell lines [10]. The chromosomal locus of the EGFR gene has been regionally assigned to chromosome 7p12-14 by in situ hybrid-ization [8]. This region is in close proximity to the chromosome 7 breakpoints demonstrated in PANC-1, T_3M_4, and COLO 357. In this connection, it is of interest that UACC 462, the cell line which demonstrated the lowest level of EGFR expression displayed only numerical alterations of chromosome 7. It is possible that chromosomal

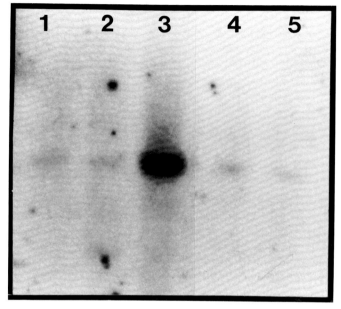

Fig. 2. Southern blot demonstrating lack of amplification of the EGFR gene in PANC-1, UACC 462, and T_3M_4 in contrast to A 431. Genomic DNA was digested with Eco RI. **Lanes 1–5** are normal lymphocytes, PANC-1, A-431, UACC 462, and T_3M_4, respectively.

rearrangement may be responsible for increased EGFR gene activity in the cell lines with the highest levels of EGFR expression. Present efforts are directed at detecting rearrangement of the EGFR gene by using gene terminal probes in combination with a variety of restriction endonucleases. Additionally, alterations in the EGFR transcript are being sought by Northern blot analysis. We anticipate that these studies will clarify the relationship of chromosome 7 alterations to EGF expression in pancreatic cancer.

ACKNOWLEDGMENTS

This work was supported in part by National Institutes of Health grants CA-29476 (J.M.T.) and CA-40162 (M.K.) Jeffrey Trent is a Scholar of the Leukemia Society of America.

REFERENCES

1. Goustin AS, Leof EB, Shipley GD, Moses HL: Cancer Res 46:1015, 1986.
2. Stoschek CM, King LE: Cancer Res 46:1030, 1986.
3. Downward J, Yarden Y, Mayes E, Scrace JG, Totty N, Stockwell P, Ullrich A, Schlessinger J, Waterfield M: Nature 307:521, 1984.
4. Hendler FJ, Ozanne BW: J Clin Invest 74:647, 1984.
5. Koprowski H, Herlyn M, Balaban G, Parmitter A, Ross A, Nowell P: Somatic Cell Mol Genet 11:297, 1985.
6. Fitzpatrick SL, LaChance MP, Schulz GS: Cancer Res 44:3442, 1984.
7. Liebermann TA, Bartal AD, Yarden Y, Schlessinger J, Soreq H: Cancer Res 44:753, 1984.
8. Merlino GT, Ishii S, Whang-Peng J, Knutsen T, Xu Y-H, Clark AJ, Stratton RH, Wilson RK, Ma DP, Roe BA, Hunts JH, Shimizu N, Pastan I: Mol Cell Biol 5:1722, 1985.

9. Korc M, Matrisian LM, Planck SR, Magun BM: Biochem Biophys Res Commun 111:1066, 1983.

10. Korc M, Meltzer P, Trent JM: Proc Natl Acad Sci USA 83:5141, 1986.

11. Trent JM: In Salmon SE (ed): "Cloning of Human Tumor Cells." New York: Alan R. Liss, Inc., 1980, p 345.

12. Scatchard G: Ann NY Acad Sci 51:660, 1949.

13. Spurr NK, Solomon E, Jannsson M, Sheer D, Goodfellow PW, Bodmer WF, Vennstrom B: EMBO J 3:159, 1984.

14. Morgan I, Woods RT, Moore, GE, Quinn LA, Gordon SG: Int J Cancer 25:591, 1980.

Cellular and Molecular Biology of Tumors and Potential
Clinical Applications 185–190 (1988)

Workshop on Chromosome Abnormalities in Cancer

Jeffrey M. Trent

*University of Arizona College of Medicine, Department of Radiation Oncology and Internal
Medicine, Cancer Center Division, Tucson Arizona 85724*

The study of chromosomal abnormalities in cancer has undergone a revolutionary change during the past five years. The emphasis has now shifted from largely descriptive studies intent upon cataloging abnormalities common to specific tumors to the study of the actual molecular events associated with chromosomal change. The Workshop[1] presentations and discussions strongly reflected this transition toward molecular analysis of chromosome change. However, it was also evident that acquiring a data base of karyotypic information on specific tumors was also of great importance and, in fact, provided information on where to commence molecular investigation. In this context, the Workshop can be divided into three major areas: 1) Primary Chromosome Alterations in Human and Experimental Cancers (F. Mitelman, C. Turc-Carel, J. Siegfried, C. Conti, and R. Muschel); 2) Molecular/Cytogenetic Analysis of Specific Chromosomal Abnormalities (G. Grosveld, C. Westbrook, B. Emanuel, J. Squire, and P. Meltzer); and 3) Cytogenetic and Molecular Biologic Examination of Amplified Cellular Genes (P. Borst, K. Alitalo, and J. Levan).

Key words: gene amplification, translocations

PRIMARY CHROMOSOME ALTERATIONS IN HUMAN AND EXPERIMENTAL CANCERS

The first area discussed at the Workshop was an update by Dr. F. Mitelman (Abst. A102) of data included within the Catalog of Chromosome Alterations in Cancer [1]. In a survey of all published cases, 610 neoplasms were reported as having only a single numeric or structural chromosome abnormality. Two major points were brought out in regards to these cancers: 1) loss or gain of chromosomes was nonrandom (with chromosomes 8, 9, 12, and 21 preferentially gained, while 7, 22, and Y were preferentially lost); and 2) structural alterations were also nonrandomly distrib-

Received March 19, 1986.

[1]A complete list of workshop participants is presented in the Appendix.

uted throughout the genome (with 97% of all neoplasms having at least 1 of 83 different bands involved in structural change). In *a presentation adding additional evidence for nonrandom chromosome change*, Turc-Carel et al (Abst. A112) discussed the interesting finding of a recurring chromosomal abnormality in a benign tumor. These data, when combined with the presentation of Siegfried et al (Abst. A111) and the molecular cytogenetic results described within the next section, strongly point to a restricted number of "cancer-associated" chromosomal regions. These results further suggest that identification of additional cancer genes is probable in the future.

A second very interesting area of discussion is related to cytogenetic evaluation of two experimental models of carcinogenesis. Interestingly, the results of the two different models lead apparently to opposite conclusions. Conti et al (Abst. A79) discussed a mouse skin model, where administration of a "two-stage" chemical carcinogen protocol (DMBA followed by TPA) led to progression over time from papillomas through metastatic squamous cell carcinoma. The results presented clearly documented that benign tumors from the earliest stages contained a high level of chromosome instability, which progressed significantly with overt development of tumors. These results contrasted sharply with the work of Muschel et al (Abst. A104), who investigated the karyotypic profile of early passage rodent cells transfected with the ras^H oncogene. Transfected cells were clearly malignant, including possessing the property of spontaneous metastasis. However, when the karyotype of the original transfected clones (or cells taken from metastatic foci) were examined, no karyotypic alterations (or only single numeric changes) were observed. The conclusion drawn by these investigators was that karyotypic alterations are probably not essential for metastatic (malignant?) behavior.

While there was insufficient time for detailed discussion of either study, the reported differences between these studies may be more apparent than real. For example, the mouse skin model is an in vivo carcinogen-generated tumor model which takes 10 wk postexposure to document evaluable papillomas (and often significantly longer [>40 wks] for animals to develop overt carcinoma). This amount of time and the carcinogen-host-tumor relationship obviously differs significantly from the rapid in vitro transformation of early passage rat embryo cells which have been transfected by an efficient transforming gene (ras^H). In summary, both methods differ so radically as to preclude direct comparison. However, both may ultimately be useful in providing insight into the possible role of chromosome alterations in the genesis of malignant (or metastic) change.

MOLECULAR/CYTOGENETIC ANALYSIS OF SPECIFIC CHROMOSOMAL ABNORMALITIES

The second major area discussed at the workshop was the molecular/cytogenetic examination of the specific breakpoint regions involved in various human cancers. The presentation of Squire et al (Abst. A113) characterized a gene (esterase D) closely linked to the loci on chromosome 13 which is known to be associated with retinoblastoma. Isolation and characterization of this sequence may be of importance in further molecular investigations of the retinoblastoma loci. The remaining studies dealt with specific malignancies, with the most fully defined system being presented by Grosveld et al (Abst. A85), describing the involvement of the c-abl oncogene in the 9;22 translocation characterizing chronic myelogenous leukemia (CML). This presentation updated the available information on cloning analysis of breakpoints fragments on both chromosomes 9 and 22. Of interest, all the breakpoints on chromosome 22 clustered to a very limited area (termed bcr), while breakpoints on chromosome 9 were scattered over a very large area (100 kilobases [kb]) upstream of the v-abl homologous sequences of the c-abl gene. Of great interest, despite the distance between the two genes on the ph[1] chromosome, cimeric mRNA linking these two genes has been recognized and attributed to RNA splicing across this considerable distance.

A second study was presented examining the possibility that c-abl was also implicated in acute leukemia, specifically those displaying a relatively common translocation involving chromosome 6 and 9 (where the breakpoint on 9 appears to involve the same region cytologically as that altered in CML). Westbrook et al (Abst. A163) presented evidence that in contrast to the translocation of c-abl in CML, results of in situ hybridization suggested that breakpoints along the t(6;9) were significantly 3' of the c-abl gene (> 18 kb as defined by Southern blotting). Also, preliminary data suggested the size and abundance of the c-abl protein was unchanged in this subset of acute leukemias (again in direct contrast to CML). Efforts to identify the sequence(s) associated with the breakpoints of t(6;9) leukemias are just underway. A study with similar intent was presented by B. Emanuel and colleagues (Abst. A84), who hoped to define the possible role of alteration of the c-ets gene (which resides on chromosome 11) and the immunoglobulin lambda light chain loci (located on chromosome 22) in the 11;22 translocations characteristic of both Ewing's sarcoma (ES) and peripheral neuroephithelioma (NE). Although it was of interest that differences between translocation breakpoint sites were observed for ES vs NE (as recognized by in situ hybridization), no firm conclusions regarding a clear-cut role for either sequence could be made from this current study.

Finally, Meltzer et al (Abst. A100) described the recent finding of alterations in the expression of the epidermal growth factor receptor gene (EGFR) in human pancreatic carcinomas. Overexpression of EGFR has previously been reported as a common feature of both squamous cell and breast carcinomas, with the most common mechanism for overexpression being amplification of the EGFR gene (which is homologous to the c-erbB oncogene). One aspect of significant interest in this current study related to the lack of evidence for c-erbB amplification, despite the fact that $> 10^6$ EGFR receptors per cell were observed in some pancreatic tumors. These results suggest that in pancreatic neoplasms, overexpression of EGFR is mediated by a mechanism other than amplification, possibly associated with alteration of chromosome 7p (the loci of the EGFR gene). Studies are currently underway to define the molecular alterations associated with the observed overexpression.

CYTOGENETIC AND MOLECULAR BIOLOGIC EXAMINATION OF AMPLIFIED CELLULAR GENES

The final area discussed at the Workshop involved the study of amplified DNA sequences in human cancers. Discussion began with an extremely intriguing presentation by Piet Borst (Abst. A77), which applied the procedure of pulsed field gradient (PFG) gel electrophoresis to elucidating the structure of double minute (DM) chromosomes. Basically, the PFG procedure makes use of lysed and deproteinized culture DM or homogeneously staining region (HSR)-bearing cells (isolated within an agarose block), which are then digested with various infrequently cutting restriction endonucleases, and fragments separated by alternating (orthogonal) current elecrtrophoresis. At present, this method has been successfully applied to studies of chromosomes in several lower eukaryotes, including yeast [2] and unicellular parasites like trypanosomes [3]; and ideally this method appears capable of rapidly establishing the structure and linkage relationships of large DNA fragments (ie amplicons) of up to 1,000 kb in mammalian cells. Borst and his colleagues have successfully modified this procedure to examine mammalian DNA, and have provided interesting and compelling evidence suggesting that the size of amplicons (contained within DMs or HSRs) are in fact extremely large (900->1500 kb). However, although progress has been made in estimating the size and complexity of amplification units, practical problems still exist with the usefulness of this method in determining linkage relationships between larger fragments (owing primarily to the added complexity of amplicon rearrangements, and the lack of a large number of enzymes which cut infrequently enough to generate large DNA fragments). Despite these current technical hurdles, this approach appears likely to provide valuable new insights into our understanding of the mechanisms of gene amplification.

The final two presentations focused on the molecular and cytogenetic examination of amplified cellular oncogenes in human and murine tumor cell lines. K. Alitalo (Abst. A74) described the analysis of molecular and chromosomal alterations associated with over-expression of myb and myc-family oncogenes in several neoplasms. Of particular interest was work regarding N-myc amplified neuroblastoma cell lines, and the failure of these tumors to show coordinate amplification of a gene residing near N-myc [ornithine decarboxylase]. These results may suggest a certain degree of specificity to the size of flanking regions co-amplified with N-myc. Although co-amplification of flanking genes has been recognized previously in other amplified domains (eg, rDNA/CAD amplification associated with PALA resistance [4]), there is reason to consider that such co-amplification of flanking sequences may be dependent on regional location of the sequence to be amplified [4], possibly leading to a "consistent" core unit of amplification [5].

Finally, Levan and colleagues (Abst. A97) reported on the relationship of amplification and overexpression of c-myc in SEWA tumor cells displaying varying degrees of tumorigenic potential. Although a weakly positive correlation appeared to be present between c-myc amplification and tumorigenicity, the current study failed to firmly establish a causal relationship between myc overexpression and increasing malignant potential. Examination of other genes potentially responsible for the malignant phenotype are currently underway.

CONCLUSIONS

The information presented at the Workshop, coupled with the accompanying discussions, clearly indicated a continuing role for molecular/cytogenetic investigations in the studies of human and experimental cancers. As recurring sites of chromosome change are uncovered by chromosome-banding analysis, "targeting" of molecular investigation is likely to provide important new information of relevance to the genesis and progression of neoplasia. Finally, it appears reasonable to suggest that the emphasis of current molecular/cytogenetic study will continue to shift from principally hematopoietic malignancies to more frequent investigation of common epithelial tumors (as additional recurrent sites of chromosome change are identified). Additionally, there is no question that "benign" neoplasms will be receiving significantly more study by both cytogenetic and molecular biologic techniques. The merging of the discipline of cytogenetics with "mainstream" molecular biology is providing a significant stimulus to both fields.

REFERENCES

1. Mitelman F: Cytogenet Cell Genet 36:1, 1983.
2. Trent JM, Thompson FH: Methods Enzymol (in press), 1986.
3. Schwartz DC, Cantor CR: Cell 37:67, 1984.
4. Van der Ploeg LHT: EMBO J 3:3109, 1984.
5. GM Wahl, L Vitto, J. Rubnitz: Mol Cell Biol 3:2066, 1983.
6. Kinzler KW, Zehnbauer BA, Brodeur GM, Seeger RC, Trent JM, Meltzer PS, Vogelstein B: Proc Natl Acad Sci USA 83:1031, 1986.

APPENDIX: WORKSHOP PARTICIPANTS

Felix Mitelman, MD
Professor and Head
Department of Genetics
University of Lund S-221-85
Lund, Sweden

Gerard Grosveld, PhD
Professor, Cell Biology & Genetics
Erasmus University
1738 Rotterdam 300 DR
The Netherlands

Carol Westbrook
Section Hematology/Oncology
University of Chicago
5841 S. Maryland Avenue
Box 420
Chicago, IL 60637

Beverly Emanuel, PhD
Assistant Professor
Children's Hospital of Philadelphia
34th & Civic Center Boulevard
Philadelphia, PA 19104

Paul Meltzer, MD, PhD
Department of Pediatrics
University of Arizona College of Medicine
Tucson, AZ 85724

Piet Borst, PhD
Molecular Biology
The Netherlands Cancer Institute
Plesmanlaan 121
Amsterdam 1066 CX
The Netherlands

Kari Alitalo, MD, PhD
Department of Virology
University of Helsinki
Haartmaninkatu 3
00290 29 Finland

Goran Levan, PhD
University of Goteborg
Department of Genetics
Box 33031
S-400 33 Goteborg
Sweden

Jill Siegfried
Carcinogenesis Section
Environmental Health
Research & Testing, Inc.
P.O. Box 12199
Research Triangle Park, NC 27709

Claude Turc-Carel
Department of Genetics and
Endocrinology
Roswell Park Memorial Institute
666 Elm Street
Buffalo, NY 14263

Jeremy Squire
Medical Biophysics
Ontario Cancer Institute
500 Sherbourne Street
Toronto M4X IK9

Dr. Ruth Muschel
Lab of Pathology
Building 10, Room 2A33
National Cancer Institute
9000 Rockville Pike
Bethesda, MD 20892

Claudio Conti, DVM, PhD
Science Park-Research Division
University of Texas System Cancer Center
P.O. Box 389
Smithville, TX 78957

Cellular and Molecular Biology of Tumors and Potential
Clinical Applications 191–202 (1988)

Domains of p60$^{\text{v-}src}$ Involved in Dissociable Transformation Parameters Induced by Rous Sarcoma Virus Variants

Richard Jove, Bruce J. Mayer, Ellen A. Garber, Teruko Hanafusa, and Hidesaburo Hanafusa

The Rockefeller University, New York, New York 10021

PA101 and PA104 are temperature-sensitive variants of Rous sarcoma virus that display dissociation of cell transformation parameters. Cells infected with the variants are fully transformed when maintained at 34°C, are stimulated to proliferate in the absence of morphological transformation or anchorage-independent growth at 37°C, and are indistinguishable from uninfected cells at 41°C. To investigate the basis for these dissociable transformation-related functions of p60$^{\text{v-}src}$, the PA101 and PA104 v-*src* genes and the corresponding gene products were characterized. The mutant v-*src* genes were molecularly cloned and sequenced, and chimeric genes were constructed by in vitro recombination with a wild-type v-*src* gene. Analysis of the cellular phenotypes induced by the chimeric genes revealed that lesions within the tyrosine kinase domain confer temperature sensitivity upon all of the dissociable transformation parameters. These lesions also are responsible for temperature sensitivity in the kinase activity of the mutant *src* proteins as assayed in vivo by the levels of phosphotyrosine in cellular protein p34. In addition, experiments with deletion mutants revealed that the amino-terminal third of p60$^{\text{v-}src}$, including the domain required for membrane association, is dispensable for the stimulation of cell proliferation. These results suggest that the tyrosine kinase domain is required for all of the transformation-related functions of p60$^{\text{v-}src}$, while the membrane binding domain is not.

Key words: avian tumor viruses, chondrocytes, myristylation, oncogenes, RNA tumor viruses, temperature sensitive mutants, anchorage independent growth, cell morphology, dissociation of transformation parameters, mitogenic activity, tyrosine kinase

The Rous sarcoma virus (RSV) v-*src* gene encodes a protein, p60$^{\text{v-}src}$, that induces cell transformation and tumor formation [1]. This transforming protein is a tyrosine protein kinase associated with the plasma membrane [2,3]. The carboxy-terminal half of p60$^{\text{v-}src}$ contains the tyrosine kinase catalytic domain [4–6], the activity of which correlates with transformation [7]. An amino-terminal domain composed of the first 14 residues is involved in myristic acid attachment and mem-

Received February 26, 1986.

brane association, which also correlate with transformation [8–10]. An additional amino-terminal domain has been proposed to have a modulatory function, perhaps in altering kinase activity or substrate specificity [11,12]. Putative cellular substrates for p60$^{v\text{-}src}$ have been identified [3], including a 34-kilodalton (kd) protein (p34) [13–15], although substrates causally related to transformation have not been demonstrated.

Infection of chicken cells with RSV results in stimulation of cell proliferation, morphological transformation, and anchorage-independent growth [1]. PA101 and PA104 are temperature-sensitive (ts) variants of RSV that originally were selected for the ability to stimulate cell proliferation without causing morphological transformation [16,17]. Moreover, it was shown that the induction of anchorage-independent growth is not required for the stimulation of cell proliferation [17]. Further analysis [18] revealed that the mutants are differentially ts in the various transformation parameters, which is manifest as the dissociation of these parameters as a function of temperature. Such mutants are potentially useful for discerning the contributions of p60$^{v\text{-}src}$ domains to the transformed phenotype.

In order to identify the domains that are involved in the dissociable transformation-related functions of p60$^{v\text{-}src}$, we molecularly cloned and analyzed the PA101 and PA104$^{v\text{-}src}$, genes. In addition, the roles of the tyrosine kinase activity and subcellular localization of p60$^{v\text{-}src}$ in the various transformation functions were investigated using these ts mutants and deletion mutants of a wild-type v-src gene. Our findings suggest that the tyrosine kinase activity is critical to all of the transformation parameters examined, although phosphorylation of different cellular substrates might be required for expression of the different parameters.

MATERIALS AND METHODS

Cells and Viruses

Cultures of chicken embryo fibroblasts (CEF) and neuroretina (NR) cells were prepared as previously described [19,20]. Chondrocytes were prepared essentially as described [21] except that the sterna of 17-day-old chicken embryos were used as the source of cells (Kato, unpublished). The isolation and characterization of the PA101 and PA104 variants of RSV have been reported [16,17]. The wild-type transforming virus (SRA) is derived from a molecular clone of Schmidt-Ruppin RSV subgroup A [19]. NYHB5 and NY501 are RSV variants that contain molecularly cloned c-src sequences in place of v-src [22]. Although the NYHB5 results are described here, similar results were obtained with NY501. The RSV variants that contain v-src deletions (see Fig. 6) have been described [8,11,12].

Recombinant DNA

Details of the molecular cloning and nucleotide sequence analyses of the PA101 and PA104 v-src genes will be presented elsewhere [18,23]. The recombinant plasmids constructed for this study are all derived from pSR-XD2 [19] by replacing the wild type v-src gene with the indicated src sequences (see Fig. 3). Standard recombinant DNA techniques were used for the in vitro constructions, and the structures of the recombinant plasmids were verified by restriction analysis. Infectious RSV variants were recovered by ligation of the pSR-XD2 derivatives to pSR-REP followed by transfection into CEF as previously described [19].

Protein Biochemistry

The metabolic labeling of cells with isotopes, preparation of cell lysates, and immunoprecipitations were performed essentially as described [11,24]. Antiserum raised against p60$^{v\text{-}src}$ synthesized in bacteria (anti-p60 serum) was used for the in vitro autophosphorylation assay as described [24,25]. Antiserum raised against cellular protein p34 purified from CEF (anti-p34 serum) was generously provided by M.E. Greenberg and G.M. Edelman [26]. Subcellular fractionation and glycerol gradient sedimentation analyses were performed as previously described [11]. Immunoprecipitates were resolved by electrophoresis through 10% polyacrylamide gels containing SDS, and labeled proteins were visualized by fluorography or autoradiography.

Assays of Transformation Parameters

Mitogenic activity was assayed using cultured chicken embryo chondrocytes by counting the numbers of cells at various time intervals. For the growth curves, chondrocytes were maintained in Ham's F-10 medium supplemented with 10% fetal bovine serum. Similar results were obtained using the NR cell system previously described [27]. Morphological transformation was assayed by focus formation in infected CEF cultures overlaid with agar containing Scherer's medium supplemented with 5% calf serum, 10% tryptose phosphate broth, and 1% beef embryo extract. Anchorage-independent growth was assayed by colony formation of infected CEF suspended in agar containing Dulbecco's modified Eagle medium supplemented with 10% calf serum, 10% tryptose phosphate broth, and 1% chick serum.

RESULTS
Molecular Clones of the PA101 and PA104 *src* Genes

PA101 and PA104 were previously shown to stimulate proliferation of cultured NR cells without causing morphological transformation [16,17]. To investigate the structural basis for this dissociation of transformation parameters, proviral DNA fragments containing the v-*src* genes of these variants were molecularly cloned from infected NR cells [18]. The cloned proviral fragments were then reconstructed into replication-competent viral DNA by in vitro recombination, and infectious viruses were recovered from the culture fluids of transfected CEF as previously described [19]. The NYPA101 and NYPA104 viruses thus obtained are reconstructed RSV variants containing the molecularly cloned v-*src* genes of PA101 and PA104, respectively. These viruses were used to verify the biological activity of the cloned genes.

NYPA101 and NYPA104 could stimulate proliferation of infected NR cells as effectively as the original PA isolates and the wild-type transforming virus, SRA (data not shown). Figure 1 shows that similar results could be obtained using chicken embryo chondrocytes, demonstrating that the mitogenic activity of p60$^{v\text{-}src}$ is not unique to the NR system. The chondrocyte system [21] is also a sensitive assay for mitogenic activity: the population doubling times (Fig. 1) of the infected cells are approximately one-half that of the uninfected cells (20 hr versus 40 hr). Other cellular phenotypes induced by NYPA101 or NYPA104 (Table I) are also indistinguishable from those induced by PA101 or PA104, respectively (data not shown). These results confirm that the molecularly cloned genes are representative of the original mutant genes.

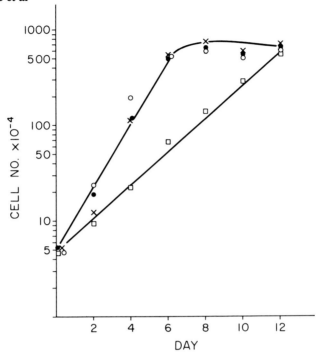

Fig. 1.   Growth curves of chicken embryo chondrocytes. Secondary cultures were infected with the indicated viruses, maintained for 1 wk to allow virus spread, and then plated on day 0 at a density of 5 × 10⁴ cells per 60-mm dish for the growth curve analysis. Culture medium was renewed daily, and cell numbers in parallel cultures were counted with a hemocytometer on the days indicated. □, mock-infected; ●, SRA-infected; ×, NYPA101-infected; ○, NYPA104-infected.

TABLE I. Cellular Phenotypes Induced by RSV Variants as a Function of Temperature

Virus	Mitogenic activity (°C)		Anchorage-independent growth (°C)			Morphological transformation (°C)		
	37	42	34	37	41	34	37	41
SRA	+	+	+	+	+	+	+	+
NYHB5	−	−	−	−	(+)[a]	−	−	−
NYPA101	+	−	+	+	−	+	(+)[b]	−
NYPA104	+	−	+	−	−	(+)[c]	−	−
NY101-SRA	+	+	+	+	+	(+)	+	(+)[d]
NY104-SRA	+	+	+	+	+	+	+	+
NYSRA-101	+	−	+	+	−	+	+	−
NYSRA-104	+	−	+	−	−	(+)[c]	−	−

[a]Experiments are under way to determine whether the colonies observed at 41° in NYHB5-infected cells are induced by variants.
[b]The transformed morphology of NYPA101-infected cells at 37°C is subtle in comparison with that of SRA-infected cells.
[c]Detection of foci at 34°C in these cultures is critically dependent on the culture conditions and varies with the embryo and the serum lot.
[d]Cells infected with NY101-SRA exhibit a fusiform morphology at all temperatures.

Infection of chondrocytes with another reconstructed RSV variant (NYHB5) that contains chicken c-src sequences in place of v-src [22] did not cause any detectable stimulation of cell proliferation (Jove and Hanafusa, unpublished results). The same result was observed in previous experiments using NR cells [25], indicating that p60^{c-src}, the cellular homologue of p60^{v-src}, does not have mitogenic activity even when it is overexpressed to high levels using the retroviral long terminal repeat (LTR) promoter. These observations are consistent with the suggestion that p60^{c-src} lacks transforming activity [22]. Moreover, the result obtained with NYHB5, which is identical in structure with NYPA101 or NYPA104 except for the src sequences, demonstrates that viral infection per se is not sufficient to stimulate cell proliferation in this system.

Genetic Analysis of the Cloned Mutant src Genes

The DNA sequences of the cloned v-src genes of PA101 and PA104 were determined and compared with that of the cloned wild-type SRA v-src gene [23,28]. The results of this analysis are summarized in Figure 2. The predicted PA104 p60 contains only two amino acid substitutions relative to the wild-type protein, both of which occur in the carboxy-terminal half. In contrast, the PA101 p60 contains a total of 19 amino acid changes relative to the SRA protein, which are scattered throughout the anino- and carboxy-terminal halves.

We wished to evaluate the respective contributions of amino-terminal and tyrosine kinase domains of these src proteins to the cellular phenotypes of cells expressing the proteins. For this purpose, chimeric genes were constructed by in vitro recombination using the cloned mutant and wild-type v-src genes [18]. This was accomplished by bisecting these genes at the Mlu I restriction site (Fig. 2) and exchanging amino- and carboxy-terminal coding halves among the various genes. The

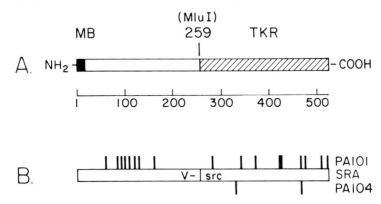

Fig. 2.   Summary of the sequence analysis of the molecularly cloned PA101 and PA104 src genes. **A:** Domains of p60^{v-src} are illustrated. The membrane binding domain (MB) is indicated by the solid box (the first 14 amino acids). The tyrosine kinase-related sequence (TKR) is represented by the hatched box (amino acids 255–516). The proposed modulatory domain is contained within the open box (including at least amino acids 81–169). The Mlu I restriction endonuclease cleavage site used for the chimeric constructs shown in Figure 3 corresponds to the codon for amino acid 259. **B:** Predicted amino acid sequences of the mutant and wild-type src proteins are compared. Amino acid substitutions in the PA101 and PA104 proteins are indicated, respectively, by the vertical lines above and below the open box representing the wild type SRA protein. Approximate positions of amino acid residues are shown on the scale.

chimeric genes were then reconstructed into replication-competent viral DNAs, and infectious viruses were recovered from transfected CEF. The designations of these viruses, and the structures of their respective *src* genes, are shown in Figure 3. With these viruses we examined the transformation phenotypes induced by the chimeric proteins in infected cells, including mitogenic activity, morphological transformation, and anchorage-independent growth.

Table I summarizes the cellular phenotypes of cells infected with the viruses and maintained at various temperatures [18]. All of the viruses, with the exception of NYHB5 discussed above, could stimulate proliferation of chondrocytes or NR cells incubated at 37°C. At 42°C, however, NYPA101 and NYPA104 exhibit temperature sensitivity in the mitogenic activity, as previously reported for PA101 and PA104 [16,17]. Furthermore, NYSRA-101 and NYSRA-104 are also ts in the mitogenic activity, whereas NY101-SRA and NY104-SRA are not (Calothy, personal communication). These results demonstrate that the ts property for stimulation of cell proliferation segregates with the carboxy terminal halves of both mutant *src* proteins.

The ability of these *src* proteins to induce morphological transformation was assessed by focus formation in infected CEF cultures (Table I). Unexpectedly, we observed that NYPA101 and NYPA104 could induce the appearance of foci in CEF maintained at 34°C. This was not anticipated from previous studies in which experiments had been conducted at temperatures above 34°C [16,17]. Therefore, the defectiveness in morphological transformation observed in cells infected with these variants is actually a manifestation of temperature sensitivity in this parameter at 37°C or 41°C. The ts property with respect to morphological transformation is also determined by the carboxy-terminal halves of the mutant *src* proteins. Although CEF infected with NYPA101 (or PA101) produce foci at 37°C, the transformed morphology of these cells is subtle in comparison with that of SRA-infected cells (data not shown). In addition, CEF infected with NY101-SRA have a fusiform morphology

PLASMID	VIRUS	SRC NH₂	COOH
pSR-XD2	SRA	V	V
pHB5	NYHB5	C	C
pXD101	NYPA101	101	101
⁾XD104	NYPA104	104	104
pXD101-SRA	NY101-SRA	101	V
pXD104-SRA	NY104-SRA	104	V
pXDSRA-101	NYSRA-101	V	101
pXDSRA-104	NYSRA-104	V	104

Fig. 3. Designations of recombinant plasmids and viruses are shown together with the structures of their corresponding *src* proteins. The vertical lines that bisect the *src* proteins into amino- (NH₂) and carboxy-terminal (COOH) halves represent amino acid 259 (see Fig. 2). All of the recombinants were derived from pSR-XD2 by substitution of the appropriate *src* sequences in vitro. The origins of the *src* sequences in the recombinants are wild-type v-*src* (V), chicken c-*src* (C), and the PA101 (101) and PA104 (104) mutant v-*src* genes. The replication-competent viruses were recovered from the culture fluids of CEF transfected with the indicated plasmid DNAs.

(data not shown), suggesting that the amino-terminal half of the NYPA101 p60 modulates expression of the transformed phenotype.

The in vitro transformation parameter that correlates most highly with tumorigenicity is anchorage-independent growth in semisolid media. The ability of the *src* proteins to stimulate colony formation by infected CEF maintained at various temperatures in soft agar was examined (Table I). As demonstrated for the mitogenic activity and morphological transformation, temperature sensitivity in anchorage-independent growth also segregates with the carboxy-terminal halves of the *src* mutants. Consistent with the colony formation data and previous tumorigenicity studies [29], NYPA101 is significantly more tumorigenic than NYPA104 in chickens (data not shown).

Table I shows that identical results were obtained with NY104-SRA or SRA and also with NYSRA-104 or NYPA104. These results are consistent with the predicted amino acid sequences of the NYPA104 and SRA p60 proteins, since both are expected to have the identical sequence in their amino-terminal halves (Fig. 2).

Biochemical Analysis of the Mutant *src* Proteins

Previous studies showed that the in vitro tyrosine kinase activities of the PA101 and PA104 p60s in immune complexes are low as measured by phosphorylation of immunoglobulin G heavy chain [27] or autophosphorylation [25]. Figure 4 shows the results obtained with an in vitro autophosphorylation assay that includes immunopre-

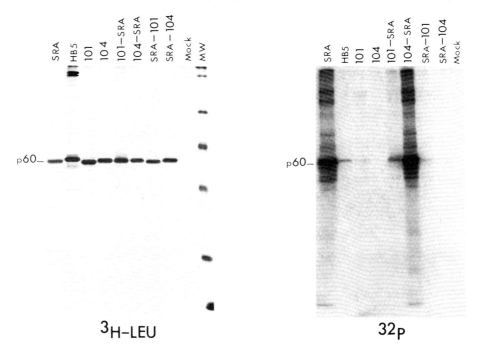

Fig. 4. In vitro kinase activity of the *src* proteins assayed by autophosphorylation in immune complexes. Infected or mock-infected CEF were metabolically labeled with [^{3}H] leucine for 4 hr and p60 proteins were immunoprecipitated from cell lysates with anti-p60 serum. One half of each immunoprecipitate was used to detect ^{3}H-labeled protein by fluorography (left panel), and the other half was used in the autophosphorylation assay with [γ^{32}P]ATP (right panel). The viruses used to infect the cells are indicated above the corresponding lanes. The molecular weight markers (MW), from top to bottom, are: 200, 97, 68, 43, and 26 kd.

cipitates from cells expressing the chimeric *src* proteins. These data demonstrate that the carboxy-terminal halves of the mutant proteins severely inhibit the autophosphorylating activity in this assay. In addition, it is evident that the amino-terminal half of the NYPA101 p60 also suppresses the kinase activity. The activity of the NY104-SRA p60 is the same as that of wild-type $p60^{v-src}$, as expected from the sequence analysis.

To investigate the in vivo kinase activities of these *src* proteins, we examined the levels of phosphotyrosine in p34 in cells infected with the variants (Fig. 5). In agreement with previous studies [27], the low levels of phosphotyrosine in p34 from cells infected with NYPA101 or NYPA104 at 37°C are abolished when these cells are shifted to 41°C. The data shown in Figure 5 demonstrate that temperature sensitivity in p34 phosphorylation segregates with the carboxy-terminal halves of the mutant *src* proteins. In addition, we examined p34 phosphorylation in infected cells incubated at 34°C [30] and found no difference between these results and those obtained with cells at 37°C, even though the cellular phenotypes are strikingly different at the two temperatures (see Table I).

It is interesting to compare the results obtained with the in vitro and in vivo kinase assays described here. The carboxy-terminal half of the NYPA101 p60 has a significantly greater inhibitory effect on autophosphorylation in vitro than on p34

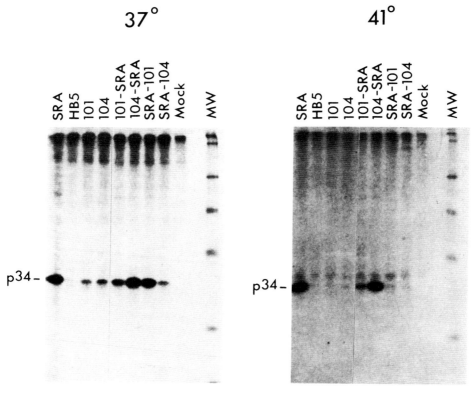

Fig. 5. Levels of cellular protein p34 phosphorylation in vivo. Infected or mock-infected CEF were metabolically labeled with $^{32}P_i$ for 4 hr, and p34 was immunoprecipitated with anti-p34 serum from cell lysates containing the same amount of radioactivity. Cell cultures were maintained at either 37°C or 41°C prior to and during the labeling. Gels were treated with 1 M KOH at 55°C for 2 hr in order to enrich for labeled phosphotyrosine in proteins. The molecular weight markers (MW) are the same shown in Figure 4, and the viruses used are indicated above the lanes.

phosphorylation in vivo at 37°C. Similarly, the amino-terminal half of the NYPA101 p60 inhibits autophosphorylation in vitro to a greater extent than p34 phosphorylation. Another difference is that while the kinase activities of both the NYPA101 and NYPA104 p60s appear to be thermolabile in vivo, only the kinase activity of the NYPA104 p60 is more thermolabile than that of wild-type p60$^{\text{v-}src}$ in vitro [27]. Moreover, in contrast to the in vitro autophosphorylation data, p60$^{\text{c-}src}$ appears to lack detectable kinase activity in vivo as assayed by p34 phosphorylation, consistent with previous results [24,25]. These apparent discrepencies between the two systems might reflect artifact, particularly in the in vitro assay, and/or the fact that different substrates are being examined.

The data discussed above indicate that the two assay systems for *src* kinase activity are not directly comparable, although the significance of the observed differences is not clear. Despite these differences, the conclusion that the kinase activities of the mutant p60s are much lower than that of wild-type p60$^{\text{v-}src}$ is further supported by other lines of evidence. The in vivo levels of phosphotyrosine in the mutant *src* proteins and in total cellular protein from cells infected with the mutants are extremely low [27] (Jove and Hanafusa, unpublished results). However, abolishment of p34 phosphorylation correlates with loss of mitogenic activity (compare Table I and Fig. 5), suggesting that retention of at least a low level of kinase activity is required for biological activity.

We also examined the subcellular distribution of the mutant *src* proteins by biochemical fractionation experiments [30]. It previously was shown that the majority of wild-type p60$^{\text{v-}src}$ in cells is plasma membrane associated [3,8]. Surprisingly, the NYPA101 and NYPA104 p60s were found to be approximately equally distributed between the membrane and soluble fractions, even though both proteins are myristylated (data not shown). Furthermore, the mutant proteins were found predominantly in fast-sedimenting complexes with cellular proteins p50 and p90 [30]. Analysis of the chimeric *src* proteins revealed that subcellular fractionation and complex formation segregate with the carboxy-terminal halves of the mutants (data not shown). However, since these properties do not detectably change as a function of temperature (from 34°C to 41°C), they evidently do not correlate with any specific cellular phenotypes [30].

Mitogenic Activity of *src* Deletion Mutants

Previous studies [8] have shown that deletions spanning the first 14 amino-terminal residues of p60$^{\text{v-}src}$ abolish myristylation, membrane association, and transformation but not kinase activity (Fig. 6). Deletion of amino acids 169 to 264 also abolishes transformation and, in addition, severely reduces kinase activity [12]. Analysis of other deletion mutants revealed that amino acids located between positions 81 and 169 are required for morphological transformation but not for anchorage-independent growth [12].

We were interested in the mitogenic activity of these *src* deletion mutants and therefore examined their capacities to stimulate proliferation of chicken embryo chondrocytes. As shown in Figure 6, all but one of the mutants retains mitogenic activity in the chondrocyte system. Of particular interest are the results obtained with the NY314 and NY315 variants, which encode soluble non-myristylated *src* proteins that are defective in all other transformation parameters examined [8]. The cellular phenotype induced by these two variants is strikingly similar to that induced by PA104

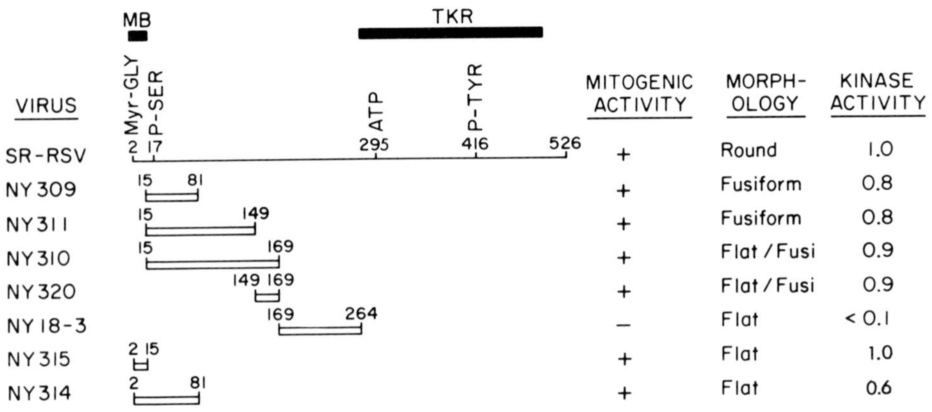

Fig. 6. Mitogenic activity of *src* deletion mutants in chicken embryo chondrocytes. The structural features of wild-type p60^{v-src} illustrated are the membrane binding domain (MB), the tyrosine kinase-related sequence (TKR), the glycine residue at position 2 that is myristylated, the major site of serine phosphorylation (serine 17), the major site of tyrosine phosphorylation (tyrosine 416), and the lysine residue at position 295 that binds ATP. The designations of the *src* deletion viruses are shown together with the corresponding deletions represented by the open boxes (amino acid numbers define limits of deletions). Mitogenic activity in chondrocytes was determined by counting cells as in Figure 1. Cellular morphology was assayed in CEF, and kinase activity (normalized to the kinase activity of the wild type protein) was measured in vitro by immunoglobulin G heavy chain phosphorylation [8,12].

at 37°C, even though the corresponding proteins have different structural defects and biochemical properties. In contrast, deletion of amino acids 169 to 264 results in the complete loss of function with respect to all of the transformation parameters examined, suggesting that the tyrosine kinase activity of this mutant might be too low to support biological activity.

Results similar to those described here also were obtained in another study using the NR cell system (Calothy, personal communication). These data demonstrate that membrane association of p60^{v-src} is not required for the stimulation of cell proliferation. Moreover, the amino-terminal third of this protein is dispensable for the mitogenic activity, although deletions extending into this region result in reduced levels of growth stimulation (data not shown).

DISCUSSION

Extensive genetic and biochemical analyses have led to the identification of three domains within p60^{v-src}: a tyrosine kinase catalytic domain, a membrane binding domain, and a modulatory domain. To understand better the roles that these domains play in the biological functions of p60^{v-src} related to transformation, we analyzed the PA101 and PA104 mutant *src* genes and proteins. These mutants are particularly attractive for such studies because they exhibit dissociation of transformation parameters as a function of temperature.

We have shown that lesions within the tyrosine kinase domains of the mutant *src* proteins confer temperature sensitivity upon all of the transformation parameters examined. Lesions in this domain also are responsible for temperature sensitivity in p34 phosphorylation in vivo. These results suggest that the tyrosine kinase activity

TABLE II. Requirements of Dissociable Transformation Parameters for p60$^{\text{v-}src}$ Domains

Domain	Mitogenic activity	Anchorage independent growth	Morphological transformation
Tyrosine kinase	+	+	+
Membrane binding		+	+
Modulatory[a]			+

[a]The proposed modulatory domain may be involved in the expression of all of the transformation phenotypes, although its function appears to be most indispensable for morphological transformation.

mediates all of the biological functions of p60$^{\text{v-}src}$, even though these functions can be dissociated.

Lesions within the amino-terminal half of the NYPA101 p60 appear to affect morphological transformation and suppress kinase activity. These lesions coincide with the proposed modulatory domain [11,12,31], and *src* deletions that extend into this region also affect morphological transformation [12,32]. The finding that amino-terminal lesions in the NYPA101 p60 suppress kinase activity is consistent with the proposed modulatory function of this domain, and suggests an interaction between the amino-terminal and tyrosine kinase domains.

Analysis of the *src* deletion mutants revealed that the amino-terminal third of p60$^{\text{v-}src}$, including the entire membrane binding domain and at least part of the modulatory domain, are not required for mitogenic activity. In contrast, previous studies showed that the membrane binding domain is required for morphological transformation and anchorage-independent growth [8]. These results raise the intriguing possibility that substrates of p60$^{\text{v-}src}$ involved in the different transformation parameters are localized in different subcellular compartments.

Table II summarizes our conclusions concerning the requirements of the dissociable transformation functions for the various domains of p60$^{\text{v-}src}$. We suggest that the expression of each transformation parameter requires the tyrosine kinase activity, and that the other domains have ancillary roles that aid the protein kinase in carrying out its functions. It seems plausible that the ancillary domains are involved primarily in determining substrate specificity for the protein kinase. As suggested by Table II, this is consistent with the possibility that phosphorylation of different substrates is required for expression of the different transformation parameters. Thus the observed dissociation of transformation-related functions might reflect altered substrate specificities of the p60$^{\text{v-}src}$ mutants.

Interestingly, p34 phosphorylation correlates to a limited extent with mitogenic activity but not with other transformation phenotypes. This suggests the p34 phosphorylation might be involved in the mitogenic activity, although it is also possible that p34 phosphorylation is not directly related to transformation. Mutants of p60$^{\text{v-}src}$ such as the ones described here might have restricted substrate specificities and therefore could facilitate the search for substrates causally related to transformation.

ACKNOWLEDGMENTS

We are grateful to G. Calothy for providing the original PA101 and PA104 isolates, Y. Kato for teaching us how to prepare chicken embryo chondrocytes, and M.E. Greenberg and G.M. Edelman for providing the anti-p34 serum. We thank R.

Williams for excellent technical assistance. R.J. is the recipient of Damon Runyon-Walter Winchell Cancer Fund Fellowship DRG-786, E.A.G. is the recipient of a Merck Fellowship, and B.J.M. is the recipient of a National Science Foundation Graduate Fellowship. This work was supported by grant MV128 from the American Cancer Society and Public Health Service Grant CA14935 from the National Cancer Institute.

REFERENCES

1. Hanafusa H: In Fraenkel-Conrat H, Wagner RR (eds): "Comprehensive Virology." New York: Plenum, 1977, pp 401–483.
2. Bishop JM, Varmus H: In Weiss R, Teich N, Coffin J (eds): "RNA Tumor Viruses." New York: Cold Spring Harbor, 1982, pp 999–1108.
3. Krueger JG, Garber EA, Goldberg AR: Curr Top Microbiol Immunol 107:51, 1983.
4. Levinson AD, Courtneidge SA, Bishop JM: Proc Natl Acad Sci USA 78:1624, 1981.
5. Brugge J, Darrow D: J Biol Chem 259:4550, 1984.
6. Hunter T, Cooper JA: In Richardson CC, Boyer PD, Dawid IB, Meister A (eds): "Annual Review of Biochemistry." Palo Alto: Annual Reviews, 1985, pp 897–930.
7. Sefton BM, Hunter T, Beemon K, Eckhart W: Cell 20:807, 1980.
8. Cross FR, Garber EA, Pellman D, Hanafusa H: Mol Cell Biol 4:1834, 1984.
9. Pellman D, Garber EA, Cross FR, Hanafusa H: Nature (Lond) 314:374, 1985.
10. Pellman D, Garber EA, Cross FR, Hanafusa H: Proc Natl Acad Sci USA 82:1623, 1985.
11. Garber EA, Cross FR, Hanafusa H: Mol Cell Biol 5:2781, 1985.
12. Cross FR, Garber EA, Hanafusa H: Mol Cell Biol 5:2789, 1985.
13. Radke K, Martin GS: Proc Natl Acad Sci USA 76:5212, 1979.
14. Erikson E, Erikson RL: Cell 21:829, 1980.
15. Cooper JA, Hunter T: Mol Cell Biol 1:394, 1981.
16. Calothy G, Poirier F, Dambrine G, Pessac B: Virology 89:75, 1978.
17. Calothy G, Poirier F, Dambrine G, Mignatti P, Combes P, Pessac B: Cold Spring Harbor Symp Quant Biol 44:983, 1980.
18. Jove R, Mayer BJ, Iba H, Laugier D, Poirier F, Calothy G, Hanafusa T, Hanafusa H: J Virol 60:840, 1986.
19. Cross FR, Hanafusa H: Cell 34:597, 1983.
20. Pessac B, Calothy G: Science 185:709, 1974.
21. Tanaka A, Parker C, Kaji A: J Virol 35:531, 1980.
22. Iba H, Takeya T, Cross FR, Hanafusa T, Hanafusa H: Proc Natl Acad Sci USA 81:4424, 1984.
23. Mayer BJ, Jove R, Krane J, Poirier F, Calothy G, Hanafusa H: J Virol 60:858, 1986.
24. Iba H, Cross FR, Garber EA, Hanafusa H: Mol Cell Biol 5:1058, 1985.
25. Iba H, Jove R, Hanafusa H: Mol Cell Biol 5:2856, 1985.
26. Greenberg ME, Edelman GM: Cell 33:767, 1983.
27. Poirier F, Calothy G, Karess RE, Erikson E, Hanafusa H: J Virol 42:780, 1982.
28. Takeya T, Feldman RA, Hanafusa H: J Virol 44:1, 1982.
29. Poirier F, Jullien P, Dezelee P, Dambrine G, Esnault E, Benatre A, Calothy G: J Virol 49:325, 1984.
30. Jove R, Garber EA, Iba H, Hanafusa H: J Virol 60:849, 1986.
31. Parsons JT, Bryant D, Wilkerson V, Gilmartin G, Parsons SJ: In Vande Woude GF, Levine AJ, Topp WC, Watson JD (ed): "Cancer Cells 2-Oncogenes and Viral Genes." New York: Cold Spring Harbor, 1984, pp 37–42.
32. Kitamura N, Yoshida M: J Virol 46:985, 1983.

Cellular and Molecular Biology of Tumors and Potential
Clinical Applications 203–212 (1988)

Mutational Analysis of *ras* Processing and Function

Douglas R. Lowy, Alex G. Papageorge, William C. Vass, and Berthe M. Willumsen

Laboratory of Cellular Oncology, National Cancer Institute, Bethesda, Maryland 20892 (D.R.L., A.G.P., W.C.V.); University Microbiology Institute, 1353 Copenhagen, Denmark (B.M.W.)

We have used linker insertion-deletion mutatgenesis to study the Harvey murine sarcoma virus v-*ras*[H] transforming protein. The mutants were characterized with respect to their ability to induce morphologic transformation of NIH 3T3 cells and the capacity of their proteins to bind guanosine nucleotides, undergo post-translational processing, and localize to the plasma membrane. One class of mutants has enabled us to show that two distinct steps can account for the post-translational changes of altered migration rate and palmitylation. We have also identified four nonoverlapping segments that are dispensable for morphologic transformation of NIH 3T3 cells, several segments that are required for transformation and guanosine nucleotide binding, and one essential segment that does not affect guanine nucleotide binding. This latter segment appears to lie on the exterior of the protein and may therefore interact with the putative *ras* target.

Key words: cell transformation, mutagenesis, oncogenes

Ras genes are widely conserved in eukaryotes, from yeast to humans [1,2]. Mammalian cells contain at least three *ras* genes: c-*ras*[H], c-*ras*[K], and c-*ras*[N]; each of these genes encodes similar 189 amino acid protein products which have been called p21 because they migrate in gels as molecules that are approximately 21 kd. The *ras* genes were first identified as the viral oncogenes of Harvey murine sarcoma virus (v-*ras*[H]) and Kirsten (Ki) MuSV (v-*ras*[K]), which are highly oncogenic versions of their normal cellular counterparts.

Members of this multigene family appear to serve essential, growth-related, physiologic functions in eukaryotes [3–5]. They have also been implicated in the pathogenesis of a variety of human and animal tumors [6]. *ras* genes can induce tumors in vivo [7] and tumorigenic transformation of tissue culture cells in vitro. The mammalian *ras* proteins can induce morphologic transformation of NIH 3T3 cells by overproduction of the normal *ras* protein product, by amino acid deletion [8], or by

Received April 15, 1986.

single amino acid substitution. In tumors, missense mutations appear to be the commonest mechanism by which the genes become activated; the v-ras^H and v-ras^K genes of Ha-MuSV and Ki-MuSV, respectively, contain two missense mutations either of which can independently activate the gene.

It has not yet been determined how the *ras* proteins carry out their normal physiological functions, nor has the pathway by which they induce cellular transformation been elucidated. Several presumably relevant features have been identified. The *ras* proteins noncovalently bind guanosine nucleotides (GDP and GTP) and possess a GTPase activity that is analogous to that of the regulatory G proteins, with which they share some sequence homology [2]. Activated versions of many *ras* proteins are associated with a significantly reduced GTPase activity. In the yeast *Saccharomyces cerevisiae, ras* apparently functions primarily by stimulating adenylate cyclase [9], but this does not seem to be the case for mammalian cells [10,11] or even for a different yeast (*Schizosaccharomyces pombe* [12]).

It has also been determined that the primary *ras* translation product (pro-p21) is synthesized in the cytosol and undergoes post-translational processing (to mature p21), leading to its translocation from the cytosol to the plasma membrane [1]. The mature p21 protein has a slightly faster mobility and contains palmitic acid linked near the C-terminus of the protein [13,14]. Genetic studies of v-ras^H have shown that both the processing and membrane association depend on a conserved cysteine residue (at amino acid 186) that in the primary translation product is located four amino acids from the C-terminus [15,16]. Mutants that encode a protein lacking cysteine-186 cannot transform NIH 3T3 cells; their proteins remain in the cytosol, do not change their migration rate, and fail to bind lipid. The biochemical nature of the processing event has not been elucidated, and it is not known if the lipid attachment and the faster migration rate are different aspects of a single event or if they represent two distinct steps.

We are carrying out structure-function studies of *ras* via a mutational analysis of the Ha-MuSV v-ras^H oncogene [15–18]. The protein encoded by v-ras^H is identical with that encoded by the normal human or rodent c-ras^H gene except for the two independently activating mutations, which are located at amino acid residues 12 and 59. These studies have enabled us to map segments in v-ras^H that are dispensable for morphologic transformation, others that are essential for this function and for guanine nucleotide binding, and one essential region that does not affect guanine nucleotide binding (see ref. 18 for a more detailed report of these results). We have also identified mutants in which the faster migration rate of the processed protein can be uncoupled from its palmitylation.

MATERIALS AND METHODS

v-ras^H Mutants and Transfection of Mouse Cells

We have previously described the technique used to generate in frame v-ras^H mutants by deletion and linker insertion mutagenesis [14]. In summary, the mutants are constructed by the combination of two sequenced parts (N-terminal front ends and C-terminal tail ends) of v-ras^H through a BclI oligonucleotide linker. This linker results in the addition of three novel amino acids within the protein at the site of the deletion, as shown in Table I for each mutant. Two eukaryotic vectors and one prokaryotic vector have been used to express the mutant genes in NIH 3T3 cells and

TABLE I. Transforming Activity of Deletion Mutants

Mutant No.	Amino acid structure[a]	Focus formation[b]	Protein processing[c]
Full-length			
pBW601	1–189	High	Com
Deletion mutants			
pBW758	1–172 PDQ 175–189	High	Com
pBW739	1–165 PDQ 180–189	High	Com
pBW757	1–172 PDQ 180–189	High	Com
pBW766	1–165 PDQ 184–189	High	Inc
pBW767	1–172 PDQ 184–189	Low	Inc
pBW768	1–180 SDQ 184–189	Low	Inc
Control for 184–189 tail end			
pBW1092	1–184 PDQ 184–189	High	Com

[a]The numbers indicate the v-*ras*[H] amino acids in front and tail ends, respectively; the letters indicate the three amino acids encoded by the oligonucleotide linker joining the front- and tail-ends.
[b]High transforming efficiency: approximately 1,000 focus forming units (ffu) per microgram DNA; low, approximately 10–50 ffu per microgram DNA.
[c]Com = complete processing, as seen with full-length protein; Inc = incomplete processing, as described in the text.

Escherichia coli$_2$, respectively. One eukaryotic vector contains the Ha-MuSV transforming region (the viral long terminal repeat (LTR) plus v-*ras*[H]) and a linked thymidine kinase (tk) gene [14]. The eukaryotic vector used for most of the mutants was developed by C. Jhappan, G. Vande Woude, and T. Robins [18a]. In this vector, the v-*ras*[H] gene (the 2.1-kilobase [kb] BamHI/EcoRI fragment) is located upstream from the simian virus 40 (SV40) sequences and neo[R] gene of pSV$_{neo}$; these two genes are flanked by the Moloney MuLV LTR. The use of the prokaryotic vector (pJCL-30), which places the *ras* mutants under control of the lambda pL promoter and initiates *ras* synthesis from its authentic initiation AUG, has been described previously [18]. The *E. coli* cells that harbor the expression vector contain a temperature-sensitive allele of the lambda repressor gene, cI857.

The NIH 3T3 cells and DNA transfection procedure have been previously described [14].

Immunoprecipitation of *ras* Proteins

For immunoprecipitation, cultures transfected with Ha-MuSV mutants were metabolically labeled with ^{35}S-methionine (250 μCi/ml) in methionine-free medium. Extracts of whole cells were prepared and precipitated as previously described with a *ras* monoclonal antibody—either Y13-238 or Y13-259 [14,15]. For cell fractionation, hypotonic swelling of the cells was followed by homogenization and low-speed centrifugation to remove nuclei. The supernatant was then fractionated into a pellet particulate fraction containing the plasma membranes and a supernatant cytosol fraction as described and subjected to immunoprecipitation. This procedure separates the cytosol-associated pro p21 from the membrane-associated mature p21. Purified bacterially synthesized *ras* proteins were assayed with antibody Y13-259 by electroblotting.

RESULTS AND DISCUSSION
Construction of Mutants

The *ras* proteins can be divided into at least three functional domains. The extreme C-terminus, which we call the membrane anchoring domain, is required for postranslational processing and membrane localization. A 20-amino-acid segment that is called the major heterogenous region lies just upstream from the C-terminus (amino acid residues 165–185); it is highly divergent among different *ras* genes. The N-terminal 160 amino acids, which are highly conserved among mammalian *ras* proteins, represents the catalytic domain of the protein.

Because of the oligonucleotide linker used in constructing the mutants, each mutated v-*ras*H gene encoded three novel amino acids at the site of the deletion. The eukaryotic vector into which the mutants were placed contained a linked selectable marker (a neomycin-resistance or thymidine kinase gene). These selectable markers enabled us to to study in NIH 3T3 cells the *ras* proteins encoded by transformation-defective (td) mutants. Representative mutants were also placed in a prokaryotic expression vector to analyze the GDP binding activities of purified mutant *ras* proteins produced in bacteria.

Mapping Domains That Are Required and Dispensable for Cell Transformation and Nucleotide Binding

The capacity of these mutant v-*ras*H genes (promoted by a viral LTR) to induce focal transformation of NIH 3T3 cells is shown in Figure 1. Some mutants were transformation-competent and induced foci with an efficiency similar to that of the wild-type v-*ras*H gene, the transforming capacity of other competent mutants was significantly reduced, and some mutants were transformation defective (any mutant whose transforming activity was more than three orders of magnitude lower than that of the wild-type gene will score as defective in this assay). The foci induced by mutants possessing a transforming efficiency less than 20% that of the wild-type gene were generally detected later and remained smaller than those mutants that induced foci with an efficiency similar to that of the wild-type gene.

Within the catalytic domain, we noted three different segments where deletions did not abolish the transforming activity of the gene (labeled A–C in Fig. 1). Each nonessential segment was quite large; A, B, and C were at least 13 (residues 64–76), 16 (93–108), and 19 (120–138) amino acids long, respectively. Segment D in Figure 1 corresponds to the majority of the heterogeneous region; the dispensable nature of this region for transformation has been documented previously.

Given the evolutionary conservation of most v-*ras*H amino acids, it might be expected that most deletions outside the heterogeneous region would abolish the transforming activity of the gene. Indeed, six different regions within the catalytic domain were apparently essential for transformation (labeled 1–6 in Fig. 1) since lesions in each region rendered the genes defective. The precise boundaries of these essential regions are not defined because the defective phenotype represents loss of a function, and we did not determine which of the variant amino acids in each mutant were responsible for the phenotype.

When the in vitro GDP binding activities of the mutants were determined (from mutant protein synthesized in bacteria [18]), proteins from three of the six essential regions (1, 5, and 6) were negative (any mutant that bound less than 1% as much

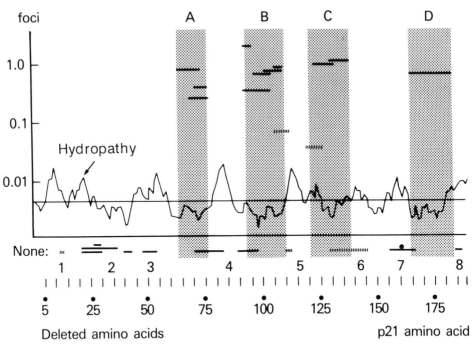

Fig. 1.   Transforming activity of representative *ras* mutants and hydropathic index of the *ras* protein [from ref. 18]. The main horizontal axis represents the amino acids (1–189) in the *ras* protein; the vertical axis represents the relative NIH 3T3 focus forming activity of the mutants. Each mutant is represented by a horizontal line (solid for those mutant proteins that bind GDP, interrupted for those mutants that do not bind detectable levels of GDP); this line corresponds to the location and extent of the deletion. Segments designated **A–D** represent sequences that are not essential for transformation. Regions designated **1–8** contain sequences that are essential for transformation. Data for mutants in A–C and 1–6 are taken from ref 18; data for mutants in D, 7, and 8, which are included for comparative purposes, are from ref 17. The hydropathic index has been plotted according to Kyte and Doolittle [21]; hydrophobic regions are above the axis of the midpoint line, hydrophilic are below.

GDP as the wild-type protein registered as negative in this assay). Two GDP-negative mutants were exceptional in that they had some biological activity, but it was markedly impaired (Fig. 1). The few mutants from essential regions 3 and 4 had low (2% of wild-type) binding activity. Mutants from essential region 2 were unusual in that they retained high GDP binding activity. These results are consistent with the hypothesis that GDP binding is necessary, but not sufficient, for efficient *ras*-mediated transformation. They also suggest that at least some of the sequence homology noted between *ras* and other nucleotide binding proteins, such as *E. coli* elongation factor Tu (EF-Tu), has functional significance, since the regions we have defined as being required for GDP binding also serve this function in EF-Tu [19,20].

When the mutant *ras* proteins in NIH 3T3 cells stably transfected with the mutants were characterized, the cells carrying transformation-defective mutants from the five essential regions in the catalytic domain other than essential region 2 did not contain detectable levels of mutant protein. Since the bacterially derived proteins encoded by these defective mutants bound antibody as well as did wild-type protein, we tentatively conclude the mutant *ras* proteins not detected in the NIH 3T3 cells are unstable in these mammalian cells. By contrast, those cells carrying mutants from essential region 2 contained readily detectable mutant protein, as had been found previously for td mutants with lesions at the C-terminus. Subcellular localization studies indicated further that these mutant proteins migrated normally to the membrane [18].

An Essential Region That May Interact With the *ras* Target

Figure 1 also plots the hydropathic index of the wild-type protein, according to the program of Kyte and Doolittle [21]. For soluble globular proteins, interior portions generally map to the hydrophobic side of the axis of the midpoint line, while exterior portions are usually found on the hydrophilic side. The required regions tend to fall on the hydrophobic side, with the notable exception of the hydrophilic region 2.

When considered in conjunction with the transforming and biochemical activities of the mutants and the *ras* model derived from EF-Tu [15, 26], the hydropathic index suggests several topological and functional features of *ras* protein. Most of the required regions appear to be hydrophobic, implying that disruption of interior portions alter the protein sufficiently to inactivate it biologically. Each of the nonessential segments correspond to hydrophilic regions, suggesting that they are located on the exterior of the protein, which correspond to external alpha-helices in the EF-Tu model.

Essential region 2, which is highly conserved among *ras* proteins, is unusual in that it apparently represents a required exterior portion of the protein. Although there is no sequence homology between *ras* and EF-Tu in this region, acylated tRNAs are believed to bind to the analogous region of EF-Tu-GTP [22]. The *ras* mutants with lesions in essential region 2 are transformation defective despite possessing all the known important biochemical features of *ras* proteins in that they synthesize a protein that is stable in NIH 3T3 cells, localizes to the membrane, and has GDP binding, GTPase, and autophosphorylating activities that are similar to that of the wild type v-*ras*[H] protein. These mutants argue for the existence of an essential *ras* function that has not yet been defined. We speculate that the region 2 mutant proteins are defective because they fail to interact with the putative target of the normal *ras* protein.

C-Termimus Mutants Show Post-Translational Processing Is More Than One Step

One class of mutants whose lesions lie in the heterogeneous region a few amino acids upstream from cysteine-186 suggest that post-translational processing can be divided into at least two distinct steps, since in these mutants the change in migration rate can be uncoupled from palmitylation of the protein. This phenomenon is seen when the proteins encoded by each of three different mutants with the same tail end (encoding amino acids 184–189; pBW766, 767, and 768) have been analyzed. As noted below, the biological results obtained with these mutants have been somewhat perplexing, although they are reproducible.

pBW766, from which amino acids 166–183 have been deleted, transformed NIH 3T3 cells almost as efficiently as did the wild-type gene (Table I). However, much lower transforming activity (by two orders of magnitude) was noted for the two other deletion mutants (pBW767 and 768) that carry the same tail end as 766 and whose deletions were smaller than the deletion in 766.

The lower transforming efficiency of these two mutants was not the consequence of different inserted amino acids in the region linking the front and tail ends (both

766 and 767 encode Pro-Asp-Gln as their novel amino acids), nor does it appear to be the result of a cloning artifact. To rule out this latter possibility, a second pair of independently derived mutants that are identical with 766 and 767 yielded transformation results that were identical with those obtained with 766 and 767. In addition, exchanging the 766 and 767 tail ends with their respective fronts resulted in the expected transformation phenotype (high for the 766-like clone and low for the 767-like clone). Finally, the highly transforming deletion mutant 757 used the same front end as 767.

Cells transformed by the three mutants were metabolically labeled with methionine and analyzed by immunoprecipitation and polyacrylamide gel electrophoresis (PAGE, Fig. 2). In PAGE, the mature wild-type v-*ras*^{H} protein in NIH 3T3 cells is seen principally as a doublet [1]. The upper band of the doublet represents a phosphorylated form of the protein in the lower band. This phosphorylation of threonine-59 is believed to result in vivo from autophosphorylation. Analysis of the protein produced by the three mutants revealed the characteristic doublet for each and migration rates of their proteins that were approximately those expected for the number of amino acids each encoded (Fig. 2). Mutant pBW766 reproducibly contained lower levels of immunoprecipitable p21 protein compared with that found in the other mutants, presumably because its protein is more active biologically.

Pulse-chase experiments carried out after ^{35}S-methionine labeling indicated that by the criterion of the change in electrophoretic migration and phosphorylation the *ras* proteins encoded by the three mutants were processed in a manner similar to full-

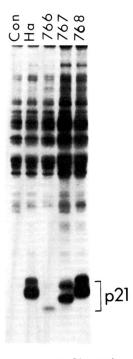

Fig. 2. Immunoprecipitation of mature mutant p21 proteins. NIH 3T3 cells transformed by the indicated plasmid DNAs were labeled overnight with methionine and immunoprecipitated. Con=control cells; Ha=full-length viral p21. The viral p21 protein is a doublet; the slower-migrating form is phosphorylated at threonine-59 [1].

length viral protein or to mutants that contain larger tail ends (Fig. 3). However, when cells transformed by the three deletion mutants were metabolically labeled overnight with methionine and the cells fractionated into a crude cytosolic supernatant and membrane pellet fractions, the processed *ras* protein in the mutants was found in both fractions, while full-length processed protein (and protein from mutants with larger tail ends) was confined to the pellet fraction (Fig. 4). Close to one-half of the p21 found in each deletion mutant with the six C-terminal amino acids was found in the cytosolic fraction, whether selected by morphologic transformation or thymidine kinase (tk) activity in tk⁻ NIH 3T3 cells. The mutant protein in both fractions migrated similarly, indicating that the protein found in the cytosol had undergone the post-translational processing associated with the faster migration rate of mature p21. When the proteins encoded by the mutants were metabolically labeled with ³H-palmitic acid and fractionated as above, the palmitylated protein was found almost exclusively in the pellet fraction (Fig. 5). This result indicates that the processed p21 found in the cytosolic fraction did not bind a significant amount of palmitic acid; thus the change in migration rate did not result from the binding of lipid to p21.

We conclude that the change in migration rate represents a step that is separate from palmitylation. Consistent with this conclusion, Chen et al have noted that removal of lipid from p21 does not restore the mobility of the mature protein to that of the precursor form [13]. We speculate that the change in migration rate results principally from cleavage of two or three amino acids from the C-terminus of the pro-p21. The mechanism underlying the phenotype observed with the three mutants remains unclear. The results obtained with pBW1092 (see Table I) strongly suggest that the incomplete processing found with 766, 767, and 768 does not result from the sequence specificity of the three novel amino acids generated by the oligonucleotide linker just upstream from the six C-terminal amino acids. Duplication mutant pBW1092 has the same tail end as the three mutants and the same three novel ami-

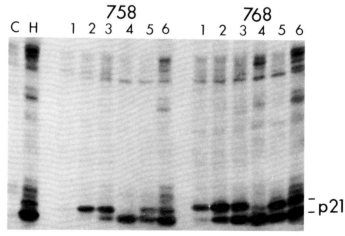

Fig. 3. Immunoprecipitation of mutants under pulse-chase conditions. **Lane 1**=10-min pulse; **lane 2**=30-min pulse; **lane 3**=60-min pulse; **lane 4**=60-min pulse and 3-h chase; **lane 5**=60-min pulse and 24-h chase; **lane 6**=24-h labelling. C=control cells; H=full-length viral p21 (24-h labelling). The slower-migrating forms in lanes 1–3 represent nonphosphorylated pro-p21; the slower-migrating forms in lanes 5 and 6 represent phosphorylated p21. Mutants 766 and 767 gave results that were similar to those obtained with 768.

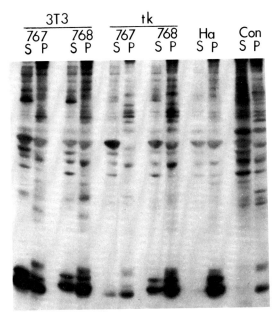

Fig. 4. Fractionation of p21 in methionine-labeled mutants. Cells were labeled overnight, fractionated as described in the Materials and Methods into a cytosolic supernatant fraction (S) and membrane pellet fraction (P), and immunoprecipitated. Con=control cells; Ha=full-length viral p21. The mutants under "3T3" were selected by morphologic transformation of NIH 3T3 cells. The mutants under "tk" were selected by thymidine kinase activity in tk⁻ cells. In other assays, mutant 766 fractionated as did 767 and 768, whereas mutants 739 and 758 fractionated as did the full-length viral p21.

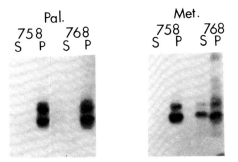

Fig. 5. Palmitylation of p21 mutants. Cultures were labeled overnight with methionine (right panel) or palmitic acid (left panel), fractionated as in Figure 4, and immunoprecipitated.

no acids as 766 and 767, but it has a front end that is intact through amino acid 184. The protein encoded by this mutant, which has the high transformation phenotype, fractionated as did full-length p21, in contrast to the results obtained with 766, 767, and 768.

ACKNOWLEDGMENTS

Parts of this work have been supported by the Danish Cancer Society (84-068), the Danish Medical Research Council (12-5345 and 12-4663), the Danish Natural Science Research Council (11-5095), and NATO (84/165).

REFERENCES

1. Shih TY, Weeks MO: Cancer Invest 2:109, 1984.
2. Gibbs JB, Sigal IS, Scolnick EM: Trends Biochem Sci 10:350, 1985.
3. DeFeo-Jones D, Tatchell K, Robinson LC, Sigal IS, Vass WC, Lowy DR, Scolnick EM: Science 228:179, 1985.
4. Kataoka T, Powers S, Cameron S, Fasano O, Goldfarb M, Brouch J, Wigler M: Cell 40:19, 1985.
5. Mulcahy LS, Smith MR, Stacey DW: Nature (Lond) 313:241, 1985.
6. Marshall C: In Weiss R, Teich N, Varmus H, Coffin J (eds): "RNA Tumor Viruses. Molecular Biology of Tumor Viruses." Supplement to 2nd edition. New York: Cold Spring Harbor Laboratory, 1985, pp 487–558.
7. Tabin CJ, Weinberg RA: J Virol 53:260, 1985.
8. Chipperfield RG, Jones SS, Lo K-M, Weinberg R: Mol Cell Biol 5:1809, 1985.
9. Broek D, Samily N, Fasano O, Fujiyama A, Tamanoi F, Northrup J, Wigler M: Cell 41:763, 1985.
10. Beckner SK, Hattori S, Shih TY: Nature 317:71, 1985.
11. Levitzki A, Rudick J. Pastan I, Vass WC, Lowy DR: FEBBS Lett 197:134, 1986.
12. Fukui Y, Kozasa T, Kaziro Y, Takeda T, Yamamoto M: Cell 44:329, 1986.
13. Chen Z-Q, Ulsh LS, DuBois G, Shih TY: J Virol 56:607, 1985.
14. Buss JE, Sefton BM: Mol Cell Biol 6:116, 1986.
15. Willumsen BM, Christensen A, Hubbert NL, Papageorge AG, Lowy DR: Nature (Lond) 310:583, 1984a.
16. Willumsen BM, Norris K, Papageorge AG, Hubbert NL, Lowy DR: EMBO J 3:2581, 1984b.
17. Willumsen BM, Papageorge AG, Hubbert NL, Bekesi E, Kung H-F, Lowy DR: EMBO J 4:2893, 1985.
18. Willumsen BM, Papageorge AG, Kung H-F, Bekesi E, Robins T, Johnsen M, Vass WC, Lowy DR: Mol Cell Biol 6:2646, 1986.
18a. Jhappan C, Vande Woude GF, Robins TS: J Virol 6:750, 1986.
19. Jurnack F: Science 230:32, 1985.
20. McCormick F, Clark BFC, La Cour TFM, Kjeldgaard M, Norskov-Lauritsen L, Nyborg J: Science 230:78, 1985.
21. Kyte J, Doolittle RF: J Mol Biol 157:105, 1982.
22. Kaziro Y: Biochim Biophys Acta 505:95, 1978.

Cellular and Molecular Biology of Tumors and Potential
Clinical Applications 213–223 (1988)

Microinjection Studies of c-*ras* Proteins and the Proliferation of Normal, Transformed, and Tumor Cells

Dennis W. Stacey

Roche Institute of Molecular Biology, Roche Research Center, Nutley, New Jersey 07110

An anti-*ras* monoclonal antibody has been found which neutralizes the activity of viral and cellular *ras* proteins within microinjected cells. When this antibody is injected into normal fibroblast and epithelial cell types, cellular proliferation is efficiently interrupted. Inhibition by the antibody occurs just prior to the initiation of S-phase. This fact, along with the observation that purified viral *ras* protein can induce DNA synthesis in the absence of growth factors, indicates c-*ras* proteins play a critical role in the control of cell proliferation. As an indication of how c-*ras* proteins function, viral oncogenes related to receptor molecules were shown to require c-*ras* proteins for activity, whereas two cytoplasmic viral oncogenes functioned independently of c-*ras*. These observations suggest that the oncogenes are involved in a signal transduction pathway with c-*ras* proteins required to transfer the proliferative signal from the cell surface to cytoplasmic effector molecules. In tumor cells inhibition of proliferation by the antibody is seldom as efficient as observed with nontransformed cells. This indicates that tumor mutations generate molecules which stimulate proliferation independently of c-*ras* activity (as with cytoplasmic viral oncogenes).

Key words: cell proliferation, antibody microinjection, oncogenes

Dramatic progress has been made over the last several years in identifying and characterizing normal genes which participate in tumor formation following mutation. The challenge now is to determine the normal biological functions of these molecules, their interactions, and how mutations alter their activity. A novel approach in these studies involves the microinjection of a neutralizing antibody into individual living cells. Data obtained in microinjection studies and summarized here provide a unique biological perspective in the study of these important biological molecules.

Our understanding of the molecules likely to be involved in cellular proliferation was aided by analysis of RNA tumor viruses which induce rapid tumor formation and the related transformation of cultured cells. These viruses were found to have recombined with host genes. The recombinant genes had altered sequence or expression

Received March 12, 1986.

characteristics and were totally responsible for transformation by the virus [1]. Sequence analysis has identified the original cellular proto-oncogenes of some of these viral oncogenes as growth factors or as growth factor receptor molecules [2–5]. While the function of other proto-oncogenes is unknown, the 20–30 viral oncogenes characterized to date often fall into related groups such as membrane-bound receptor-like molecules with tyrosine kinase activity, cytoplasmic serine/threonine kinases, or nuclear molecules [1]. In addition to these broad categories, the *ras* gene family contains three closely related, membrane-bound proteins with little homology to other oncogenes [6]. It is generally assumed that proto-oncogenes play an important role in normal cellular proliferation and that they function similarly to the viral genes derived from them. The studies described here with the *ras* gene provide support for both these hypotheses.

The importance of the *ras* gene family was demonstrated by the observation that perhaps 10% of all human tumors contain a mutation in a cellular *ras* (c-*ras*) gene creating a transforming oncogene analogous to that observed in *ras*-containing RNA tumor viruses [7–9]. The 21-kilodalton (kD) *ras* protein is a GTP-binding and GTP-hydrolyzing protein [10–12] with biochemical and structural similarities to the G-proteins involved in regulating adenyl cyclase [13].

ras Protein Injections

Microinjection studies, in collaboration with H.-F. Kung, first involved purified v-*ras* protein which had been synthesized in bacterial cells. When this protein was solubilized and injected into NIH3T3 cells, the recipient cells exhibited a transformed morphology between approximately 12 and 30 hr after injection. Quiescent NIH3T3 cells were also induced to enter a round of DNA synthesis in the absence of added growth factors. As evidence that the oncogene and proto-oncogene proteins function similarly, purified c-*ras* protein was also able to induce morphologic transformation and induce DNA synthesis, but only at approximately ten-fold greater concentration than required for the viral protein [14].

Anti-*ras* Antibody Analysis

Identification of a biologically active *ras* protein provided a means to screen anti-*ras* antibodies and identify one able to neutralize intracellular *ras* function. The monoclonal antibodies screened were originally prepared by Furth et al [15] against viral *ras* protein. Purified viral protein was mixed with each monoclonal antibody and the mixture injected into NIH3T3 cells. Cells injected with *ras* protein along with antibody Y13-259 were not transformed, indicating that the antibody had neutralized *ras* protein transforming activity. Antibody Y13-238, on the other hand, did not neutralize the activity of coinjected *ras* protein. These antibodies were further ana-lyzed by injection into NIH3T3 cells transformed by a *ras* oncogene. As expected, those transformed cells injected with antibody 259 reverted to a normal morphology between approximately 14 and 30 hr after injection and stopped proliferating during that time. Antibody 238 had no effect upon the morphology or proliferation of injected cells [16].

The above results suggest that antibody 259 recognizes and neutralizes *ras* protein within a living cell. The results could, however, result from anti-*ras* binding to another cellular protein. Two lines of evidence suggest that it is *ras* proteins which are recognized and neutralized by the injected antibody. First, studies with tumor cells to be described later show a strong correlation between the effect of the antibody and the presence of a mutant, transforming *ras* gene in the tumor [17]. Second, D.R. Lowy and collaborators have obtained deletion mutants of viral *ras* protein that are no longer recognized by antibody 259 but retain the ability to transform cultured cells. In NIH3T3 cells transformed by these mutant *ras* genes, injected antibody 259 did not alter the transformed phenotype and produced little inhibition of proliferation [18]. This strongly suggests that it is *ras* protein which is recognized by the injected antibody.

It is interesting to note that antibody 259 is known to bind all three members of the *ras* gene family from a variety of species. It is therefore clear that in the mutant-*ras* transformed cells described above, c-*ras* proteins would be neutralized by the injected antibody 259. Proliferation of the cells following antibody injection must therefore rely upon the activity of mutant viral *ras* proteins. Since proliferation occurred normally, and in view of results to next be described, it is clear that the viral *ras* proteins substituted functionally for c-*ras* proteins during cell proliferation [18]. This provides further support for the idea that oncogenes function similarly to their cellular counterparts.

ras Activity in Normal Cells

The identification of a neutralizing and specific anti-*ras* monoclonal antibody made it possible to remove *ras* activity transiently from a living cell and determine the resulting effect upon the cells. NIH3T3 cells were first analyzed after rendering them quiescent by serum starvation or density arrest. Antibodies 259 or 238 were injected into the nonproliferating cells after which they were induced to reenter the cell cycle by the addition of fresh serum. The cells injected with neutralizing antibody 259 were efficiently inhibited from entering a new S-phase and incorporating thymidine, while those injected with non-neutralizing antibody 238 were unaffected and incorporated thymidine as well as uninjected cells [19]. These observations indicate that cellular *ras* proteins play a critical role in NIH3T3 cell proliferation.

To characterize further the requirement for c-*ras* during proliferation, rapidly proliferating, nonsynchronized NIH3T3 cells were injected with antibody 259 and pulsed with thymidine at various times thereafter. Cells labeled between 1 and 11 hr after injection were unaltered in thymidine incorporation, while those labeled between 11 and 22 hr were approximately 90% inhibited [19]. This result indicates that the antibody does not interfere with DNA synthesis itself, but rather with the initiation of a cycle of DNA synthesis. Cells labeled soon after injection were likely to have been in S-phase at the time of injection. The antibody apparently did not interfere with thymidine incorporation in these cells. A cycle of DNA synthesis in progress at the time of injection would normally terminate within 11–15 hr. In order for injected cells to incorporate label after that time they would have to initiate a new cycle of DNA synthesis after antibody injection and were apparently inhibited from doing so by the neutralizing anti-*ras* antibody.

To determine carefully the kinetics of anti-*ras* inhibition, we rendered NIH3T3 cells quiescent by serum deprivation. Fresh serum was then added to the cultures, and at various times thereafter the cultures were injected with antibody 259 (or labeled to determine the proportion of cells synthesizing DNA). Injected antibody efficiently blocked thymidine incorporation until approximately 8 hr after serum addition, which is the time at which cells in the culture started entering S-phase [19].

Anti-*ras* antibody therefore is apparently inhibitory until just prior to the initiation of cellular S-phase, as one might expect if a molecule that functions in the control of proliferation were affected. It is not known if c-*ras* proteins are also required earlier during serum stimulation. It is clear, however, that c-*ras* proteins are required for the proliferative action of each growth factor present in serum since no component in fresh serum could efficiently override the inhibition of anti-*ras* antibody.

The kinetic studies indicate that the requirement for c-*ras* proteins can be tested in any rapidly proliferating cell culture. For such an analysis the injection must be followed by sufficient time to allow the completion of any cycle of DNA synthesis in progress at the time of injection prior to thymidine labeling. In the studies to follow, cells were given a 3-hr pulse of thymidine between 15 and 24 hr after injection. To identify injected cells positively, the labeled cultures were washed, fixed, and stained with a fluorescent antibody able to react with the injected immunoglobulin within the cells. This procedure also ensures that the injected antibody remains within the cell throughout the labeling period. Furthermore, the exact time of labeling was varied to ensure that the results obtained were not dependent upon a specific labeling protocol.

Interrelationship of Oncogenes

As previously described, several different viral oncogenes are structurally related to growth factor receptors or in the case of the *sis* oncogene—for example, the platelet-derived growth factor molecule itself [2–5]. Since serum growth factors apparently depend upon c-*ras* proteins to stimulate proliferation, it was of interest to determine if the growth factor-related oncogenes also require c-*ras* proteins to exert their transforming potential. To make this determination NIH3T3 cells were transformed by various viral oncogenes either by transfection with the cloned viral genome or by infection with the virus. The transformed cells then received injections of anti-*ras* antibody. Cells were pulsed, fixed, and stained as described above (between 15 and 21 hr after injection).

NIH3T3 cells transformed by three oncogenes related to growth factor receptor molecules (*src*, *fms*, and *fes*) along with *sis* were first analyzed. In each case, the injected cells reverted from the rounded, refractile appearance of transformed cells to the more flattened morphology of nontransformed cells (Fig. 1B,D). This reversion to the normal phenotype was first observed 12–15 hr after injection and continued for up to 20 hr until cells gradually reverted to their previous transformed morphology (as injected antibody protein disappeared from the cells). In addition, thymidine incorporation in each type of transformed cell was inhibited by nearly 80% following injection of anti-*ras* 259 (Fig. 1A,C). An inhibition by injected antibody of approximately 85% was observed with NIH3T3 cells transformed by viral *ras* itself. There was no effect upon these cells by control antibody 238 [20]. As with the normal growth factors and their receptors, these oncogenes depended upon c-*ras* activity to exert their transforming potential. This observation not only provides a third line of evidence described here that oncogenes and their cellular homologues function similarly, it establishes a critically important interrelationship between several viral oncogenes and reemphasizes the central role played by c-*ras* during cellular proliferation.

As previously noted, viral oncogenes commonly fall into separate groups. Two oncogenes of a second type were next analyzed. The *mos* and *raf* oncogenes are soluble proteins with serine/threonine kinase activity [21–23]. NIH3T3 cells transformed by these molecules were also recipients of neutralizing anti-*ras* 259. In

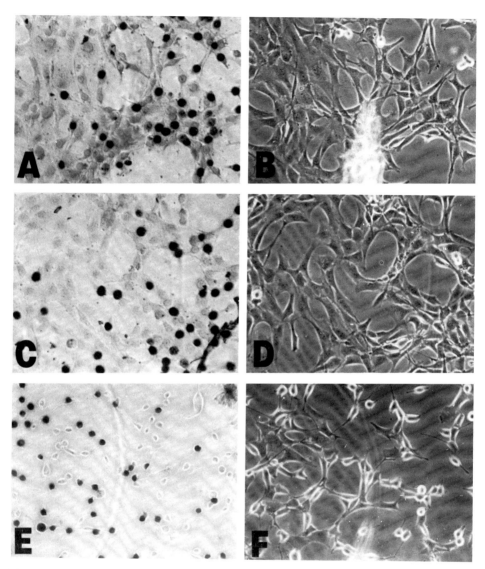

Fig. 1.   Anti-*ras* antibody microinjection into cells transformed by other oncogenes. These NIH3T3 cells were transformed by the *fms* (**A,B**), *fes* (**C,D**), or *mos* (**E,F**) oncogenes [20]. Neutralizing anti-*ras* antibody 259 was injected into all cells within an area designated by a mark on the back of the coverslip. These photographs were taken so that cells in the left half of each frame were injected while those at the right were uninjected. At 14 hr after injection, phase-contrast photographs (right) were taken. The cells were then labeled with thymidine, autoradiography was performed, and photographs were again taken of the same cellular area (left). It is clear that *fms* and *fes* transformed cells become more flattened and less refractile following injection (phase-contrast photographs), whereas the *mos* transformed cells were not morphologically altered by injected anti-*ras* antibody. In addition, the proportion of *fms* and *fes* transformed cells able to incorporate label was reduced by the injection, while *mos* transformed cells were uninhibited in proliferation by the antibody.

contrast to the previous results, these transformed cells were not affected noticeably by the injected antibody (Fig. 1F). The transformed morphology was not altered and thymidine incorporation was reduced by less than 10% [20] (Fig. 1E). The biological function of the proto-oncogenes corresponding to these two viral molecules is not known. The *raf* proto-oncogene is commonly expressed in many or all proliferating tissues while that for *mos* is not expressed in adult tissues [23]. The differential sensitivities to injected anti-*ras* antibody of the two types of viral oncogenes must relate to their distinct functions and modes of action within the cell and will be of critical importance in understanding how these various types of regulatory molecules interrelate. For the purpose of further study, however, the most critical point is that anti-*ras* injection can discriminate between the actions of two classes of oncogenes.

Tumor Cell Studies

It is believed that multiple alterations are involved in tumor initiation and progression [24,25]. Mutations and chromosomal aberrations in many tumors have been carefully analyzed. While these mutations are most likely critical to the process of tumor formation, it is not clear what role they play in the maintenance or development of the tumorous state, or what other mutations might also be present in the cell. Anti-*ras* antibody injection provides a means to classify the molecules within a tumor cell which directly affect its proliferation. This information will help establish the role of specific mutations, will help identify unknown alterations, and will indicate if an alteration was involved only during the early stages of tumor progression or if it retains a function in the mature tumor cell.

Initially, 14 carcinoma cell lines from the colon, lung, breast, and bladder were studied. Each cell line had previously been analyzed in other laboratories for the presence of a mutant, transforming *ras* oncogene. Of the nine carcinoma cell lines without a mutant c-*ras* gene, seven were not noticeably inhibited by neutralizing anti-*ras* antibody 259 in thymidine incorporation. Antibody staining confirmed that the antibody remained at high levels within each cell type during the analysis. Several different labeling times were tested. The other two carcinomas without an activated *ras* gene along with all five of those containing a mutant *ras* gene were reduced in proliferation by the injected antibody. Inhibition ranged between 60% and 90%, but in only one case (a colon line containing a mutant *ras* gene) was the extent of inhibition comparable to that observed with uninfected NIH3T3 cells [17].

It might appear obvious from these data that most of the tumor cells analyzed contained mutations or alterations in genes which, like *mos* and *raf*, function independently of c-*ras* proteins. This conclusion, however, assumes that normal epithelial cells do require c-*ras* during proliferation as do NIH3T3 cells. To analyze the dependence of normal epithelial cell proliferation upon c-*ras* proteins, primary mouse skin keratinocytes were prepared with the aid of S. Yuspa and colleagues, and normal mammary epithelial cells were provided by M. Stampfer. Anti-*ras* antibody 259 was injected into each cell type. Of more than 1,000 cells analyzed for each cell type in numerous separate experiments fewer than 5 injected cells incorporated thymidine. With non-neutralizing antibody 238 injected epithelial cells displayed little or no difference in thymidine incorporation compared to uninjected cells (20–50% thymidine labeling; unpublished data). Thus at least these two types of epithelial cells are profoundly sensitive to anti-*ras* injection. It therefore appears likely that the reduced dependence upon c-*ras* proteins observed in the carcinoma cell lines tested was a consequence of tumor formation. Unfortunately, it cannot be formally proven that tumor formation involves reduced c-*ras* protein involvement in proliferation because it is not possible to positively identify and test that specific cell type at the appropriate developmental state from which the tumor originates. Therefore an attempt was made to analyze other normal cell types and related tumors to determine if reduction in c-*ras* protein involvement in proliferation is a common characteristic of tumor formation.

Fibroblast Cells and Sarcomas

Sarcomas arise from connective tissue cells as do fibroblasts. Six sarcoma cell lines along with four separate normal fibroblast preparations were next analyzed for sensitivity of proliferation to anti-*ras* antibody injection. Of the six sarcoma lines four were fibrosarcomas and two were rhabdosarcomas; two of the six contained an activated *ras* oncogene. Inhibition of thymidine incorporation was less than 30%, except for the two sarcomas with activated c-*ras* oncogenes which were inhibited by 70%. In contrast, the normal fibroblast lines including human diploid lung and skin fibroblasts along with murine embryo fibroblasts in secondary culture were all inhibited by at least 90% in thymidine incorporation by neutralizing antibody 259. Control antibody 238, as before, had little effect on thymidine incorporation [17]. Again, it is not known if any of the four normal fibroblast cell types are related to the cells from which any of the six tumors developed. It is clear as before, however, that normal cells are much more likely to be sensitive to anti-*ras* antibody than tumor cells, particularly tumor cells without an activated *ras* oncogene.

Each of the tumor cells tested had been established in permanent culture. It is therefore likely that these cells will display at least subtle differences from the tumors from which they were obtained. It is possible that the insensitivity to anti-*ras* antibody might be related to the establishment in culture. To test this possibility six cell lines derived from normal epithelial tissues or tumor cells which have been maintained in culture for long periods of time were tested for sensitivity to injected anti-*ras* antibody. Of the six cell lines tested only one was insensitive to the injected antibody. Each of the other cell lines was inhibited by 60–80% in thymidine incorporation [17]. While it will be necessary to test fresh tumor cells in the future, studies with epithelial cell lines indicate that establishment in culture is not necessarily responsible for insensitivity to the antibody displayed in the tumor cells tested. The indication is that tumor formation often involves reduced dependence upon c-*ras* proteins during proliferation.

DISCUSSION

The experiments described rely upon the action within a living cell of monoclonal antibody 259 (originally prepared by Furth et al [15]). Whereas various antibodies have previously been microinjected [26], an understanding of their behavior within cells is incomplete. This uncertainty is a factor in the interpretation of the results described. Careful analysis, however, suggests that the anti-*ras* antibody does specifically neutralize the biological function of cellular *ras* proteins. The antibody neutralized the transforming potential of coinjected, purified *ras* protein and transiently abolished the transformed phenotype of viral *ras*-transformed cells. The strongest evidence for the specificity of anti-*ras* action comes from study of tumor cells and viral gene mutants. Of the 13 tumor lines studied without mutant, transforming *ras* genes 11 exhibited less than 30% inhibition in proliferation following antibody injection. All seven of those with a mutant *ras* gene were inhibited by over 60% [17]. This correlation between genotype and cellular phenotype strongly suggests cellular *ras* proteins are directly involved in the action of the injected antibody. In addition, mutants of the *ras* gene have been obtained from which the epitope recognized by the neutralizing antibody had been eliminated. Cells transformed by these *ras* gene mutants were unaffected by the antibody, indicating that neutralization of a cellular protein other than *ras*-protein is probably not responsible for the results seen [18]. Finally, a related monoclonal antibody without the ability to neutralize *ras* protein activity was without inhibitory effect, indicating that a nonspecific effect of the injected immunoglobulin cannot be responsible for inhibition of proliferation. Notwithstanding the rigor of these controls, there remains an uncertainty in these studies resulting from the unproven nature of this approach. Even in the light of this uncertainty, however, the studies with neutralizing anti-*ras* antibody injection constitute a unique and powerful approach to the study of proteins involved in cellular proliferation.

Injection of neutralizing anti-*ras* antibody indicates that c-*ras* proteins play a central role in the proliferation of normal cells. Of the six normal epithelial and fibroblast cell types analyzed, thymidine incorporation in each was inhibited at least 90%. Incorporation in the two normal epithelial cell types was profoundly inhibited by the antibody. Inhibition in NIH3T3 cells occurred just prior to the initiation of S-phase, but the process of DNA synthesis itself was not affected by the antibody [19].

Anti-*ras* antibody injections were also found to distinguish between the actions of separate classes of viral oncogenes. Those related to membrane receptors for growth factors required c-*ras* activity to induce the phenotype of transformation, while those related to cytoplasmic serine kinases were not dependent upon c-*ras* activity. Since there is evidence that oncogenes act similarly to their related normal genes, this observation might aid in understanding intracellular proliferative signal transduction. It is important to point out that present data do not distinguish between many possible signal transduction mechanisms. It seems most likely, however, that c-*ras* proteins act to transmit the proliferative signal generated by receptor molecules into the cell where cytoplasmic kinases affect the biological response to that signal [20]. While this scheme is hypothetical, it appears plausible chiefly because of its simplicity, its consistency with these data, and the remarkable similarity it bears to the cAMP signal transduction pathway [13]. According to the model (Fig. 2), a receptor molecule would require c-*ras* protein to induce proliferation even if it were mutated to the extent that it functioned actively without appropriate stimulation. No such requirement would exist for the cytoplasmic kinase.

In addition to the results described, the nearly universal expression of c-*ras* proteins in proliferating tissues suggest that they have an important role in cell division. There is evidence that c-*raf* proteins are also widely expressed [23] (whereas c-*mos* is highly restricted in its expression), suggesting that c-*raf* also has a common role in cellular proliferation. If the proliferative scheme described above is correct, it is possible that c-*raf* might be an integral part of this pathway. A molecular study of c-*raf* proteins might provide further evidence for its participation in a proliferative pathway and aid in understanding the nature of the proposed proliferative signal transduction mechanism.

If the hypothesis described above and in Figure 2 were correct, it might be tempting to assume that a proliferative signal originating at a membrane receptor and

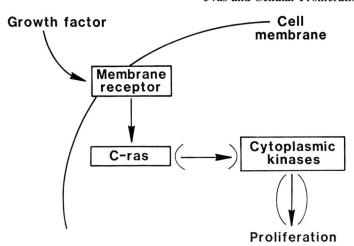

Fig. 2.   Model of cellular oncogene action. As one explanation for the data presented it is proposed that cellular genes important in proliferation are involved in a signal transduction mechanism. Membrane tyrosine kinases such as growth factor receptors receive the initial proliferative signal at the cell surface. Cellular *ras* proteins are involved in transfer of this signal to cytoplasmic serine kinases. The cytoplasmic kinases which are presumably activated in this process phosphorylate the cellular molecules which function in the cellular proliferative response. In this way the membrane receptor-like oncogenes require c-*ras* proteins to relay their proliferative signal, whereas cytoplasmic oncogenes, which act subsequently to c-*ras* proteins, do not depend upon them for activity. Since most tumor cells are able to proliferate following anti-*ras* injection, this scheme would postulate that they contain activating alterations which operate subsequently to c-*ras*. Normal tissues, which depend upon an external proliferative signal, rely upon c-ras to relay this signal into the cell. Consequently normal cells rely upon c-*ras* for proliferation (as do tumors with mutations in c-*ras* itself or molecules which act prior to c-*ras* in this proposed pathway).

passing through c-*ras* proteins to the cytoplasmic kinase molecule might then proceed to the nucleus and to nuclear oncogenes such as c-*myc*, c-*fos*, and the P-53 molecule. This possibility, however, is likely to be an oversimplification. The induction of nuclear oncogenes occurs during mitogenic stimulation much before the initiation of S-phase [27,28] when c-*ras* is required. Microinjection of anti-p53 antibody indicates that this molecule is required during the G0-G1 boundary [29], whereas c-*ras* proteins continue to be required until the G1-S transition. It is therefore likely that two biochemical pathways are involved. Since both are induced by growth factors, possibly even the same growth factors, they might be closely connected functionally. Both pathways appear necessary for cellular proliferation since oncogenes from both appear necessary during transformation [30]. It is clear that tumor formation, proliferation, and differentiation state are all interconnected and that the nuclear oncogenes including c-*myb* are likely to play critical roles during cellular differentiation. It is therefore proposed that nuclear oncogenes function at least in part to prepare the cell to respond to a subsequent proliferative signal.

The proposed mechanism by which cellular oncogenes interrelate (Fig. 2) may help visualize the results described here with tumor cells, but the hypothetical mechanism is not critical to the general conclusion reached. In fact, the conclusions reached in tumor cell studies do not even depend upon the specificity of c-*ras* neutralization. By whatever mechanism it functions, it is clear that the injected antibody 259 can distinguish between the action of two separate classes of viral oncogenes. When injected into tumor cells this distinction is made upon those molecules actually controlling cell proliferation. Such information is totally independent of molecular studies of genome structure and mutations but may help explain the biological significance of these genomic alterations.

While all six normal cell types were dramatically inhibited by anti-*ras* antibody, only 1 of 22 tumor cell lines exhibited similar inhibition. This raises the important possibility that the antibody is able to distinguish between the proliferative properties of most normal and tumor cells. This distinction relies upon the activity of a cellular protein which is known from separate injection experiments to be critical in normal cell proliferation and therefore is likely to relate to the fundamental alterations responsible for uncontrolled tumor cell proliferation. Antibody injection studies further indicate that in most tumor cells proliferation is controlled by a molecule which functions in the presence of injected antibody as do cytoplasmic viral oncogenes. The suggestion that c-*ras* activity is able to distinguish normal from tumor cell proliferation might have important practical significance. If it became possible to interfere pharmacologically with c-*ras* activity, DNA synthesis in normal tissues would be specifically yet temporarily blocked. Treatment with toxic deoxyribonucleotide analogues would be targeted to noninhibited tumor cells.

The opportunity to look critically at the proliferative capacity of normal and tumor cells may have great significance in our understanding of tumor formation. It is, for example, clear that c-*ras* proteins retain a role in proliferation even in the mature tumor cell since all tumor lines with a mutant *ras* gene were inhibited by the antibody. The fact that in five of six cases this inhibition was not as dramatic as observed in normal cells further indicates that activated c-*ras* genes are not alone responsible for proliferation of the mature tumor (although there is evidence that the mutation might be present at the time of tumor initiation) [31]. While further work is required for a more thorough interpretation of the results obtained, it is apparent that antibody injection studies are likely to play an important role in our understanding of molecular control over proliferation in normal and tumor cells. As neutralizing antibodies to other cellular oncogenes are described along with alternative means of eliminating cellular gene activity, these studies can be broadened and further verified.

ACKNOWLEDGMENTS

Steven DeGudicibus, Mark Smith, Linda Mulcahy, and H.F. Kung participated in these studies. I thank Michael Sherman and David Webb for critical reviews of this manuscript, and Janet Hansen for technical assistance in its preparation.

REFERENCES

1. Bishop JM: Cell 42:23–38, 1985.
2. Doolittle RF, Hunkapiller MW, Hood LE, Devare SG, Robbins KC, Aaronson SA, Antoniades HN: Science 221:275–277, 1983.
3. Downward J, Yarden Y, Mayes E, Scrace G, Totty N, Stockwell P, Ullrich A, Schlessinger J, Waterfield MD: Nature 307:521–527, 1984.
4. Waterfield MD, Scrace GT, Whittle N, Stroobant P, Johnsson A, Wasteson A, Westermark B, Heldin C-H, Huang JS, Deuel TF: Nature 304:35–39, 1983.
5. Sherr CJ, Rettenmier CW, Sacca R, Roussel MF, Look AT, Stanley ER: Cell 41:665–676, 1985.
6. Ellis RW, DeFeo D, Shish TY, Gonda MA, Young HA, Tsuchida N, Lowy DR, Scolnick EM: Nature 292:506–511, 1981.

7. Santos E, Tronick SR, Aaronson SA, Pulciani S, Barbacid M: Nature 298:343–347, 1982.
8. Parada LF, Tabin CJ, Shih C, Weinberg RA: Nature 297:474–478, 1982.
9. Reddy EP, Reynolds RK, Santos E, Barbacid M: Nature 300:149–152, 1982.
10. Sweet RW, Yokoyama S, Kamata T, Feramisco JR, Rosenberg M, Gross M: Nature 311:273–275, 1984.
11. McGrath JP, Capon DJ, Goeddel DV, Levinson AD: Nature 310:644–649, 1984.
12. Manne V, Bekesi E, Kung H-F: Proc Natl Acad Sci USA 82:376–380, 1985.
13. Gilman A: Cell 36:577–579, 1984.
14. Stacey DW, Kung H-F: Nature 310:508–511, 1984.
15. Furth ME, Davis LJ, Fleurdelys B, Scolnick EM: J Virol 43:294–304, 1982.
16. Kung H-F, Smith MR, Bekesi E, Manne V, Stacey DW: Exp Cell Res 162:363–371, 1986.
17. Stacey DW, DeGudicibus SJ, Smith MR: Exptl Cell Res (in press).
18. Papageorge AG, Willumsen BM, Johnsen M, Kung H-F, Stacey DW, Vass WC, Lowy DR: Mol Cell Biol 6:1843–1846, 1986.
19. Mulcahy LS, Smith MR, Stacey DW: Nature 313:241–243, 1985.
20. Smith MR, DeGudicibus SJ, Stacey DW: Nature 320:540–543, 1986.
21. Moelling K, Heimann B, Beimling P, Rapp UR, Sander T: Nature 312:558–561, 1984.
22. Papkoff J, Nigg EA, Hunter T: Cell 33:161–172, 1983.
23. Rapp UR, Bonner TI, Moelling K, Jansen HW, Bister K, Ihle J: Recent Results Cancer Res 99:221–236, 1985.
24. Foulds L: "Neoplastic Development, Vol. 1." London: Academic, 1969.
25. Crawford BD, Barrett JC, Ts'o POP: Mol Cell Biol 3:931–945, 1983.
26. Stacey DW, Allfrey VG: J Cell Biol 75:807–817, 1977.
27. Greenberg ME, Ziff EB: Nature 311:433–438, 1984.
28. Muller R, Bravo R, Burchhardt J, Curran T: Nature 312:716–720, 1984.
29. Mercer WE, Avignolo C, Baserga R: Mol Cell Biol 4:276–281, 1984.
30. Ruley HE: Nature 304:602–606, 1983.
31. Zarbl H, Sukumar S, Arthur AW, Martin-Zanca D, Barbacid M: Nature 315:382–385, 1985.

Cellular and Molecular Biology of Tumors and Potential
Clinical Applications 225–237 (1988)

Role of the Proto-Oncogene *fos* During Growth and Differentiation

Richard L. Mitchell, Wiebe Kruijer, David Schubert, Charles Van Beveren,
and Inder M. Verma

The Salk Institute, San Diego, California 92138

During pre- and postnatal development of the mouse, expression of the proto-oncogene *fos* is highest in specific tissues, particularly in amnion, yolk sac, and midgestation fetal liver and bone marrow. Macrophage cell lines and peritoneal macrophages also express high levels of *fos* transcripts. Within minutes after the initiation of phorbol ester (tetradecanoylphorbol-13-acetate [TPA])-induced differentiation of HL-60 or U-937 promyelocyte or promonocyte cell lines to macrophages, c-*fos* gene expression is dramatically increased. In U-937 cells, transcripts of *fos* are detectable for at least 240 hr following TPA treatment, but at a level 3–4-fold lower than the highest levels, which are seen within 30 min of TPA addition. In contrast, *fos* protein is detectable for only 90–120 min postinduction. Differentiation of PC12 cells to neurites following treatment with nerve growth factor (NGF) is also accompanied by the rapid and transient expression of *fos* mRNA and protein, but *fos* transcripts become undetectable within 120–240 min after the addition of NGF. Following the mitogenic stimulation of quiescent mouse fibroblasts, expression of *fos* is one of the earliest detectable events. We discuss the complex regulation of the *fos* gene in the context of its role in normal cells and its ability to induce cellular transformation in vitro.

Key words: macrophage, neurite, fibroblast, transformation

Structural similarities between retroviral oncogenes and their cellular homologs (proto-oncogenes) supports the hypothesis that proto-oncogenes may be critically involved in cellular growth control. The products of at least three proto-oncogenes are related to normal cellular proteins known to regulate cellular growth. The c-*sis* gene probably encodes the β-chain of platelet-derived growth factor (PDGF) [1,2]; the c-*erb*-B gene is a truncated form of the epidermal growth factor (EGF) receptor gene [3,4]; and the c-*fms* gene product is related to or identical with the receptor for macrophage colony-stimulating factor (CSF-1) [5]. Extensive phylogenetic conserva-

Received April 18, 1986.

Wiebe Kruijer's present address is Hubrecht Laboratorium, Uppsalalaan, 8, 3584 CT, Utrecht, The Netherlands.

tion and tissue- and stage-specific expression of many proto-oncogenes lends further support to the notion that these genes are involved in normal cellular processes [6,7]. An extensive survey of the expression of proto-oncogenes has been compiled [8]. In this manuscript, we report the unique structural features of proto-oncogene *fos* and its expression in a variety of cell types.

MATERIALS AND METHODS
Cell Cultures and Inductions

We have previously described the conditions for maintenance of human leukemia cell lines U-937 and HL-60 [9], PC12 cells [10], and NIH-3T3 cells [11]. A fresh solution of each inducer was prepared for each experiment from stock solutions of 12-O-tetradecanoylphorbol-13-acetate (TPA, Sigma), [1 mg/ml in dimethyl sulfoxide (DMSO)] or 1-oleoyl-2-acetyl-*rac*-glycerol (diacylglycerol, Sigma) [100 mg/ml in DMSO]. Addition of PDGF (essentially homogeneous, purified through phenyl-Sepharose, dissolved in 1 mM acetic acid containing 1 mg/ml BSA) or an equal volume of 1 mg/ml BSA in 1 mM acetic acid was made directly to the medium. Other inducers were added directly to the culture medium in the DMSO solvent, and DMSO at the final concentration of 0.2% in the growth medium as used in the experiments did not affect the expression of the various differentiation markers. The protein synthesis inhibitor cycloheximide (10 mg/ml in H_2O) and the transcription inhibitor actinomycin D (10 mg/ml in H_2O) were added directly to cultures to achieve final concentrations of 10 μg/ml each.

Isolation and Analysis of Total Cellular RNA

Total cellular RNA was isolated by the method of Chirgwin et al [12] and analyzed by electrophoresis of 15-μg samples through 1% agarose formaldehyde gels [13] followed by Northern blot transfer to nitrocellulose [14] and hybridization to radiolabeled probes. Oncogene-specific probes were isolated from agarose gels by electroelution onto NA45 membrane filters, then labeled with [α^{32}P]-dCTP (>3,000 Ci/mmol, New England Nuclear, Boston, MA) by nick translation [15]. Nitrocellulose filters were pretreated, hybridized in 50% formamide, and washed according to published procedures [16] before autoradiography. RNA protection experiments were performed as described previously [10]. The size of the protected fragments was determined relative to denatured TaqI fragments of pBR322 end-labeled with ^{32}P.

Analysis of *fos* Protein Expression

Immunoprecipitates were analyzed by SDS-PAGE. Except where noted, confluent 35-mm-dish cultures of 3T3 cells were incubated in 1 ml of Dulbecco's modified eagle medium (DME) containing methionine at 1% of the regular concentration and 0.5% calf serum for 40–48 hr, and ^{35}S-methionine (100 μCi of <1,000 Ci/mmol; Amersham/Searle, Arlington Heights, IL) was added directly to the medium. Cultures were lysed after washing with cold Tris-buffered saline by adding 0.5 ml of RIPA buffer (0.15 M NaCl, 1% Nonidet P-40, 5% sodium deoxycholate, 0.5% SDS, 2 mM EDTA, 100 U/ml Trasylol, 10 mM sodium phosphate, pH 7.0) and scraping. Lysates were clarified at 20,000g for 60 min at 4°C. IgG or antisera were added as indicated. After 1 hr at 0°C, 1 mg of Pansorbin (Calbiochem, La Jolla, CA) was added for a further 1 hr. Immunoprecipitates were centrifuged through a solution of

10% sucrose in RIPA, then washed repeatedly by centrifugation in RIPA. When required, separation into cytoplasmic and nuclear fractions was performed as described before [10]. Briefly, after washing with Tris-saline, the cells were scraped from the dish in 1.0 ml of 1 mM dithiothreitol (DTT), 10 mM HEPES (pH 7.4), and 10 U/ml Trasylol and homogenized in a Teflon/glass homogenizer. Half of the sample was removed, and the remainder was centrifuged at 600g for 5 min at 4°C. One volume of twice-concentrated RIPA buffer was added to each fraction. Homogenate, supernatant, and pellet fractions are identified in the figure legends. For immunoprecipitations with rat antitumor serum or normal rat serum, goat antiserum to rat IgG was added 30 min prior to Pansorbin. Immunoprecipitates were dissociated by incubation at 100°C for 2 min in 2% SDS, 20% β-mercaptoethanol, 10% glycerol, and 0.1 M Tris-HCl (pH 6.8); and one-half of each sample was analyzed by SDS-PAGE (12.5% acrylamide, 0.10% bis-acrylamide). Gels were stained to visualize marker β-galactosidase, phosphorylase, BSA, ovalbumin, and carbonic anhydrase and impregnated with diphenyloxazole. Dried gels were exposed to presensitized film at $-70°C$.

RESULTS

Structure of the *fos* Gene

Before the nature of *fos* gene expression was known, the complete molecular structure of the gene had been determined. This was fortunate, since this knowledge helped us to grasp the subtle and complex regulation of its expression.

The c-*fos* gene is the cellular homolog of the transforming gene carried by FBJ murine sarcoma virus (FBJ-MSV) and FBR-MSV [17,18]. The complete nucleotide sequences of c-*fos* and of the proviral DNAs of FBJ-MSV and FBR-MSV have been determined [19,20]. Figure 1 is a diagram of the organization of viral and cellular *fos* genes and the protein products deduced from their sequences. The salient features can be summarized as follows:

1. FBJ-MSV proviral DNA contains 4,026 nucleotides, including the two long terminal repeats (LTRs) of 617 nucleotides each, 1,639 nucleotides of acquired cellular sequences (v-*fos*), and a portion of the envelope (*env*) gene.

2. Both the initiation and termination codons of the v-*fos* protein are within the acquired sequences that encode a protein of 381 amino acids, having a molecular weight of 49,601.

3. In cells transformed by FBJ-MSV, a phosphoprotein with an apparent M_r of 55,000 (p55) on SDS-PAGE has been identified as the transforming protein [21]. The discrepancy between the observed size and the size predicted by sequence analysis is likely due to the unusual amino acid composition of the *fos* protein (10% proline), since the v-*fos* protein expressed in bacteria has a similar relative mobility [22].

4. The sequences in the c-*fos* gene that are homologous to those in the v-*fos* gene are interrupted by four regions of nonhomology, three of which represent bona fide introns.

5. The 104-nucleotide-long fourth region, which is present in both mouse and human c-*fos* genes, represents sequences that have been deleted during the biogenesis of the v-*fos* gene. (The additional 104 nucleotides in the c-*fos* gene transcripts do not increase the predicted size of the c-*fos* proteins, because of a switch to a different reading frame.)

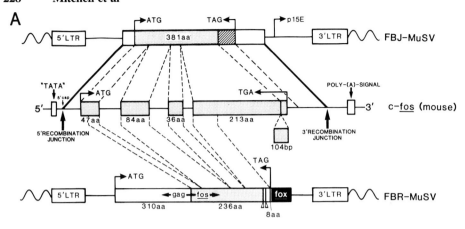

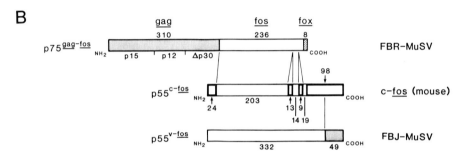

Fig. 1.   **A**: Molecular architecture of FBJ-MSV (top) and FBR-MSV (bottom) proviral DNAs and the c-*fos* gene (middle). **Top**: The large, stippled box indicates the acquired cellular sequences; solid, vertical bars indicate the initiation and termination codons of v-*fos* proteins; the hatched region indicates the carboxyterminal 49 amino acids of the v-*fos* protein encoded in a different reading frame owing to deletion of 104 bp of c-*fos* sequences. **Middle**: The stippled boxes are the exons; the number of amino acids encoded by each exon is given. The 104-bp sequence that has been deleted in the v-*fos* sequence is indicated with a box below the line. Unlike the v-*fos* protein, the c-*fos* protein terminates at a TGA codon. **Bottom**: Broken lines indicate the portions of the exons acquired from the c-*fos* gene; small open triangles indicate deletions from FBR-MSV as compared with the c-*fos* gene. Details of the structure of FBR-MSV proviral DNA have previously been described [19]. **B**: A schematic comparison of p75$^{gag\text{-}fos}$ (**top**), p55$^{c\text{-}fos}$ (**middle**), and p55$^{v\text{-}fos}$ (**bottom**) proteins. In p75, the *gag*-encoded portion is indicated with a stippled box; and that encoded by v-*fox* is shown by the hatched box. The regions of p55$^{c\text{-}fos}$ indicated by thickened boxes and vertical arrows are those portions deleted in p75$^{gag\text{-}fos}$. The hatched regions in p55$^{v\text{-}fos}$ is the carboxyterminal portion, which differs from that of p55$^{c\text{-}fos}$. The numbers refer to the number of amino acids encoded by each region.

6. The c-*fos* protein is 380 amino acids in length, which is remarkably similar to the size of the v-*fos* protein (381 amino acids).

7. In the first 332 amino acids, the v-*fos* and mouse c-*fos* proteins differ at only five residues, while the remaining 48 amino acids of the c-*fos* protein are encoded in a different reading frame from that in the v-*fos* protein. Thus the v-*fos* and c-*fos* proteins, though largely similar, have different carboxyl termini (Fig. 1B).

8. Despite their different carboxyl termini, both the v-*fos* and c-*fos* proteins are located in the nucleus. Still, the c-*fos* protein undergoes more extensive modifications than the v-*fos* protein.

9. The mouse and human c-*fos* genes share greater than 90% sequence homology, differing in only 24 residues out of a total of 380 amino acids [23].

10. FBR-MSV proviral DNA contains 3,791 nucleotides (specifying a genome of 3,284 bases) and encodes a single *gag-fos* fusion product of 554 amino acids.

11. The *fos* portion of the genome lacks sequences that encode the first 24 and the last 98 amino acids of the 380 amino acid mouse c-*fos* gene product (Fig. 1B). In addition, the coding region has sustained three small in-frame deletions, one in the p30*gag* portion and two in the *fos* region as compared with sequences of AKR-MLV and the c-*fos* gene, respectively [19].

12. The gene product terminates in sequences termed *fox* (Fig. 1A) which are present in normal mouse DNA at loci unrelated to the c-*fos* gene. The c-*fox* gene(s) is expressed as an abundant class of polyadenylated RNA in mouse tissues.

Expression During Prenatal Development

We have previously shown that many proto-oncogenes are not only expressed in specific tissues during prenatal mouse development, but, moreover, their expression is temporally regulated as well [6,8]. Some oncogenes, like *fos* and *fms*, are expressed early during development, while others, like *abl*, are expressed at the highest levels during midgestation. Proto-oncogene *ras*[Ha] is expressed at all stages of development. An extensive evaluation of the expression of *fos* and *fms* genes reveals that these genes are expressed at the highest levels in extraembryonal tissues (placenta, amnion, and yolk sac) [8]. The levels of *fms* expression are found to be low in day 10–12 extraembryonal membranes but increase approximately sixfold between day 12 and day 18 to a level that is slightly higher than that observed in the placenta. A detailed analysis of the microsurgically isolated components of the late-gestation extraembryonal membranes showed that the levels of *fos* transcripts are higher in visceral yolk sac (endoderm and mesoderm), as compared to placenta. Furthermore, the highest levels of c-*fos* are observed in day 18 amnion. These levels are close to those of v-*fos* transcripts in FBJ-MSV transformed cells. The nuclear *fos* protein is detected in amnion cells, both by immunoprecipitation as well as by immunofluorescence with specific antisera [24].

Expression During Hematopoiesis

In postnatal tissues, we initially found the highest levels of *fos* expression in neonatal bone [8]. Subsequent analysis revealed that *fos* expression was confined primarily to bone marrow tissue present in our neonatal bone preparations. Although macrophages constitute only a small percentage of the bone marrow cell population, initial experiments revealed c-*fos* transcripts in macrophage cell lines and in peritoneal exudates enriched for macrophages. Since this indicated that *fos* might have a role in macrophage differentiation, we studied the expression of c-*fos* during the differentiation of several hematopoietic cell lines.

Our results showed that c-*fos* expression is rapidly induced during TPA-induced differentiation of HL-60 or U-937 promyelocyte or promonocyte cell lines to macrophages [25]. The highest levels of c-*fos* transcripts are detected within 30–60 min of TPA treatment, followed by a decline of 4–5-fold to a level that is maintained for at least 10 days. Despite the persistence of the mRNA, c-*fos* protein is detectable for only 120 min after TPA treatment. In contrast, no c-*fos* is expressed during dimethylsulfoxide (DMSO)-induced differentiation of HL-60 cells to granulocytes.

By run-off transcription analysis, we have recently shown that *fos* expression is regulated primarily at the transcriptional level following TPA treatment [25]. In the presence of cycloheximide (CH), c-*fos* mRNA is superinduced by TPA. The super-induction of *fos* by TPA in the presence of CH is primarily due to an increased stability of the mRNA, since the half-life of c-*fos* mRNA is increased from less than 30 min in the absence of CH to more than 4 h in the presence of CH [25]. Degradation of *fos* mRNA is characterized by a slow, progressive cleavage of about 200 nucleotides, followed by a more rapid complete degradation of the molecule (Fig. 2A; ref. 25). We do not yet know from which end of the molecule the progressive shortening occurs, but one attractive possibility is the selective loss of sequences at the 3' end which have been implicated in the stability of c-*fos* mRNA [26].

Is the expression of c-*fos* necessary for macrophage differentiation or is it merely a coincidental effect of the agents which induce differentiation of HL-60 and U-937 cells? Two lines of evidence suggest that *fos* expression results from activation of C-kinase and is unnecessary for the expression of most macrophage markers. First, certain agents that activate C-kinase such as diacylglycerol [25] or the calcium ionophore A23187 (Fig. 2B) invariably induce transient *fos* expression, yet fail to induce the differentiation of U-937 or HL-60 cells. In fact, when rat 208F cells are treated with TPA for 60 hr to down-regulate C-kinase, they fail to express *fos* when stimulated with diacylglycerol, lending support to the notion that C-kinase activation is crucial for *fos* expression (Fig. 2C). Second, studies on TPA-resistant HL-60 cell variants demonstrated differentiation to macrophages in the absence of detectable *fos*

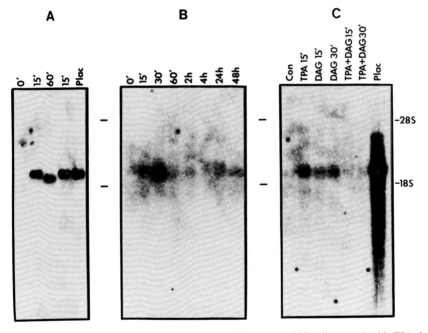

Fig. 2.   **A**: Size of *fos* transcripts in human placenta (Plac), or U-937 cells treated with TPA for 15 min (two aliquots, 15′) and cultivated an additional 60 min in the presence of actinomycin D (60′). **B**: Expression of *fos* transcripts at indicated intervals following treatment of U-937 cells with A23187. **C**: *fos* transcripts detected in rat 208F cells (Con) or, as indicated in the figure, treated with TPA (TPA) or diacylglycerol (DAG) for the times indicated, or treated with diacylglycerol (TPA+DAG) for the times indicated after 60 hr of preincubation in the presence of TPA.

expression after treatment with the vitamin D_3 metabolite $1,25\text{-}(OH)_2D_3$ [25]. It is intriguing that these TPA-resistant HL-60 cell variants which fail to express *fos* also fail to become growth arrested when induced to differentiate. Perhaps *fos* expression has a role in the growth arrest that normally accompanies differentiation of HL-60 cells.

Expression During Neuronal Differentiation

To investigate further the role of the *fos* gene in differentiation, we have studied the induction of its expression by nerve growth factor (NGF) in the clonal rat pheochromocytoma cell line PC12. In the presence of NGF, PC12 cells acquire properties of sympathetic neurons, including neurite outgrowth, increased electrical excitability, and changes in neurotransmitter synthesis [27,28]. NGF may also act as a weak mitogen in these cells [29]. Figure 3A shows that *fos* gene transcripts can be detected 5 min after addition of NGF, are maximally abundant after 30 min, and that their levels decrease thereafter. Synthesis of the p55/65 *fos* protein parallels the expression of *fos* mRNA (Fig. 3B) and the induced *fos* proteins are located in the nucleus (Fig. 3C).

Binding of NGF to its cell surface receptor causes a rapid (within min) and transient increase in intracellular cyclic AMP (cAMP) [30]. Figure 4A shows that dibutyryl cAMP also induces *fos* gene transcription upon addition to PC12 cells, although with slightly slower kinetics than NGF. Exogenous K^+ induces neurite outgrowth without a detectable increase in the level of intracellular cAMP [30]. It

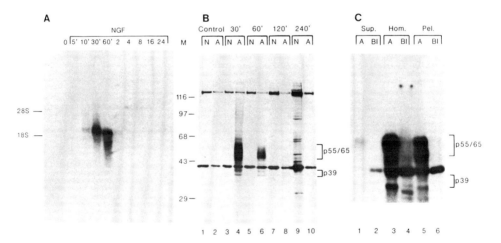

Fig. 3. **A:** *fos* expression in NGF-induced PC12 cell line—Northern blot analysis of total RNA (15 μg/lane) isolated at the indicated times after addition of 50 ng/ml of NGF. After electrophoresis and Northern transfer, *fos*-specific sequences were detected by hybridization to ^{32}P-labeled v-*fos* probe. **B:** Characterization of *fos* proteins—kinetics of *fos* synthesis. PC12 cells were induced for the times indicated, followed by labeling with ^{35}S-methionine (New England Nuclear, 600–1,000 Ci/mmol) for 20 min. RIPA lysates were immunoprecipitated with normal rabbit serum (N, **lanes 1,3,5,7,9**) or with affinity-purified M2 peptide antiserum (A, **lanes 2,4,6,8,10**). The position of *fos* and p39 proteins is indicated. M; molecular weight standards. **C:** Subcellular localization of *fos* proteins—PC12 cells were induced with 50 ng/ml NGF for 30 min and labeled for 20 min in 5 ml of N2 (low methionine) medium with 0.1 mCi/ml of ^{35}S-methionine. Half of the total homogenate (**lanes 1,2**), supernatant (**lanes 3,4**), and pellet (**lanes 5,6**) were immunoprecipitated with M2 peptide antiserum (lanes 1,3,5) or M2 peptide antiserum preincubated with excess M peptide (lanes 2,4,6).

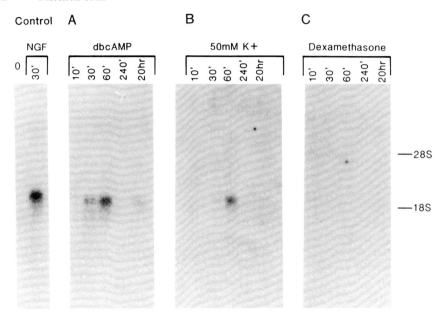

Fig. 4.   Induction of *fos* mRNA by dbcAMP, 50 mM K$^+$, and dexamethasone. Subconfluent PC12 cells were induced with NGF (50 ng/ml), dbcAMP (1 × 10^{-3} M), K$^+$ (50 mM), or dexamethasone (1 × 10^{-6} M), for the times indicated.

causes an influx of Ca^{++} ions, which can directly stimulate neurite extension in PC12 cells. Although it does not lead to enhanced cAMP levels, 50 mM K$^+$ depolarization does induce *fos* expression (Fig. 4B). In addition to NGF, cAMP and elevated K$^+$, TPA, and epidermal growth factor (EGF) also induce *fos* [10]. All of these reagents also rapidly stimulate the phosphorylation of PC12 tyrosine hydroxylase at one or more of four distinct sites in the enzyme [31]. The phosphorylation of only one site is stimulated by TPA, but the TPA-stimulated site is also phosphorylated in response to cAMP, EGF, NGF, and K$^+$ depolarization. Since TPA is a fairly specific activator of C-kinase, and since all conditions which cause the C-kinase-specific phosphorylation of tyrosine hydroxylase peptides also increase *fos* expression, it again follows that C-kinase may be involved in the induction of *fos* expression.

PC12 cells have some degree of developmental plasticity in that they can be induced to differentiate into cells with characteristics of sympathetic ganglion cells by NGF treatment, and into cells that resemble chromaffin cells when treated with corticosteroids [32]. Neither *fos* mRNA nor *fos* proteins were detected up to 5 days after the addition of dexamethasone, indicating that the expression of the *fos* gene is correlated with the pathway of differentiation induced by NGF but not corticosteroids (Fig. 4C).

Expression During Cell Growth

It has previously been shown that when quiescent mouse fibroblasts are treated with serum or growth factors like PDGF, EGF, or TPA, the proto-oncogene *fos* is rapidly induced [10,33–35]. The salient features of these observations are shown in a composite figure (Fig. 5) and can be summarized as follows: 1) Within 2–3 min of stimulation of growth, c-*fos* transcripts can be detected as measured by hybridization with ^{32}P-labeled complementary RNA (cRNA [10]). 2) Maximal levels of induction (20-fold) occur within 20 min of the exposure of cells to 0.83 nM purified PDGF. The levels declined by 60 min, and by 240 min little or no c-*fos* transcript could be detected. 3) Addition of cycloheximide resulted in a 50-fold induction, suggesting stabilization of c-*fos* mRNA transcripts. 4) We estimate that after a 20-min exposure to PDGF, 0.0001% of NIH/3T3 cell RNA (0.005% of mRNA) is c-*fos* mRNA. Assuming a cellular RNA content of about 6 pg, this corresponds to about 5–10 copies of *fos* mRNA per cell. 5) Exposure to PDGF for a time as short as 30 min induces the synthesis of *fos* protein which can be detected by immunoprecipitation with *fos*-specific peptide antisera. 6) At least 6–8 polypeptides are identified by immune precipitation, most of which represent modified forms of *fos* protein; however, some non-*fos* polypeptides are also precipitated. One possibility is that some of them may be related to *fos* and may react with peptide antisera [33]. 7) c-*fos* protein synthesis was maximal with PDGF concentrations that saturate PDGF binding sites at 37°C (1.0 nM) and half-maximal at 0.3–0.5 nM. 8) It appears that c-*fos* is transiently induced in response to a variety of mitogens in addition to inducers of differentiation.

DISCUSSION
Regulation of *fos* Expression

fos is a multifaceted gene, the product of which may play a role during development, cellular differentiation, and cell growth. Since the products of both the viral and cellular *fos* genes can induce the transformation of fibroblasts in vitro, it is puzzling that the expression of *fos* protein in vivo and the induced expression of *fos* in vitro do not result in transformation. It is possible that some cell types, such as peritoneal macrophages or macrophages in culture, are refractory to transformation by *fos*, even during sustained expression of *fos* mRNA. Perhaps fibroblasts and other cells that are normally susceptible to c-*fos*-induced transformation are not transformed because the expression of the *fos* protein is only transient.

The synthesis of the *fos* gene product displays an exquisite regulation. Our previous findings have led us to believe that *fos* protein synthesis may be regulated post-transcriptionally, or even more likely, at the first translational level. Two sets of observations favor this notion. First, when the intact proto-oncogene c-*fos* is transcribed constitutively, it is unable to transform fibroblasts and only very low levels of the *fos* protein are detected [36]. The *fos* gene becomes transforming when a short stretch of only 67 base pairs (bp) located 527 bp downstream of the termination codon and 123 bp upstream of the poly(A) addition site, is removed [31]. We hypothesize that the *fos* protein may regulate its own synthesis, possibly by binding to the 67-bp region and altering the translational efficiency of the c-*fos* mRNA. Second, and perhaps related, is the observation that promonocytes induced to differentiate into macrophages following treatment with TPA continue to express *fos* mRNA for at least 10 days, even though the *fos* protein is only detected for 10–120 min following treatment with the inducer [9].

We have no firm grip on the mechanism of such a translational control. We have been unable to demonstrate any homologies or complementarity between the 67-bp stretch and the rest of the gene. In addition, there are at least two pitfalls in our hypothesis of a translational control mechanism. First, it is possible that the c-*fos*

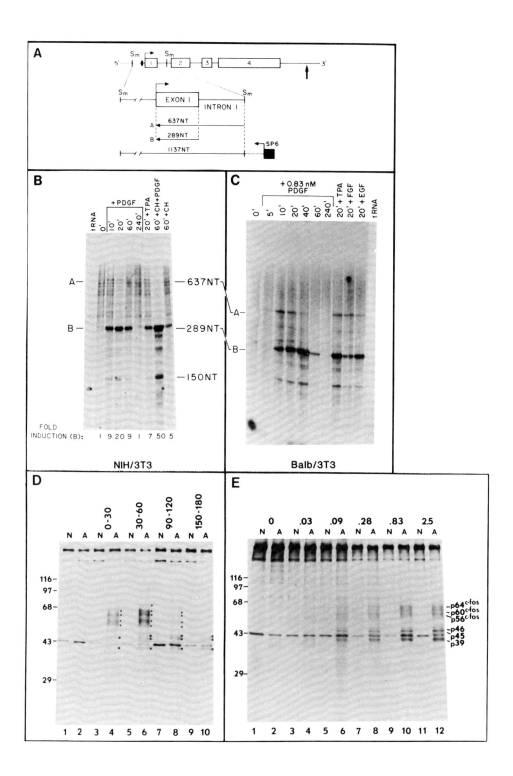

protein is made in cells carrying the nontransforming construct, but we are unable to detect the protein with our *fos* antisera because of extensive protein modifications. Second, the *fos* protein appears to be exclusively nuclear, at least by immunofluorescence, yet a direct translational control mechanism would likely require some cytoplasmic *fos* protein. Regardless of the molecular mechanism controlling *fos* at the transcriptional or post-transcriptional level, we believe that the natural expression of the c-*fos* protein does not transform cells because the expression of the protein is only transient. In contrast, v-*fos* escapes this regulation of *fos* protein synthesis due to its altered C-terminus, and hence induces transformation.

Transcriptional Regulation of *fos* Synthesis

Sequences required for efficient functioning of a gene are likely to be conserved during evolution. A transcriptional enhancer element of proto-oncogene *fos* has been identified in such a conserved region [26,37]. It lies between -60 to -400 nucleotides upstream of the 5' cap nucleotide. A dot matrix analysis of identities between the promoter and 5' flanking regions of the human and mouse *fos* genes indicates two regions of striking similarity; one surrounding the cap site and TATAA box and another stretching from -250 to -475, the region identified as the transcriptional enhancer [37]. The same two regions also bear a DNAase I hypersensitive site, another hallmark of a region involved in regulation of transcription. The precise nature of the essential sequences in the enhancer region and the molecular mechanism underlying their functioning remains to be established. The proto-oncogene *fos* could be a housekeeping gene, since it is transcribed at low levels in most if not all cells. One would thus expect the *fos* enhancer to be non-tissue-specific, a notion borne out by our observations that enhancer activity assays, as well as the mapping of DNAase I hypersensitive sites, give similar results in different cell types [37].

Fig. 5. Analysis of PDGF-stimulated c-*fos* RNA and proteins. **A**: Diagram of the molecular structure of the mouse c-*fos* gene, based on nucleotide sequence analysis. Expected sizes of the protected c-*fos* mRNA transcripts are indicated. Positions of putative 5'-cap (rightward-bent arrow), polyadenylation signal (↑), TATAA Box (■), exon (□), intron (——), SP6 phage promoter (filled box with leftward-bent arrow), and vector (......) are indicated. **B,C**: Analysis of c-*fos* transcripts. Total RNA from PDGF-treated cells was used for RNA protection experiments. Times of induction (min) and types of treatment are indicated. As a control for self-hybridization of the probe, one hybridization contained 10 μg for tRNA in place of cellular RNA. The expected size of fragment A was 637 nucleotides (nt), and that of fragment B was 189 nt. For experimental details, see [10]. **D**: Time course of c-*fos* protein synthesis. BALB/c 3T3 cell cultures were treated with 0.67 nM pure PDGF for 0 min (**lanes 3, 4**), 30 min (**lanes 5, 6**), 90 min (**lanes 7, 8**), or 150 min (**lanes 9, 10**) before the addition of 100 μCi ^{35}S-methionine. Another culture received an equivalent volume of bovine serum albumin (BSA) in 1 mM acetic acid for 30 min before labeling (**lanes 1, 2**). After a further 30 min of incubation, cultures were washed, lysed, and one-third volumes were immunoprecipitated with 1 μg of IgG equivalent of nonimmune rabbit serum (N; lanes 1, 3, 5, 7, 9) or 1 μg of affinity-purified IgG to M peptide (A; lanes 2, 4, 6, 8, 10). Immunoprecipitates were analyzed by SDS-PAGE. Closed circles, proteins related to p55$^{c\text{-}fos}$; open circles, unrelated proteins. A band of 43 kilodaltons, observed in all samples, is most likely actin. **E**: Dose dependence of c-*fos* protein synthesis. NIH-3T3 cells were exposed to PDGF at final concentrations of 0 nM (**lanes 1, 2**), 0.03 nM (**lanes 3, 4**), 0.09 nM (**lanes 5, 6**), 0.28 nM (**lanes 7, 8**), 0.83 nM (**lanes 9, 10**), or 2.5 nM (**lanes 11, 12**). Each lysate was immunoprecipitated with nonimmune rabbit serum (N; lanes 1, 3, 5, 7, 9, 11) or 1 μg of affinity-purified IgG to M peptide (A; lanes 2, 4, 6, 8, 10, 12). Exposure times: (D) 10 days; (E) 4 days.

What role does *fos* play in development, growth, and differentiation? Perhaps *fos* is expressed as a general anabolic response of cells to specific stimuli. If this is the case, such an explanation must account for the expression of *fos* in response to only a subset of differentiation inducers. Indeed, *fos* is expressed during differentiation of cells of the monocytic lineage to macrophages, but not granulocytes, though its expression is unnecessary for the expression of most macrophage markers. Similarly, *fos* is induced when PC12 cells differentiate into neurites with NGF, but not when they differentiate into chromaffin cells when treated with steroids. One way to establish the role of the *fos* gene in differentiation will be to introduce the gene into cells and determine if the expression of the introduced gene induces differentiation in the absence of other inducing agents. Another approach to study the role of the *fos* gene will be to block *fos* protein synthesis in cells treated with differentiation inducers using eukaryotic vectors expressing anti-sense *fos* mRNA.

ACKNOWLEDGMENTS

We thank Liza Zokas for excellent technical assistance and J. Deschamps and F. Meijlink for their sustained interest in this work.

This work was supported by grants from the National Institutes of Health, the American Cancer Society, and the Muscular Dystrophy Association of America. R.L.M. was supported by a National Institutes of Health postdoctoral fellowship (08-F32GM 10161A). W.K. was supported by a fellowship from the Dutch Queen Wilhelmina Fund.

REFERENCES

1. Doolittle RF, Hunkapiller MW, Hood LE, Devare SG, Robbins EC, Aaronson SA, Antoniades HN: Science 221:275, 1983.
2. Waterfield MD, Scrace GT, Whittle N, Stroobant P, Johnsson A, Wasteson A, Westermark B, Heldin C-H, Huang JS, Deuel TF: Nature 304:35, 1983.
3. Downward J, Yarden Y, Mayes E, Scrace G, Totty N, Stockwell P, Ullrich A, Schlessinger J, Waterfield MD: Nature 307:521, 1984.
4. Ullrich A, Coussens L, Hayflick JS, Dull TJ, Gray A, Tam AW, Lee J, Yarden Y, Libermann TA, Schlessinger J, Downward J, Mayes ELV, Whittle N, Waterfield MD, Seeburg PH: Nature 309:418, 1984.
5. Scherr CJ, Rettenmier CW, Sacca R, Roussel MF, Look AT, Stanley ER: Cell 41:665, 1981.
6. Muller R, Slamon DJ, Tremblay JM, Cline MJ, Verma IM: Nature 299:640, 1982.
7. Shilo BZ, Weinberg RA: Proc Natl Acad Sci USA 78:6789, 1981.
8. Muller R, Verma IM: Curr Top Microbiol Immunol 112:73, 1984.
9. Mitchell RL, Zokas L, Schreiber RD, Verma IM: Cell 40:209, 1985.
10. Kruijer W, Schubert D, Verma IM: Proc Natl Acad Sci USA 82:7330, 1985.
11. Kruijer W, Cooper JA, Hunter T, Verma IM: Nature 312:711, 1984.
12. Chirgwin M, Przybyla AE, MacDonald RJ, Rutter WJ: Biochemistry 18:5294, 1979.
13. Lehrach H, Diamond D, Wozney JM, Boedtker H: Biochemistry 16:4763, 1977.
14. Thomas PS: Proc Natl Acad Sci USA 77:5201, 1980.
15. Rigby PWJ, Dieckmann M, Rhodes C, Berg P: J Mol Biol 113:237, 1977.
16. Meinkoth J, Wahl G: Anal Biochem 138:267, 1984.
17. Finkel MP, Biskis BO, Jinkins PB: Science 151:698, 1966.
18. Finkel MP, Reilly CA, Jr, Biskis BO, Greco IL: Colston Res Soc Proc Symp 24:353, 1973.
19. Van Beveren C, Enami S, Curran T, Verma IM: Virology 135:229, 1984.
20. Van Beveren C, van Straaten F, Curran T, Muller R, Verma IM: Cell 32:1241, 1983.
21. Curran T, Peters G, Van Beveren C, Teich NM, Verma IM: J Virol 44:674, 1982.

22. MacConnel WP, Verma IM: Virology 131:367, 1983.
23. van Straaten F, Muller R, Curran T, Van Beveren C, Verma IM: Proc Natl Acad Sci USA 80:3183, 1983.
24. Curran T, Miller AD, Zokas LM, Verma IM: Cell 36:259, 1984.
25. Mitchell RL, Henning-Chubb C, Huberman E, Verma IM: Cell 45:497, 1986.
26. Treisman R: Cell 42:889, 1985.
27. Dichter MA, Tischler AS, Greene LA: Nature 268:501, 1977.
28. Green LA, Tischler A: Proc Natl Acad Sci USA 73:2424, 1976.
29. Boonstra J, Moolenaar WH, Harrison PH, Moed P, van der Saag PT, De Laat SW: J Cell Biol 97:92, 1983.
30. Traynor A, Schubert D: Dev Brain Res 14:197, 1984.
31. Meijlink F, Curran T, Miller AD, Verma IM: Proc Natl Acad Sci USA 82:4987, 1985.
32. Schubert D, LaCorbiere M, Klier FG, Steinbach JH: Brain Res 109:67, 1980.
33. Cochran BM, Zullo J, Verma IM, Stiles CD: Science 226:1080, 1984.
34. Greenberg ME, Ziff EB: Nature 311:433, 1984.
35. Muller R, Bravo R, Buckhardt J, Curran T: Nature 312:716, 1984.
36. Miller AD, Curran T, Verma IM: Cell 36:51, 1984.
37. Deschamps J, Meijlink F, Verma IM: Science 230:1174, 1985.

Cellular and Molecular Biology of Tumors and Potential Clinical Applications 239–246 (1988)

Structure and Differential Regulation of the *myb* Proto-Oncogene in Murine B-Lymphoid Tumors

Timothy P. Bender and W. Michael Kuehl

National Cancer Institute, NCI-Navy Medical Oncology Branch, Naval Hospital, Bethesda, Maryland 20814–2015

We have examined the steady-state levels of c-*myb* mRNA in a series of murine B-lymphoid tumor cell lines representative of the pre-B-cell, immature and mature B-cell, and plasma cell stages of development. The pre-B-cell lymphomas all express equivalent high levels of c-*myb* mRNA. In contrast, the B-cell lymphomas and plasmacytomas all express detectable but low steady-state levels of c-*myb* mRNA which were 0.05 to less than 0.005 units relative to the pre-B-cell lymphomas. This suggests that c-*myb* mRNA is expressed at high levels in pre-B-cell stage of development. The 7OZ/3.12 bacterial lipopolysaccharide (LPS) inducible pre-B-cell lymphoma line and hybrid B-lymphoid cell lines were used to examine events at the pre-B-cell/B-cell junction. These experiments clearly correlate high levels of c-*myb* mRNA expression with the pre-B-cell phenotype and demonstrate differential regulation of this expression. To begin examination of this regulation we have recently reported the structure and nucleotide sequence of c-*myb* mRNA in a murine pre-B-cell lymphoma line. We show that the 5′ end of c-*myb* mRNA is very heterogeneous in both nuclear and cytoplasmic RNA preparations, suggesting multiple transcription initiation sites.

Key words: oncogene expression, B-cell development, 5′mRNA heterogeneity, mRNA structure

Murine B-lymphoid development progresses through a series of discrete stages from a presumed committed stem cell to a terminally differentiated plasma cell [1]. These stages have been defined based on criteria including immunoglobulin gene rearrangement and expression [2,3], J-chain expression [4], and the expression of cell surface markers including Ia antigens [5]. The earliest identifiable cells in the B-lymphoid lineage are pre-B-cells which have rearranged their heavy chain locus (IgH) and express cytoplasmic mu heavy chain protein though rearrangement of the light chain locus has not yet occurred [3]. Subsequently, L-chain gene rearrangement takes place. Pre-B-cells do not express Ia antigen on the cell surface nor make J-chain. The intermediate B-cell stage is characterized by the presence of membrane-bound im-

Received March 25, 1986.

munoglobulin. Initially, immature B-cells express membrane-bound IgM (mIgM) [6] but not Ia antigen or J-chain [4,5]. During subsequent B-cell maturation, mIgD [7] and Ia antigen [5] appear on the cell surface; and still later immunoglobulin secretion and J-chain production begin [4]. The final phase of B-cell development is represented by the terminally differentiated plasma cell. Plasma cells greatly increase immuno-globulin production, which shifts from membrane-bound to secreted immunoglobulin [3,8]; J-chain production increases; and the cells become Ia negative [9].

The c-*myb* proto-oncogene, which encodes a nuclear DNA binding protein [10,11], has been reported to be expressed predominantly in normal tissue and tumor cells of hematopoietic origin [12–15]. In each lineage examined, the steady-state levels of c-*myb* mRNA expression are highest in immature cells. We have recently described the structure and sequence of c-*myb* mRNA in a murine pre-B-cell lym-phoma [16], and now report that the expression of c-*myb* mRNA correlates with the developmental phenotype of murine B-lymphoid tumors. Specifically, we show that movement from the pre-B-cell to the B-cell stage of development results in at least a 20-fold decrease in steady-state levels of c-*myb* mRNA expression.

RESULTS AND DISCUSSION
Expression of c-*myb* mRNA in Murine B-Lymphoid Tumors

We have examined a series of B-lymphoid tumor cell lines which represent different stages of B-cell development. The HAFTL-1 cell line may be a tumor of a pre-B-cell progenitor because it expresses the B220 early B-cell surface marker and its H-chain genes are in a germline configuration, although they spontaneously rearrange at a high frequency upon subcloning (J. Pierce, personal communication). Pre-B-cells are represented by the LS8.T2 and 1881.B4 Abelson virus-transformed cell lines [17] and the carcinogen-induced 7OZ/3.12 cell line [18]. The intermediate B-cell stage, which includes immature B-cells (eg, WEHI-231) and mature B-cells (eg, A20.2J), is represented by eight B-cell lymphoma cell lines [19–21]. Four classical plasmacytoma cell lines, such as S107, are representative of plasma cells [22]. Total cellular RNA was prepared by the guanidinium thiocyanate method [23] from the tumor cell lines shown in Figure 1. The RNA was fractionated on 0.8% agarose gels containing 0.22 M formaldehyde [24], transferred to nitrocellulose, and hybridized to a nick-translated 592-base pair (bp) Smal/EcoR1 murine c-*myb* cDNA probe [16].

The pre-B-cell lymphoma lines examined all express similar high levels of steady-state c-*myb* mRNA. In contrast, the B-cell lymphoma and plasmacytoma cell lines were found to express very low detectable levels of c-*myb* mRNA. Tumor lines that made levels of c-*myb* mRNA which were difficult to detect in total cellular RNA are clearly visible in polyA + mRNA preparations (see Fig. 1). The relative levels of c-*myb* mRNA were measured by scanning densitometry. The pre-B-cell lymphomas express 1.1–0.75 units of c-*myb* mRNA relative to the HAFTL-1 cell line, while the B-cell lymphomas and plasmacytomas contain levels of steady-state c-*myb* mRNA ranging from 0.05 to less than 0.005 units relative to HFTL-1. These results show that all of the B-lymphoid cell lines examined express detectable levels of c-*myb* mRNA but that cell lines representing later stages of B-cell development express steady-state levels of c-*myb* message that are at least 20-fold lower than in pre-B-cells. Furthermore, this experiment suggests that some event or events involving differen-

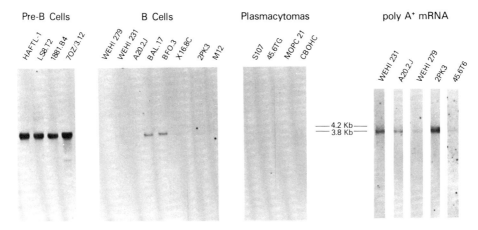

Fig. 1.   Expression of c-*myb* mRNA in murine B-lymphoid tumor cell lines. Ten micrograms of total cellular RNA isolated from each tumor cell line was fractionated in 0.8% agarose gels containing 0.22 M formaldehyde, transferred to nitrocellulose, and hybridized to a 592 bp Sma1/EcoR1 murine c-*myb* cDNA probe. In some cases 2–5 μg of polyA$^+$ mRNA was also examined as indicated. After hybridization the filters were washed twice for 30 min in 0.1X SSC/0.1% SDS at 58°C, dried, and exposed to Kodak XAR-5 film at -70°C with an enhancer screen for 15 hr.

tiation at the pre-B-cell/B-cell junction down-regulates the production of c-*myb* mRNA. Since all of these cell lines grow continuously in culture, down-regulation of c-*myb* mRNA probably is not due to changes in the growth properties of the cells, but rather correlates with maturation beyond the pre-B-cell stage of development.

Steady-State Levels of c-*myb* mRNA Decrease During LPS Induction of a Pre-B-Cell Lymphoma Line

The 7OZ/3.12 cell line is a carcinogen-induced pre-B-cell lymphoma [18]. Though it has productive rearrangements of both H- and kappa L-chain genes, only the H-chain gene is transcribed and expressed as cytoplasmic mu H-chain [18,25]. Treatment of 7OZ/3.12 with LPS reversibly induces transcription of the kappa locus, resulting in mIgM expression on >90% of the cells and thus a phenotype similiar to that of an immature B-cell [18]. We have utilized this cell line to examine events more carefully at the pre-B-cell junction.

Parallel cultures of 7OZ/3.12 were established by seeding 5×10^5 cells/ml in RPMI 1640 with 10% fetal calf serum (FCS) and 10 μM 2 mercaptoethanol. One set of cultures was treated with LPS at a final concentration of 10 μg/ml. At the time points shown in Figure 2, induced and uninduced cultures were harvested and total cellular RNA was prepared, fractionated electrophoretically, transferred to nitrocellulose, and sequentially hybridized to nick-translated probes specific for murine c-*myb*, c-*myc*, and kappa L-chain. Over this time course there was no difference in the growth rates of LPS-induced and uninduced cultures.

Hybridization of Northern blots to a 3.8-kilobase (kb) Xbal/BamH1 murine kappa L-chain constant region probe shows that upon induction with LPS kappa L-chain mRNA expression rapidly and markedly increases (Fig. 2). After 12 hr postinduction this expression does not change. No kappa mRNA was detected in uninduced cultures. By contrast, c-*myb* mRNA levels decrease approximately 12-fold (0.08 units relative to time zero) during LPS induction, while no change in c-*myb* message

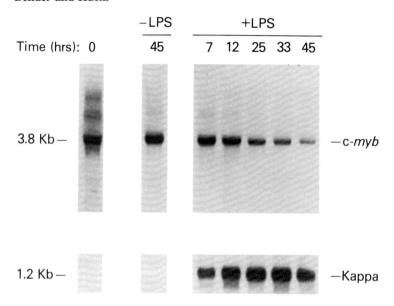

Fig. 2. Expression of c-*myb* and kappa L-chain mRNA during LPS induction of 7OZ/3.12. Total cellular RNA was isolated from LPS-induced and uninduced cultures of 7OZ/3.12 (see Results and Discussion for details). Time points are hours after beginning induction with LPS. The RNA was fractionated electrophoretically and transferred to nitrocellulose filters which were sequentially hybridized to the 592-bp Sma1/EcoR1 murine c-*myb* cDNA probe and a 3.8 kb Xba1/BamH1 murine genomic kappa L-chain probe. Filters were washed twice for 30 min at 58°C in 0.1XSSC/0.1% SDS, dried, and exposed for 15 hr (c-*myb*) or 6 hr (kappa L-chain) to Kodak XAR-5 film at −70°C with an enhancer screen.

expression was noted in uninduced cultures. It is noted that the down-regulation of c-*myb* mRNA levels takes place later in the time course than the rapid increase in kappa mRNA expression. Over the same time course c-*myc* mRNA expression did not change (data not shown). Thus, as the 7OZ/3.12 cell line is induced to progress from a pre-B-cell to a state phenotypically resembling an immature B-cell, the steady-state level of c-*myb* mRNA decreases to a level nearly within the range seen in B-cell lymphomas.

Correlation of c-*myb* mRNA Levels Phenotype in Hybrid Cell Lines

To further examine the regulation of c-*myb* mRNA expression and to correlate it with phenotype, we have constructed two types of hybrid cell lines by somatic cell fusion [26]. First, a group of pre-B-cell lymphoma × plasmacytoma hybrids (PBP) was made by fusing the hypoxanthine phosphoribosyl transferase negative (HPRT⁻) plasmacytoma 45.6TG with the thymidine kinase negative (TK⁻) pre-B-cell lymphoma 7OZ-3B. Second, a group of pre-B-cell lymphoma × B-cell lymphoma hybrids (PBB) was made by fusing 7OZ/3B to the mature B-cell lymphoma A20.2J (HPRT⁻). The characteristics of these parental cell lines and the PBB hybrids are shown in Table I.

Pre-B-cell lymphoma × plasmacytoma hybrids have previously been characterized and used to analyze various aspects of immunoglobulin biosynthesis [26,27]. These studies have concluded that hybrid cell lines of this type phenotypically resemble the terminally differentiated plasmacytoma parent in terms of the level of immunoglobulin expression, immunoglobulin secretion, and J-chain production. All

TABLE I. Characterization of Hybrid B-Lymphoid Cell Lines

Cell line	Ig[a]			J-chain mRNA[b]	Ia[c]	Ig[a] secretion	c-*myb*[d] mRNA
	μ	γ2b	κ				
70Z/3B	+	−	−	−	−	−	1.00
45.6TG	−	+	+	+	−	+	<0.005
A20.2J	−	+	+	+	+	+	0.01
PBB hybrids							
3	+	+	+	−	−	−	0.92
4	+	+	+	−	−	−	0.85
6	+	+	+	−	−	−	0.87
9	+	+	+	−	−	−	0.96
10	+	+	+	−	−	−	1.05
11	+	+	+	−	−	−	0.84
20	+	+	+	−	−	−	0.88

[a]Expression and secretion of H- and L-chain was determined by metabolic labeling, immunoprecipitation, and polyacrylamide gel analysis.
[b]J-chain mRNA expression determined by Northern blot analysis (a murine cDNA J-chain probe was a gift of Dr. M. Koshland).
[c]Expression of Ia antigen determined by FACS analysis (performed by Dr. D. McKean).
[d]Relative levels of c-*myb* mRNA expression determined by Northern blot analysis and compared by scanning densitometry to 70Z/3B.

five PBP hybrid lines examined secrete immunoglobulin bearing the H-chain isotype of each parental line and make abundant J-chain mRNA. Also, very low levels of c-*myb* mRNA expression were found which were indistinguishable from the plasmacytoma parent (data not shown). Thus, these hybrid cell lines phenotypically resemble the parental 45.6TG plasmacytoma line, including low levels of c-*myb* mRNA expression.

Detailed analysis of pre-B-cell × B-cell hybrids will be reported elsewhere [28]. Southern blotting data showed that the rearranged H- and L-chain genes from the 7OZ/3B and A20.2J parental lines were present in each of the hybrids examined (data not shown). The IgG$_{2a}$ expressed by A20.2J includes both membrane and secreted forms, with the latter being quantitatively secreted. In contrast, 7OZ/3B cells express cytoplasmic mu H-chain but no L-chain, and do not secrete immunoglobulin. As shown in Table I, although H-chain protein of each parental isotype and kappa L-chains encoded by each parent is expressed in each hybrid line, no secretion of immunoglobulin bearing either isotype was detected by immunoprecipitation and SDS-polyacrylamide gel electrophoresis. We have not yet determined whether the immunoglobulin produced is retained in the cytoplasm or inserted in the cell membrane. In contrast to A20.2J, which makes abundant J-chain mRNA and is Ia$^+$ by fluorescence-activated cell sorter (FACS) analysis, the hybrids—like the 7OZ/3B pre-B cell lymphoma parent—do not make detectable levels of J-chain mRNA and are Ia$^-$. Northern blot analysis shows that the high levels of c-*myb* mRNA in the hybrid lines are indistinguishable from those of the 7OZ/3B pre-B-cell lymphoma parent. Thus, the phenotype of these cells closely resembles that of the 7OZ/3B pre-B-cell parent (summarized in Table I).

These studies of hybrid cell lines show that, in contrast to the terminally differentiated plasma cell phenotype, which is consistently dominant in cell fusion experiments between B-lymphoid tumors [26,27], the mature B-cell phenotype is reversible when fused to the 7OZ/3B pre-B-cell tumor line. This includes the low steady-state level of c-*myb* mRNA expression associated with mature B-cell lymphomas. These experiments clearly correlate high levels of c-*myb* mRNA expression with the pre-B-cell stage of differentiation.

The 5′ End of c-*myb* mRNA Is Very Heterogenous in B-Lymphoid Tumors

To begin examination of a potential role for c-*myb* in the regulation of B-cell development, we have recently reported the structure and sequence of murine c-*myb* cDNA clones derived from 7OZ/3B mRNA [16]. These clones contain sufficient nucleotides to account for a c-*myb* mRNA of approximately 3.6 kb, which is smaller than the predominant mRNA of 3.8 kb seen in 7OZ/3B pre-B-cell lymphomas. However, as shown in Figure 3, when a 5′ 824-bp probe (probe A) was used in s1-nuclease protection studies, five closely spaced bands of approximately 710–820 nucleotides in length were detected in 7OZ/3B total cellular RNA. To localize this

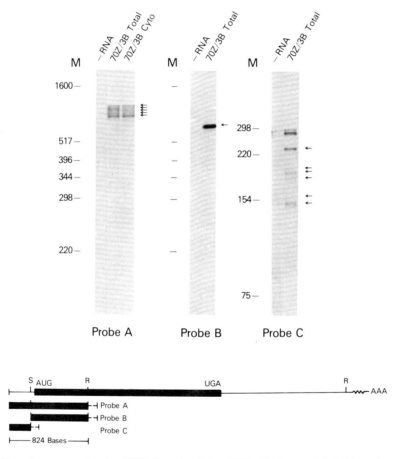

Fig. 3. S1-nuclease protection by 7OZ/3B total cellular RNA. Single-stranded DNA probes were prepared by primer extension of M13 clones [29] carrying either the 824-bp EcoR1 fragment (probe A), the 592-bp Sma1/EcoR1 3′ fragment (probe B), or the 236-bp EcoR1/Sma1 5′ fragment (probe C). The probes are shown relative to the recently reported structure of the murine c-*myb* mRNA from 7OZ/3B [16]. Probes A and B carry the 17 base primer at their 5′ ends as indicated by dashes. Probe C carries 35 bases of the M13mp10 polylinker plus the 17 base primer at its 5′ end. Specifically protected species are marked by small arrows. Molecular weight markers (M) are Hinf1-digested pBR322.

heterogeneity a convenient Smal site (see Fig. 3) was used to make a 592-bp 3′ probe (probe B) and a 236-bp 5′ probe (probe C) from probe A. When probe B was annealed to total cellular RNA from 7OZ/3B, a single protected species was found, indicating that the detected heterogeneity was located 5′ of both the Sma1 site and the translation initiation codon. When probe C was annealed to total RNA, at least six distinct protected fragments, containing 145–236 nucleotides, were detected. None of these species were seen in minus RNA controls. Thus, the 5′ end of c-*myb* mRNA appears to be hetereogeneous.

To investigate further the heterogeneity of c-*myb* mRNA, we have cloned and sequenced a 1.1-kb BamH1 genomic clone which includes bases 1–287 of our reported mRNA sequence ([16] and Fig. 3), 50 bp of intron, and 799 bp of putative 5′ untranslated region and flanking sequence. Use of this fragment in S1-nuclease protection studies has indicated at least 13 protected products. The largest product, when combined with the appropriate regions of our c-*myb* mRNA sequence, is sufficient to account for a 4.2-kb transcript. The other protected species would derive from transcripts of about 3.5–4.0 kb. Thus, the major 3.8-kb mRNA species seen on Northern blots may represent an average of multiple species.

Independent RNA preparations have been examined from other pre-B-cell lymphomas (18-81.B4 and LS8.T2) as well as tumors representing B-cells (BFO.3, A20.2J and BAL-17) and plasma cells (CBOHC). The same protected fragments were detected regardless of the source of RNA. Therefore, we do not find significant differences in this 5′ heterogeneity between tumors of different developmental phenotypes. In addition, the same protected fragments were found in cytoplasmic and nuclear RNA preparations from 7OZ/3B (data not shown), indicating that cytoplasmic mRNA processing does not cause the 5′ heterogeneity. Although the mechanism and biological relevance of this extreme c-*myb* mRNA 5′ heterogeneity is not readily apparent, we are presently analyzing the 1.1-kb BamH1 genomic clone for potential promotor/regulatory sequences.

REFERENCES

1. Kincaide PW: Adv Immunol 31:177, 1981.
2. Wall R, Kuehl WM: Annu Rev Immunol 1:393, 1983.
3. Alt FW, Yancopoulos GD, Blackwell TK, Wood C, Rosenberg N, Tonegawa S, Baltimore D: EMBO J 3:1209, 1984.
4. McHugh Y, Yagi M, Koshland M: In Klinman N, Mosier D, Scher I, Vitetta E (eds): "B Lymphocytes in the Immune Response: Functional, Developmental and Interactive Properties." New York: Elsevier 1981, pp 467–474.
5. Kearney JF, Cooper MD, Klein J, Abney ER, Parkhouse RME, Lawton AR: J Exp Med 146:297, 1977.
6. Vitetta ES, Uhr J: Science 189:946–968, 1975.
7. Vitetta ES, Melcher F, McWilliams M, Lamm ME, Phillips-Quagliata J, Uhr JM: J Exp Med 141:206, 1975.
8. Rogers J, Early P, Carter C, Calame K, Bond M, Hood L, Wall R: Cell 20:303, 1980.
9. Okumura K, Julius MH, Tsu T, Herzenberg LA, Herzenberg LA: Eur J Immunol 6:467–472, 1976.
10. Klempnauer K, Symonds J, Evan GI, Bishop JM: Cell 37:537–547, 1984.
11. Boyle WJ, Lampert MA, Lipsick JS, Baluda MA: Proc Natl Acad Sci USA 81:4265–4269, 1984.
12. Westin EH, Gallo RC, Arya SK, Eva A, Sauza LM, Baluda MA, Aaronson SA, Wong-Staal F: Proc Natl Acad Sci USA 79:2194–2198, 1982.
13. Gonda TJ, Sheiness DK, Bishop JM: Mol Cell Biol 2:617–624, 1982.
14. Roy-Berman P, Devi BG, Parker JW: Int J Cancer 32:185–191, 1983.

15. Gonda TJ, Metcalf D: Nature 310:249–251, 1984.
16. Bender TP, Kuehl WM: Proc Natl Acad Sci USA 83:3204, 1986.
17. Alt FW, Rosenber N, Lewis S, Thomas E, Baltimore D: Cell 27:391, 1981.
18. Paige CJ, Kincade PW, Ralph P: J Immunol 121:641–647, 1978.
19. Goding JW: Contemp Top Immunobiol 8:203–243, 1978.
20. Laskov R, Kim JK, Asofsky R: Proc Natl Acad Sci USA 76:915–919, 1979.
21. Sitia R, Kikutani H, Rubartelli A, Bushkin Y, Stavnezer J, Hammerling U: J Immunol 128:712–716, 1982.
22. Potter M: Physiol Rev 52:632–719, 1972.
23. Chirgwin J, Aeybyle A, McDonald R, Rutter W: Biochemistry 18:5294–5299, 1979.
24. Lehrach H, Diamond D, Wozney JM, Boedtker H: Biochemistry 16:4743, 1977.
25. Maki R, Kearney J, Paige C, Tonegawa S: Science 209:1366–1369, 1980.
26. Riley SC, Brock EJ, Kuehl WM: Nature 289:804–806, 1981.
27. Yoshida N, Watanabe T, Sakaguchi N, Kikutani H, Kishimoto S, Yamamura Y, Kishimoto T: Mol Immunol 19:1415–1423, 1982.
28. Bender TP, Kuehl WM: Manuscript in preparation.
29. Battey J, Moulding C, Taub R, Murphey W, Stewart T, Potter H, Lenoir G, Leder P: Cell 34:779–787, 1983.

Cellular and Molecular Biology of Tumors and Potential
Clinical Applications 247–259 (1988)

Complex Formation Between the p53 Cellular Tumor Antigen and Nuclear Heat Shock Proteins

Dan Michalovitz, Orit Pinhasi-Kimhi, Daniel Eliyahu, Avri Ben-Zeev, and Moshe Oren

*Departments of Chemical Immunology (D.M., O.P.-K., D.E., M.O.) and Genetics (A.B.-Z.),
The Weizmann Institute of Science, Rehovot 76100, Israel*

In cells overproducing p53, a protein of ca 70 kilodaltons (p68) is coprecipitable
with p53. We report here that p68 forms a specific physical complex with p53,
which can be dissociated upon heating under denaturing conditions. Furthermore,
p68 is actually the HSP70 heat-shock protein cognate, and a similar complex can
also be formed between p53 and the related, highly inducible HSP68 following
hyperthermia. Sucrose-gradient sedimentation analysis suggests that virtually all
the p53 in such an overproducer line is in oligomeric forms containing HSP70,
sedimenting as a broad peak of ca 10–14 S. Finally, rats bearing tumors induced
by such cells make antibodies against HSP70. It is suggested that interactions with
heat-shock proteins may be involved in determining the stability of p53 and that
the former proteins may share some properties with the SV40 large T antigen.

Key words: p53 oncogene, protein stabilization, HSP70, stability, complex with cellular proteins

One of the distinctive features of the p53 cellular tumor antigen, a protein
capable of participating in neoplastic transformation [1–3], is its ability to form tight
specific complexes with the large T antigen of Simian virus 40 (SV40) [4–6]. In
SV40-transformed cells, this interaction results in the stabilization of p53 [7,8] and
may contribute to the transforming potential of the virus [9]. Significant increases in
the stability of p53, with a concomitant elevation in the cellular levels of this protein,
have been observed in a variety of non-SV40-transformed cell lines [10–12]. This
suggested that in such transformants p53 may be stabilized by interaction with a
cellular protein, the action of which was mimicked by the large T antigen. Nevertheless, early studies did not seem to support the existence of such a putative p53 binding
protein. More recently, however, a polypeptide of 68–70 kilodaltons (kd), referred to
as p68 by us [13], was shown to be precipitated by anti-p53 monoclonal antibodies in
several different systems [12–14], raising the possibility that this was indeed the

Received March 18, 1986.

putative p53-stabilizing cellular protein [12,13]. We now report that p68, which indeed appears to form a specific complex with p53, is in fact the semiconstitutive heat-shock protien HSP70, which can be found in elevated levels in a p53-overproducing cell line. Furthermore, upon heat-shock treatment of such overproducers, p53 can also form a complex with the highly inducible HSP68. Finally, animals bearing tumors induced by cells in which the complex is manifested make antibodies against the nuclear heat-shock proteins.

MATERIALS AND METHODS

Cells and Cell Cultures

Rat-1 is a non-transformed rat fibroblast cell line. Clone 6 is a cell line derived from a transformed focus generated by cotransfecting primary rat embryo fibroblasts with activated Ha-*ras* and the p53-overexpression plasmid pLTRp53cG [1,16]. Both cell lines were maintained in Dulbecco modified Eagle's medium (DMEM) supplemented with 10% fetal calf serum.

Cell Labeling, Preparation of Extracts, and Immunoprecipitation

Prior to labeling, cells were prestarved for 45 min in methionine-free DMEM supplemented with 2% dialyzed fetal calf serum. Labeling was carried out by incubation for 4 hr in the same type of medium containing [^{35}S]methionine (50 μCi per 60-mm or 90-mm dish). Extracts for immunoprecipitation were prepared by the Nonidet P-40 (NP40) method and processed as described before [17]. When such extracts had to be denatured [18], an aliquot was made 5% in β-mercaptoethanol and 0.5% in SDS, heated to 100°C for 5 min, cleared at 12,500g for 10 min, and the supernatant was taken for immunoprecipitation. Total cell extracts were made by resuspending the cell pellet in a small volume (50–100 μl) of 50 mM Tris·Cl, pH 8.0, 5 mM EDTA, 150 mM NaCl, 0.5% NP40, 0.5% SDS, and 5% β-mercaptoethanol, followed by boiling for 5 min and clearing at 12,500g for 10 min.

Hyperthermia

To induce the heat-shock response, cells were incubated for 10 min at an elevated temperature, as indicated in the corresponding figure legend. This was done at the end of the prestarvation period (last 10 min before addition of the radioactive methionine) by placing the dishes in a water-bath adjusted to the desired temperature [19]. Following this heat shock, labeling medium was added, and the dishes were incubated at 37°C for another 4 hr before harvesting.

Gel Electrophoresis

One-dimensional gel electrophoresis was performed on a 12.5% SDS-polyacrylamide gel as described previously [13]. For two-dimensional gel-electrophoresis, samples (in standard SDS-gel protein sample buffer) were made 9.5 M in urea and 2% in β-mercaptoethanol and analysed in accordance with the procedure of O'Farrell et al [20]. The first dimension employed isoelectric focusing in the presence of 2% ampholites (LKB, 1.6% pH 5.0–7.0, 0.4% pH 3.5–10.0). The second dimension was an 8% SDS-polyacrylamide gel. Unless otherwise mentioned, all gels were subjected to fluorography [21] before being exposed to x-ray film.

Protein Analysis by Partial V8 Proteolysis

A 90-mm dish of clone 6 cells was labeled for 6 hr with 200 μCi [^{35}S] methionine. Following immunoprecipitation with PAb421, the reacting polypeptides were resolved on a 12.5% SDS-polyacrylamide gel, which was then dried without prior fixation. The p68 and p53 bands, visualized by autoradiography, were cut out of the dry gel and subjected to V8 proteolytic analysis as previously described [13,22].

Sucrose Gradient Sedimentation Analysis

A 60-mm dish of clone 6 cells was labeled at 37°C with 200 μCi [^{35}S]methionine for 4 hr, extracted as above, and sedimented through a 4.7-ml 5–20% (w/v) sucrose gradient containing 0.14 M NaCl, 10 mM Tris·Cl (pH 8), 10 mM dithiothreitol (DDT), 1% aprotinin, and 300 μg/ml phenylmethylsultonylfluoride (PMSF), including a 0.4 ml 60% sucrose pad. Sedimentation was in a Beckman SW 50.1 rotor at 48,000 rpm for 3 hr at 4°C. Fractions (0.21 ml, 23 fractions per gradient) were collected from the bottom of the tube following puncturing with a needle.

Aliquots (10 μl) were mixed with sample buffer and directly analysed on a 12.5% SDS-polyacrylamide gel. The rest of the material was subjected to immunoprecipitation with monoclonal antibody PAb421 and similarly analysed. Rat ribosomal RNA was sedimented through a parallel gradient, and the positions of the respective size species were determined with the aid of a spectrophotometer and confirmed by electrophoresis on a formaldehyde-agarose gel.

RESULTS

p68 Is not a Cross-Reactive Protein

For the studies reported here, we utilized clone 6, a cell line derived by cotransformation of rat embryo fibroblasts with a combination of p53 plus activated Ha-*ras* (Eliyahu et al, in preparation). These transformed rat cells are marked overproducers of mouse p53. p53 is greatly stabilized in such cells, possessing a half-life of about 4 hr as compared to 20 min in the untransformed embryo fibroblasts (Eliyahu et al, in preparation). Upon immunoprecipitation of labeled clone 6 proteins with anti-p53 monoclonal antibodies (Fig. 1, lane 2), one observes a prominent p53 band, along with a coprecipitating band of approximately 70 kilodaltons (kd), previously referred to as p68 [13]. The presence of such a polypeptide in the immunoprecipitate could be accounted for by one of the following explanations: a) p68 is an irrelevant protein accidentally sharing an epitope with p53; b) p68 is a modified slower-migrating form of p53; c) p68 forms a specific physical association with p53. If the first possibility were right, one would not expect p68 to react with two different monoclonal antibodies directed against different epitopes. However, as seen in Figure 1, lanes 4,5, this is clearly not the case, since p53 is brought down by both PAb421 [23] and RA3-2C2 [24], which bind to different domains of the p53 molecule [25,26]. Furthermore, both antibodies displayed a similar apparent affinity for p53 and p68, since both proteins were cleared with the same efficiency upon repeated rounds of immunoprecipitation (compare lanes 2 and 5). These data clearly rule out the first explanation—namely, that a random cross-reactivity is involved.

To further probe the relationship between p53 and p68, a labeled clone 6 extract was reduced in the presence of SDS prior to incubation with anti-p53 monoclonal

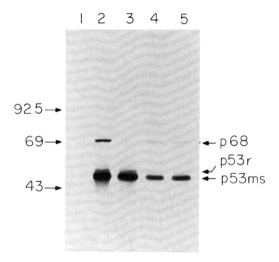

Fig. 1.   Analysis of p53–p68 interaction. [^{35}S]-labeled proteins were extracted [17] from cells of clone 6, derived by transformation of rat embryo fibroblasts by p53 plus Ha-*ras* (Eliyahu et al, in preparation). Equal amounts of TCA-insoluble radioactivity (1.4 × 10^6 cpm) were reacted with either nonimmune serum (**lane 1**) or anti-p53 monoclonal antibody PAb 421 (**lane 2**). An identical sample was heated under reducing conditions [18] and similarly reacted with PAb421 (**lane 3**). The supernatant (unreacted material) of the immunoprecipitate shown in lane 2 was divided in two halves and incubated again with either the anti-p53 monoclonal antibody RA3-2C2 [24] (**lane 4**) or PAb421 (**lane 5**). Numbers on the left denote the sizes and positions of coelectrophoresed molecular-weight markers. p53ms = mouse p53; p53r = endogenous rat p53.

antibodies. If a noncovalent complex between p53 and p68 does exist, it should be dissociated under these conditions. As seen in Figure 1, lane 3, such treatment totally abolished the immunoprecipitation of p68, while having no effect on the reactivity of p53. These results are highly consistent with p68's forming a physical complex with p53 rather than being a modified form of p53 reacting directly with the monoclonal antibodies. Nevertheless, the latter possibility could not be ruled out completely since one could argue that the putative chemical modification rendered p68 very labile and thus resulted in its disappearance from the immunoprecipitate upon boiling under reducing conditions. Although this seemed very unlikely, a direct comparison of the two polypeptides was undertaken. Both bands were isolated from an SDS gel and subjected to partial proteolysis with the V8 protease [22]. As displayed in Figure 2, the patterns of resulting proteolytic fragments were totally different between p68 and p53, clearly demonstrating that these are not closely related polypeptides. Hence, the presence of p68 in the immunoprecipitate can only be accounted for by its being in physical association with p53, thus forming part of an anti-p53 reactive complex, as is also the case for the SV40 large T antigen [4–6].

In experiments such as that shown in Figure 1, there appears to be much more p53 than p68 in the precipitate. This could suggest that only a minor fraction of p53 is tightly associated with p68. However, such experiments employ a rather short radiolabeling period (3–4 hr). Previous pulse-chase analysis [13] suggested that p53 is substantially more labile than p68, raising the possibility that p53 is misleadingly overrepresented in the radiolabeled extract owing to its relatively rapid turnover rate. To address this issue, radiolabeled polypeptides immunoprecipitated with PAb421

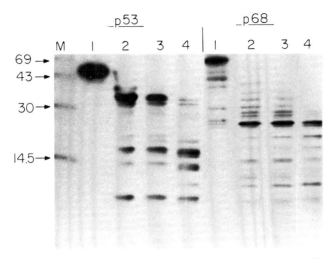

Fig. 2.   Comparative analysis of p53 and p68 by partial proteolytic cleavage. [^{35}S]-labeled p53 and p68 were incubated with increasing amounts of V8 protease and analysed by SDS-polyacrylamide gel electrophoresis. The following amounts of enzyme were used: **lane 1**, no enzyme; **lane 2**, 20 ng; **lane 3**, 50 ng; **lane 4**, 150 ng. Radiolabeled molecular weight markers are displayed on the left.

were visualized by Coomassie-blue staining. The results (Fig. 3) clearly demonstrate that p68 is indeed present in large quantities in the immunoprecipitate, consistent with (but not proving) a stoichiometric interaction between the two proteins. Furthermore, since the material applied represented one-sixth of a 90-mm dish, both proteins must be fairly abundant in clone 6 cells (see also Fig. 4), whereas p53 is normally a very minor protein.

p68 Is a Heat-Shock Protein

The finding that p53 was in complex with p68 raised the possibility that the latter protein may be related to the transforming activity of p53. It was therefore of interest to determine the precise nature of p68. Towards that end, an immunoprecipitate of clone 6 cells was subjected to two-dimensional electrophoresis. Results of a preliminary experiment (data not shown) revealed that the position of p68 was very similar to that of the ca 70-kd rodent heat-shock proteins [19,27,28]. Furthermore, at least in one system, that of the SV40-transformed COS cells, two polypeptides of approximately 68 and 70 kd were observed to coprecipitate with p53 [13], reminiscent of the heat-shock protein doublet reported in various mammalian species [19,27,29]. To determine the possible relationship between p68 and the heat-shock proteins, clone 6 cells were subjected to brief periods of hyperthermia, which are known to induce the heat-shock response efficiently [19], followed by radiolabeling for 4 hr and protein analysis. In parallel, a similar treatment was performed on Rat-1 cells, which are nontransformed established rat fibroblasts [15], producing rather low amounts of p53 [16]. The autoradiogram of the SDS-polyacrylamide gel. (Fig. 4), demonstrates that the coprecipitating p68 indeed comigrated with a major heat shock protein, the semi-inducible HSP70. Moreover, upon increased hyperthermia, increasing amounts of a slightly faster migrating polypeptide became prominent in the immunoprecipitate. This polypeptide exactly comigrated with the highly inducible HSP68, and its appearance in the precipitate precisely coincided with that of HSP68 in the total cell extract.

(a)   (b)

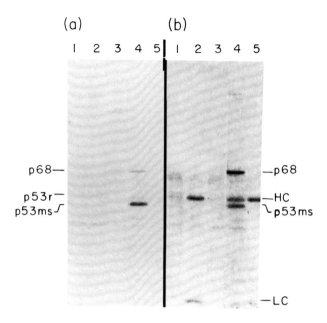

Fig. 3.   Comparison of stained and radiolabeled p53 and p68. Radiolabeled extracts of rat embryo fibroblasts (**lanes 1,2**) or clone 6 cells (**lanes 3,4**) were prepared as described under Materials and Methods. Aliquots containing equal amounts of TCA-insoluble radioactivity were reacted with 50 μl of unused culture medium (lanes 1,3) or PAb421 culture medium (lanes 2,4). In **lane 5**, 50 μl of PAb421 was reacted with extraction buffer only (no cell extract). The autoradiogram of the unfluorographed gel is shown in **a**; the Coomassie-blue staining pattern of the same gel is displayed in **b**. p53r and p53 ms refer to rat and mouse p53, respectively. HC - immunoglobulin heavy chain, LC - light chain.

Furthermore, both polypeptides were absent from immunoprecipitates of reduced samples (data not shown), indicating that this highly heat-inducible protein was also in complex with p53. None of the two ca 70-kd bands was convincingly detectable in immunoprecipitates of heat-shocked Rat-1 cells (data not shown). Based on these results, it seemed highly probable that p68 was indeed a heat-shock protein, the rat equivalent of the mouse HSP70. To establish this conclusion more firmly, appropriate immunoprecipitates were resolved on two-dimensional gels and compared with total extracts from cells which had either been exposed to hyperthermia or kept at 37°C (Fig. 5). The pertinent heat-shock proteins are most easily identified in total extracts from Rat-1 cells (panels E,F): HSP70 is well detectable at 37°C but is severalfold overproduced at 46°C, whereas HSP68 can only be seen after hyperthermia. In clone 6, on the other hand, there is hardly any increase in HSP70 after heat shock (Fig. 4; Fig. 5C,D), while HSP68 displays the same pattern as in Rat-1. Most importantly, comparison of the total cell extracts with the immunoprecipitates reveals that p68 indeed precisely comigrates with HSP70, while the other polypeptide corresponds to HSP68. This is most obvious in Figure 5G, in which an immunoprecipitate was mixed and coelectrophoresed with a small amount of total cell extract, to allow a better alignment of the coprecipitating polypeptides with the HSPs.

To better characterize the complex, a clone 6 extract was subjected to sucrose gradient sedimentation (Fig. 6). While most cellular proteins were in monomeric form (fractions 20–23), there was hardly any monomeric p53. Rather, p53 was found in oligomers sedimenting as a relatively broad peak of 10–14S, with a small proportion

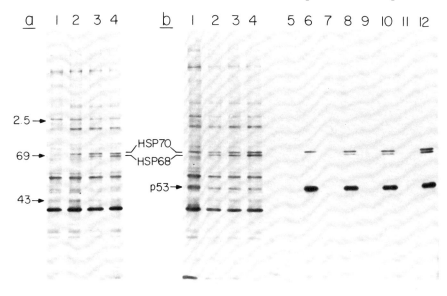

Fig. 4.   Analysis of p53 coprecipitating proteins following heat shock. Nontransformed Rat-1 cells (**a**) or clone 6 cells (**b**) were subjected to increasing temperatures followed by radiolabeling and extraction. Equal amounts of TCA-insoluble radioactivity (31,000 cpm) were analysed directly by gel electrophoresis (**lanes 1–4**). Parallel but larger aliquots (7.2 × 10^5 cpm) were reacted with either non-immune serum (**lanes 5,7,9,11**) or anti-p53 monoclonal antibody PAb421 (**lanes 6,8,10,12**). Hyperthermia was performed at the following temperatures: 37°C (lanes 1,5,6), 44°C (lanes 2,7,8), 45°C (lanes 3,9,10), or 46°C (lanes 4,11,12). The positions of the major rat heat-shock proteins HSP70 and HSP68 are indicated.

of larger complexes. HSP70 was clearly associated with p53 throughout the gradient, and the ratio between the two polypeptides appeared to be constant. Unlike p53, a substantial fraction of HSP70 was in monomers or low-molecular-weight oligomers (Fig. 6B).

Tumor-Bearing Animals Make Antibodies Against Nuclear Heat-Shock Proteins

Animals bearing SV40-induced tumors which contain conspicuous levels of the large T-p53 complex often produce antibodies against p53 [30], despite the fact that the latter is a normal cellular protein. This could either reflect the fact that the complexed form is differently recognized by the immune system, or could be due to the breaking of self-tolerance by exposure to huge quantities of an otherwise very minor polypeptide species. The latter is probably the case for Abelson virus-transformed cells, in which no complex has been reported [24]. It was therefore of interest to determine whether animals bearing p53-overproducing tumors made antibodies to any relevant cellular protein. To that end, syngeneic Fisher rats were injected with cell lines derived by cotransformation of primary rat embryo fibroblasts with p53 plus activated Ha-*ras* [1]. Two cell lines were employed: clone 31 [1] and clone 6, described in this communication. Rats were bled 2 wk after inoculation, and their sera were assayed by immunoprecipitation against a radiolabeled extract of heat-shocked rat embryo fibroblasts. Surprisingly, these sera were found to precipitate HSP70 and HSP68 (Fig. 7). Since those cells contain very little p53 [1] and no detectable p53-HSP70 complex (data not shown), these antibodies must have been

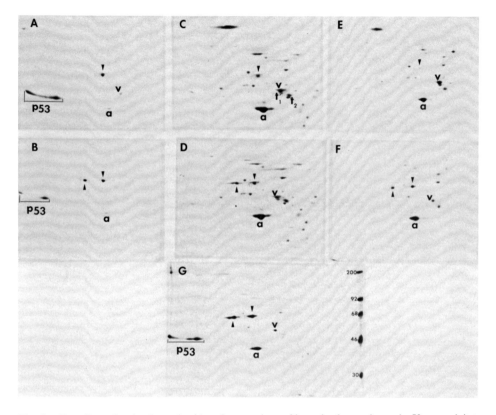

Fig. 5. Two-dimensional polyacrylamide gel comparison of heat-shock proteins and p53-coprecipitating polypeptides. Clone 6 and Rat-1 cells were either maintained at 37°C (**A,C,E**) or exposed to 46°C for 10 min (**B,D,F,G**). Clone 65 lysates containing equal amounts of acid-insoluble radioactivity (2 × 10^6 cpm) were immunoprecipitated with monclonal antibody PAb421 and analysed by 2-dimensional gel electrophoresis (A,B). Aliquots of the radiolabeled total cell extracts (3.7 × 10^5 cpm) were also taken directly for a similar analysis. C-clone 6, 37°C; D-clone 6, 46°C; E-rat-1, 37°C; F-Rat-1, 46°C. G displays a mixture of an immunoprecipitate identical with the one in B with an aliquot of unprocessed clone 6, 46°C lysate (similar to that shown in D but representing only 35,000 acid-insoluble cpm). Upward pointing arrowhead=HSP68; downward pointing arrowhead=HSP70; a=actin; t_1=tubulin; t_2=tubulin; v=vimentin. Direction of migration in the first dimension (isoelectric focusing) was from left to right. Numbers on the right of panel G indicate the positions and sizes (in kilodaltons) of coelectrophoresed protein molecular weight markers.

directly specific for these heat-shock proteins. It is noteworthy that the titer of anti-HSP antibodies strictly correlated with the state of development of the tumor at least early after injection. Thus, the lack of a palpable tumor was concomitant with the absence of detectable anti-HSP70 reactivity in the serum. Furthermore, as tumors developed later on in the seemingly negative animals, seropositivity for HSP70 also became manifest (data not shown). At later times, however, (4 wk or longer), the antibody titer actually began to decrease (data not shown), either representing the reestablishment of tolerance or the sequestration of circulating anti HSP70 antibodies by large quantities of HSP70 released from the rapidly necrotizing tumor mass.

Not surprisingly, the positive sera usually contained also anti-p53 antibodies, as evidenced by a longer exposure of the gel in Figure 7 or by incubation with a denatured clone 6 extract (data not shown). This was anticipated, both because of the

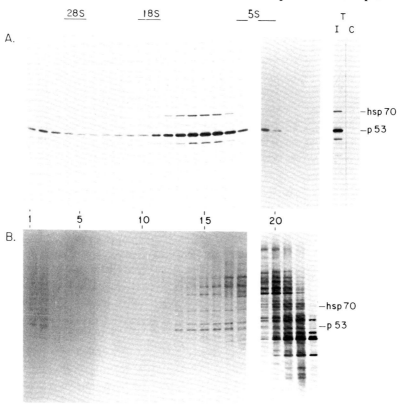

Fig. 6.   Cosedimentation of p53 and HSP70 on a sucrose gradient. A labeled cellular extract was fractionated on a sucrose gradient, and each fraction was assayed for the presence of p53 and coprecipitating HSP70. **A** displays the polypeptides immunoprecipitated with an anti-p53 monoclonal antibody. Fraction numbers are shown below with No. 1 representing the bottom of the gradient; the positions of ribosomal RNA markers, sedimented in a parallel tube, are shown on top. T represents the proteins precipitated from an aliquot of the total (unfractionated) extract by either control (c) or anti-p53 monoclonal antibodies (I). **B** displays the electrophoretic pattern of aliquots of each fraction subjected directly to gel analysis. The identification of HSP70 and p53 in B is tentative. Please note that fractions 19–23 were electrophoresed on a separate gel and that the migration distances of individual polypeptides differed slightly between the two gels; we attempted to align the gels at the tentative position of the p53 band. The bands migrating ahead of p53 most probably represent proteolytic cleavage products of this protein, present in variable quantities in different experiments and generated at least in part during the immunoprecipitation process [45].

above-cited precedents and because the rats were presented with a vast excess of a heterologous (mouse) species of p53. The anti-HSP70 reactivity, however, was less expected, since normal cells carry substantial amounts of this protein [19,27–29]. This suggests that the form of HSP70 found in complex with p53 may not be a normal occurrence and may thus not be recognized by the immune system as "self."

CONCLUSIONS

We have demonstrated here that p53 can associate in a specific manner with at least two rat heat-shock proteins, the equivalents of the mouse HSP68 and HSP70

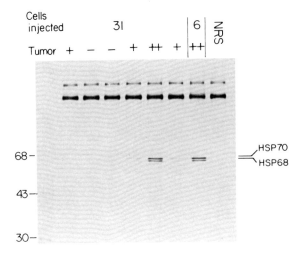

Fig. 7.   Detection of anti-heat-shock protein antibodies in tumor-bearing rats. Fisher rats were injected subcutaneously with 2×10^6 cells of clone 6 or clone 31. Two weeks later animals were bled and serum prepared. An aliquot (5 μl) of each serum was reacted with a portion of a radiolabeled cell extract prepared from primary rat embryo fibroblasts exposed to hyperthermic shock at 46°C. The presence and relative size of a palpable tumor in the individual rats at the time of bleeding is indicated on top. NRS = normal rat serum.

[19,27,28]. A similar doublet is also discernable in other mammalian species [29], and is probably also associated with p53 in monkey cells transiently overproducing mouse p53 [13]. More importantly, a similar interaction appears to exist in a variety of transformed mouse cells which overproduce p53 owing to a naturally occurring event rather than to in vitro transfection [14]. It is therefore plausible that this complex is of physiological importance, at least in such transformants, and may even be related to the transformation process.

One obvious concern is that the p53-HSP70 complex may be generated only during extraction while not being present in the living cell. Although it is hard to disprove such a claim, the inability to detect a comparable complex in p53-containing untransformed Rat-1 cells, even after heat-shock treatment (data not shown), strongly militates against it. Furthermore, even if some interaction does occur during extraction, the very specific nature of the complex is by itself very good evidence of the nonrandom association between these two proteins. Interestingly, a specific association has also been shown to take place between another heat-shock protein, HSP90, and the pp60[src] oncogene product [31]. Given the very different nature of pp60[src] and p53, it is very unlikely that both complexes arise via the same mechanism. However, it is tempting to speculate that the existence of these two types of complexes is not a mere coincidence but rather may reflect a more general involvement of heat-shock proteins in processes affecting the regulation of cell proliferation.

Is such a complex present also in normal cells? So far we have been unable to detect with confidence coprecipitating polypeptides in such cells, even after heat-shock induction which results in high cellular levels of HSP70 and HSP68 (data not shown). This may imply that the complex is not formed in normal cells. In this case, that may be related to the fact that in heat-induced cells, both heat-shock proteins have a predominantly nuclear location [32,33]. If a nuclear site is necessary for the specific association to take place, the apparent absence of p53 from nuclei of normal cells [34] may account for the inability of a complex to form. In that case, the nuclear accumulation of p53 in a variety of transformed cells [35] may lead to complex formation. Alternatively, the association between p53 and HSP70 may be a normal physiological process, except that under such conditions the complex is very unstable and dissociates rapidly, and only in abnormal situations does it accumulate to detectable levels. Such abnormal conditions could be the mere overproduction of p53, as seems to be the case in the system described above, or structural changes in either HSP70 or p53 which would result in a more stable complex. The latter may be relevant for Meth A cells, which appear to contain very elevated p53 levels as compared to nontransformed fibroblasts [35], while possessing only twice the amount of the corresponding mRNA [11]. Such cells, which do exhibit a p53-HSP70 complex [12,13] as well as a relatively stable p53 [11,12], indeed seem to carry a mutated p53 gene encoding an altered protein product [36]. Whether or not this mutant p53 has a higher affinity for HSP70 still remains to be determined.

Based on the data presented here, we would like to propose that the apparent stabilization of p53 in cells transformed by agents other than DNA tumor viruses is related to complex formation with HSP70 either as a cause or a consequence. In this respect, the SV40 T antigen could be mimicking the action of a normal cellular protein, HSP70. Is there anything else in common between the two types of complexes that p53 can form with other proteins? That this may be the case is suggested by previous studies employing the expression of mouse p53 in SV40-transformed monkey COS cells [13]. In those studies, immunoprecipitation of cell extracts with anti-p53 monoclonal antibodies brought down both complexed T antigen and a 70-kd doublet, presumably HSP68 and HSP70. However, when SV40 T antigen-specific antibodies were employed, only p53 was coprecipitated with no evidence of HSP (Fig. 8). The simplest interpretation is that p53 can either associate with T antigen or with HSP 70 but not with both together, suggesting that these two latter proteins may be competing for the same or very close sites on the p53 molecule. Although final proof will depend on the construction of mutant p53 molecules incapable of complex formation, this observation suggests that T antigen may be following a mechanism which is sometimes utilized by HSP70. The significance of such a finding can probably be assessed only once more is learned about the functions of the heat-shock proteins. However, some suggestive similarities do exist between HSP70 and the SV40 T antigen. Aside from having a nuclear affinity [32,33,37], both proteins are capable of binding ATP [32,37]. The SV40 T antigen possesses ATPase activity [37]. Such an activity has not been demonstrated for the HSP70 [29], but is indeed exhibited by the structurally related *Escherichia coli* heat-inducible DNA K protein [38,39]. Interestingly, this bacterial protein is involved in the replication of bacteriophage DNA in host cells [38], as is T antigen in the replication of SV40 in mammalian cells [37]. Studies in the *Drosophila* system revealed that HSP70 is found in ribonucleoprotein complexes [40], suggesting that it may be involved in mRNA processing or RNA stabilization. If the complex with p53 reflects a common cellular site of action, this raises the possibility that p53 may also have functions related to RNA metabolism.

Finally, as indicated in Figures 4 and 5, the p53-overproducing clone 6 possesses a markedly elevated level of HSP70 prior to heat-induction. This suggests that the production of this protein may be positively regulated by p53. This overproduction could merely result from stabilization of HSP70 in the complex. However, it is

T   P

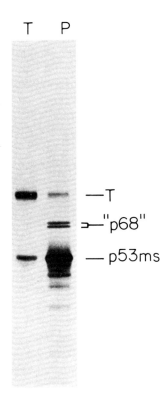

—T

⊃—"p68"

— p53ms

Fig. 8. Immunoprecipitation of proteins from infected COS cells overproducing mouse p53. COS cells were infected with recombinant SV40 virions carrying a mouse p53-specific cDNA segment inserted into the early region of the viral DNA. Extracts of infected cells were reacted either with the anti-p53 monoclonal antibody PAb421 (P) or with the anti-large T antigen monoclonal antibody clone 412 (T). p53ms=mouse p53; T=SV40 large T antigen; "p68" refers to the putative HSP68 and HSP70 bands. For further details see [13].

equally likely that it reflects transcriptional activation of the corresponding HSP gene. The latter possibility is of particular interest in light of the recent demonstration that the human HSP70 gene(s) appears to be expressed in a cell-cycle-dependent manner [41], which is in keeping with the notion that p53 may be a cell-cycle control protein [42,43]. Thus, p53 may be considered a candidate for the Ela-like cellular protein implicated in the control of heat-shock gene expression [41]. It is most noteworthy that direct evidence already exists for the ability of the *myc* oncogene product to trans-activate the *Drosophila* HSP70 promoter [44]. In light of the many analogies between p53 and *myc* [1,2,36], it is quite conceivable that both proteins may exert a similar effect on the expression of some HSP genes as part of their normal regulatory function. Clearly, further work is needed before such a conclusion can be made with confidence.

ACKNOWLEDGMENTS

We would like to thank M. Tainovitch for technical assistance, and Drs. O. Bensaude and B. Geiger for stimulating discussions. This work was supported in part by the Minerva Foundation, Munich, and by the Leo and Julia Forchheimer Center for Molecular Genetics at the Weizmann Institute. M.O. is a Leukemia Society of America, Inc., Scholar.

REFERENCES

1. Eliyahu D, Raz A, Gruss P, Givol D, Oren M: Nature 312:646, 1984.
2. Parada LF, Land H, Weinberg RA, Wolf D, Rotter V: Nature 312:649, 1984.
3. Jenkins JR, Rudge K, Currie GA: Nature 312:651, 1984.
4. Crawford LV, Lane DP, Denhardt DT, Harlow ER, Nicklin PM, Osborn K, Pim DC: Cold Spring Harbor Symp Quant Biol 44:179, 1980.
5. McCormick F, Harlow E: J Virol 34:213, 1980.
6. Lane DP, Gannon J, Winchester G: Adv Virol Oncol 2:23, Raven Press, New York, 1982.
7. Oren M, Maltzman W, Levine AJ: Mol Cell Biol 1:101, 1981.
8. Mora PT, Chandrasekaran K, Hoffman JC, McFarland VW: Mol Cell Biol 2:763, 1982.
9. May E, Lasne C, Prives C, Borde J, May P: J Virol 45:901, 1983.
10. Oren M, Reich NC, Levine AJ: Mol Cell Biol 2:443, 1982.
11. Reich NC, Oren M, Levine AJ: Mol Cell Biol 3:2143, 1983.
12. Gronostajski RM, Goldberg AL, Pardee AB: Mol Cell Biol 4:442, 1984.
13. Pinhasi O, Oren M: Mol Cell Biol 4:2180, 1984.
14. Ruscetti SK, Scolnick EM: J Virol 46:1022, 1983.
15. Steinberg B, Pollack R, Topp W, Botchan M: Cell 13:19, 1978.
16. Eliyahu D, Michalovitz D, Oren M: Nature 316:158, 1985.
17. Maltzman W, Oren M, Levine AJ: Virology 112:145, 1981.
18. Curran T, Van Beveren C, Ling N, Verma IM: Mol Cell Biol 5:167, 1985.
19. Morange M, Diu A, Bensaude O, Babinet C: Mol Cell Biol 4:730, 1984.
20. O'Farrell PZ, Goodman HM, O'Farrell PH: Cell 12:1133, 1977.
21. Bonner WM, Laskey RA: Eur J Biochem 46:83, 1974.
22. Cleveland D, Fisher S, Kirschner M, Laemmli UK: J Biol Chem 252:1102, 1977.
23. Harlow E, Crawford LV, Pim DC, Williamson NM: J Virol 39:861, 1981.
24. Rotter V, Witte ON, Coffman R, Baltimore D: J Virol 36:547, 1980.
25. Rotter V, Friedman H, Katz A, Zerivitz K, Wolf D: J Immunol 131:329, 1983.
26. Crawford LV: Adv Virol Oncol 2:3, Raven Press, New York, 1982.
27. Bensaude O, Morange M: EMBO J 2:173, 1983.
28. Lowe DG, Moran LA: Proc Natl Acad Sci USA 81:2317, 1984.
29. Welch WJ, Feramisco JR: Mol Cell Biol 5:1229, 1985.
30. Linzer DIH, Levine AJ: Cell 17:43, 1979.
31. Opperman H, Levinson W, Bishop JM: Proc Natl Acad Sci USA 78:1067, 1981.
32. Welch WJ, Feramisco JR: J Biol Chem 259:4501, 1984.
33. Velasquez JM, Lindquist S: Cell 36:655, 1984.
34. Rotter V, Abutbul H, Ben-Zeev A: EMBO J 2:1041, 1983.
35. DeLeo AB, Jay G, Appela E, Dubois GC, Law LW, Old LJ: Proc Natl Acad Sci USA 76:2420, 1979.
36. Bienz B, Zakut-Houri R, Givol D, Oren M: EMBO J 3:2179, 1984.
37. Tooze J (ed): "DMA Tumor Viruses, Part 2." Cold Spring Harbor, N.Y.: Cold Spring Harbor Laboratory, 1982.
38. Zylicz M, Georgopoulos: J Biol Chem 259:8820, 1984.
39. Bardwell JCA, Craig E: Proc Natl Acad Sci USA 81:848, 1984.
40. Kloetzel PM, Bautz EKF: EMBO J 2:705, 1983.
41. Kao HT, Capassa D, Heintz N, Nevins JR: Mol Cell Biol 5:628, 1985.
42. Mercer WE, Nelson D, DeLeo AB, Old LJ, Baserga R: Proc Natl Acad Sci USA 79:6309, 1982.
43. Kaczmarek L, Oren M, Baserga R: Exp Cell Res 162:268, 1986.
44. Kingston RE, Baldwin AS, Sharp PA: Nature 312:280, 1984.
45. Oren M, Levine AJ: Proc Natl Acad Sci USA 80:56, 1983.

Cellular and Molecular Biology of Tumors and Potential
Clinical Applications 261–268 (1988)

Molecular Genetic Analysis of Mouse B Lymphocyte Differentiation

Jan Jongstra and Mark M. Davis

Department of Medical Microbiology, Stanford University School of Medicine, Stanford, California 94305-5402

Using subtractive hybridization methodologies, we have isolated cDNA clones which are expressed in a variety of B lymphocyte cell lines but not in T lymphocyte cell lines. Several cDNA clones encoding the immunoglobulin lambda 1 light chain constant region and MHC class II proteins were isolated and used as probes on Northern blots. We find that four out of six pre-B cell lines express all four major MHC class II genes and the gene for the Ia-associated invariant chain, but only one of these cell lines expresses Ia antigens on the cell surface. We also find that five out of six pre-B cell lines express an RNA transcript derived from an unrearranged lambda light chain allele. In addition, we have isolated two previously unidentified B-lineage-specific cDNA clones the characterization of which should add to our knowledge of the differentiation and function of these cells.

Key words: B cell specific genes

During B lymphocyte differentiation, cells mature from a pluripotent stem cell through a series of discrete intermediary stages into terminally differentiated cells. These intermediary stages of development have been defined using a combination of morphological, serological, and molecular data [for review see 1]. For instance, the rearrangement and expression of the immunoglobulin (Ig) genes underlies the division of the B lymphocyte pathway in three stages. The first identifiable stage is the surface Ig$^-$ (sIg$^-$) pre-B cell, which is characterized by the expression of the Ig heavy chain gene but not of the light chain genes [2–6]. During subsequent maturation to the B-cell stage, there is a concurrent appearance of Ig and Ia molecules on the cell surface [7,8]. The final stage of the B lymphocyte pathway is the Ig-secreting plasma cell. In addition to the studies on expression of the Ig and MHC class II genes coding for the Ia antigens, there exists a large body of data on the differential expression of serological markers on the surface of B lymphocytes [1,9–12]. Thus, the study of genes and gene products of which the expression is restricted almost exclusively to

Jan Jongstra's present address is Toronto Western Hospital, McLaughlin Pavilion, Rm 13-419, 399 Bathurst Street, Toronto, Ontario M5T 2S5, Canada.

Received June 10, 1986.

cells of the B lineage has contributed greatly to our understanding of the cellular and molecular biology of B lymphocyte development.

It has recently been determined that sequences which are expressed in B cells but not in T cells make up $2\% \pm 0.5\%$ of the total cytoplasmic mRNA present in B cells [13]. Part of this difference can be accounted for by the known differential expression of the well-studied Ig and MHC class II genes, which code for effector proteins through which B cells fulfill their unique function in the immune system. Little is known about the structure and function of other B-lineage-specific genes. However, we expect that part of these specifically expressed genes are involved in regulating B-cell-specific functions such as the expression of Ig and MHC class II genes, or are involved in the regulation of the differentiation processes which drive B lymphocytes from one stage to a next more mature one.

This paper describes our analysis of the pre-B- to B-cell transition of mouse lymphocytes using a variety of in vitro tumors and Abelson leukemia virus (AbLV)-transformed cells lines. We have concentrated on this transition, since at that point the B lymphocyte undergoes a number of easily measured phenotypic changes—ie, from a sIg$^-$, sIa$^-$ pre-B cell to a sIg$^+$, sIa$^+$ B cell. Our results suggest that the induction of sIa expression during the pre-B- to B-cell transition is not solely due to transcriptional activation of the MHC class II genes, since a number of sIa$^-$ pre-B cell lines express levels of MHC class II RNA similar to those found in sIa$^+$ B cell lines. In addition to this unexpected expression of MHC class II genes, we also detect an RNA transcript related to the Ig lambda light chain constant region in five out of six pre-B cells tested. Finally, we have isolated two novel B-lineage-specific genes. Northern analysis shows that one clone is expressed throughout B lymphocyte development, while the second represents a gene expressed only in the B-cell and plasma cell stages.

RESULTS
Strategy for Isolation of B-Cell-Specific cDNA Clones

To isolate cDNA sequences representing genes differentially expressed during B lymphocyte development, we screened a B-T-subtracted cDNA library with a ^{32}P-labeled B-T-subtracted cDNA probe (B*-T). This cDNA library [14] was prepared using cDNA from the sIgM$^+$/sIgD$^+$ lymphoma cell line BAL 17 and was enriched for B-cell-specific sequences by subtraction with RNA from the T-cell lymphoma BAL 4. This subtracted cDNA was then made double-stranded and cloned into pBR322. This gave rise to approximately 9,000 independent colonies enriched approximately 25-fold for B-cell-specific sequences [as reported in 14]. This library was screened twice with different subtracted B*-T probes (specific activity 10^8 cpm/μg). The first probe was prepared from BAL 17 cells and subtracted with RNA from BAL 4, and the second probe was prepared from the B lymphoma WEHI 231 and subtracted with RNA from the T lymphoma BW5147. In total we isolated 64 positive colonies. Of these positive clones, 25 have been screened using the inserts as probes on Northern blots with RNA extracted from a variety of B- and T-cell lines. As can be seen in Table I, which summarizes the results of these cloning experiments, nine clones represent B-lineage- specific genes, indicating the substantial enrichment for B-lineage-specific genes obtained using the subtractive hybridization technique.

Isolation of MHC Class II and Lambda Light Chain cDNA Clones

Two of the nine B-lineage-specific clones represent MHC class II genes (Table I). This was expected since class II genes are expressed mainly on mature B cells and macrophages but not on terminally differentiated plasma cells or on T cells [15]. Figure 1A shows the results of a Northern blot containing total cytoplasmic RNA from a series of B- and T-lineage cells, using an A_β cDNA clone as a probe. Surprisingly, we found that four out of six pre-B cells expressed A_β mRNA (positive results for line 230.238 not shown, see also Table II). Similar results were obtained using A_α, E_α, or E_β cDNA clones as probes. We also tested the expression of RNA coding for the Ia-associated invariant chain [Ii,16]. Figure 1B shows that the pre-B cell lines expressing MHC class II RNA also express Ii RNA. In the mouse, pre-B cells are sIa$^-$ [9,12]. We therefore asked the question whether the pre-B cell lines

**TABLE I. Screening a B-T-Subtracted cDNA
Library With B*-T cDNA Probes**

Positive colonies	64
B-lineage-specific	
MHC class II clones	2
Ig lambda light chain related clones	5
novel B-lineage-specific clones	2

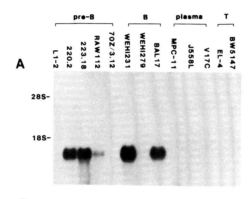

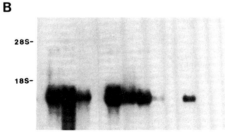

Fig. 1. Northern blot analysis of lymphoid cell lines. Each lane contains 10 μg of total cytoplasmic RNA fractionated on a 1.2% agarose-formaldehyde gel and transferred to nitrocellulose paper and hybridized with plasmid DNA labeled with ^{32}P by nick translation. The names of the cell lines used to prepare RNA are indicated above each lane. Groups of samples from cell lines representing similar stages of lymphoid development are indicated by brackets. The positions of the 28S and 18S ribosomal RNA species are indicated at the left. **A:** Probed with a cDNA clone of A_β^d in pBR322 (gift of Dr. P. Estess). **B:** Probed with cDNA clone pIi representing the gene for the Ia-associated invariant chain ([16] obtained from Dr. Dobberstein through Dr. J. Danska)

TABLE II. Northern Analysis of the Expression of B-Lineage-Specific Genes

	Cell lines			
	Pre-B	B	Plasma	T
MHC class II	4/6[a]	2/3	0/3	0/4
pJJ55 ($C_{\lambda 1}$)	5/6	N.A.	N.A.	0/2
pJJ32	6/6	3/3	2/3	0/4
pMD4	0/2	1/3	2/3	0/2

[a]No. positive/No. tested.

expressing class II RNA also expressed class II protein on the cell surface. Using monoclonal antibodies and ^{125}I-labeled protein A, we found that all pre-B cells were sIg$^-$, H-2$^+$, but only line 223.18 expressed Ia antigens on the cell surface (results not shown). It appears, therefore, that in a randomly chosen sample of six pre-B cell lines, four express class II RNA, but only one line expresses class II protein on the cell surface which can be recognized by the monoclonal antibody used in the typing experiments. This indicates that in the early stages of B lymphocyte development the surface expression of class II antigens is not solely regulated on the transcriptional level but may depend on other factors as well.

Five of the nine B-lineage-specific clones represent a lambda 1 Ig light chain transcript present in BAL 17 cells (Table I). When a Northern blot was probed with the longest of these five clones, pJJ55, we found to our surprise that five out of six pre-B-cell lines express a low level of RNA hybridizing to this cDNA clone. The only negative line, 223.18, was subsequently shown to express a similar low level of kappa Ig light chain related RNA (results not shown). pJJ55 does not hybridize to RNA extracted from four T-cell lines (Table II). It is thought that the kappa light chain locus rearranges before the lambda locus during B-cell development [17,18]. Indeed, when we probed EcoRI-restricted DNA isolated from pre-B cells, a B cell, a plasma cell, and from the myelomonocytic leukemia line WEHI 3 with pJJ55, we detected lambda gene rearrangements only in the B cells and plasma cells, but not in the six pre-B cells used in this study or in the line WEHI 3 (results not shown). This raised the question of whether the lambda-related transcript found in pre-B-cell lines derives from the unrearranged lambda variable region or constant region. To answer that question, we prepared a lambda V- and J-region-specific probe and a lambda C-region-specific probe by isolating appropriate restriction fragments from pJJ55 and hybridized duplicate Northern blots containing RNA from 6 pre-B-cell lines with each probe. The results show that the lambda-related transcript in five out of six pre-B cells derives from a lambda C region (Fig. 2). Due to sequence homology between C lambda 1 and C lambda 4, it is not possible to conclude from these data whether the transcripts derive from C lambda 1 or C lambda 4. The lambda RNA transcript present in BAL 17 cells is derived from a rearranged allele and thus hybridizes with both probes. From these data we conclude that the pre-B cells studied here all express an Ig light chain transcript, either lambda related (lines L1-2,220.2,70Z/3.12, RAW112,230.238) or kappa related (line 223.18). We do not as yet know whether the kappa-related transcript in 223.18 contains both V, J, and C region sequences; but this line, as well as all the other pre-B-cell lines used in this study, is sIg$^-$.

Isolation of Novel B-Cell-Specific cDNA Clones

One clone, pJJ32, which hybridizes to a 1.6-kilobase(kb) mRNA species represents a gene which is expressed in a variety of B-lineage cell lines representing the

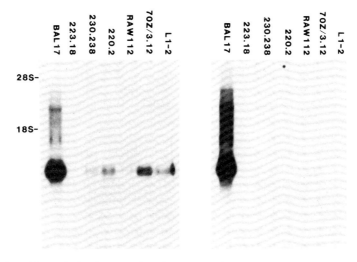

Fig. 2.   Northern blot analysis of pre-B cells. The names of the cell lines used are indicated above each lane. All cell lines except BAL 17 are sIg⁻ pre-B cells. BAL 17 is a sIgM⁺/sIgD⁺ B-cell line. Each lane contains 5 μg of polyA⁺ RNA prepared by oligo-dT selection of total cytoplasmic RNA. The RNA was fractionated on a 1.2% agarose-formaldehyde gel, transferred to nitrocellulose paper, and hybridized with DNA fragments representing different parts of the cDNA insert from pJJ55, then labeled with ³²P using the hexamer labeling procedure described in Feinberg and Vogelstein [28]. The positions of the 28S and 18S ribosomal RNA species are indicated on the left. **Left:** Probed with a 250-base pair (bp) fragment containing only lambda 1 constant region sequences. **Right:** probed with a 213-bp fragment containing part of the lambda 1 V region, the complete J region, and 53 bp of lambda 1 constant region sequences.

pre-B-cell, B-cell, and plasma cell stages, but not in four T cell lines tested (results not shown, see Table II). We have determined the nucleotide sequence of a 1.4-kb cDNA insert isolated from a pre-B-cell cDNA library prepared in phage lambda gt10, using pJJ32 as a probe. The DNA sequence of this clone does not show any significant homology with any sequence in the GenBank database. It appears, therefore, that clone pJJ32 represents a novel B-cell-specific gene expressed throughout B lymphocyte development.

To facilitate the identification of cDNA clones representing genes differentially expressed during B lymphocyte development in a manner less time-consuming than testing each clone individually as a probe on a Northern blot, we screened the 64 clones initially identified in the BAL 17-BAL 4 library as positive with a B*-T cDNA probe in the following manner. Plasmid DNA was prepared from 4-ml cultures of these 64 colonies, and after gel electrophoresis was transferred to nitrocellulose. This filter was then hybridized with a subtracted cDNA probe made from BAL 17 cDNA subtracted with RNA from uninduced 70Z/3.12 cells. In this manner all 64 clones could be screened at once, and this procedure was thus much less time-consuming than the Northern analysis used to screen the first 25 clones. In this way, we identified clone pMD4, which hybridizes to three species of mRNA with lengths of 2.0, 2.4, and 3.5 kb. Its expression pattern differs from pJJ32, since RNA hybridizing to this clone can be detected only in myeloma lines and in a late-stage B lymphoma BAL 17 but not in the less mature B lymphomas WEHI 231 or WEHI 279.12 (Table II).

DISCUSSION

We have restricted our genetic analysis of B lymphocyte development to B-lineage-specific genes for two reasons.

First, cDNA clones representing B-lineage- or stage-specific genes can be used as molecular probes to study their expression during B-cell development. These genetic markers will complement existing studies which have used a collection of differentially expressed cell surface markers and the state and expression of known genes such as the Ig or MHC class II genes to further define stages in B-cell development. This will be especially useful for the early stages of B-cell development for which no satisfactory serological markers are available and Ig gene rearrangements have not yet taken place. Examples of such clones are pJJ32 and pJJ55.

Second, our understanding of B-cell development depends on our knowledge of the genes and gene products which are involved in the regulation of development. We assume that such regulatory genes are, at least in part, expressed in a B-lineage- or stage-specific manner. To identify possible regulatory genes we adopted the following criteria. First, the gene should be expressed in a B-lineage-specific manner; that is, it should not be expressed in cells of other hematopoetic lineages or other cell types. Second, its expression pattern should be established previsely in vitro and if possible in vivo to determine during which developmental stage the expression of a given B lineage specific gene is activated. Third, we will use the nucleotide sequence of a given B-lineage-specific cDNA clone to predict the amino acid sequence and some characteristics of its gene product. For instance, it should be possible to predict whether the protein is secreted or membrane bound. Such genes are not obvious candidates for being regulatory genes, although they might be involved in other aspects of B-cell development such as cell-cell interactions. Fourth, the cDNA clone should code for a protein which accumulates in the nucleus. One possible assay for nuclear localization involves the synthesis of radioactively labeled protein from in vitro generated RNA transcripts [19], and injection of this protein into frog oocytes. At various times after injection the oocyte is enucleated and the distribution of the injected protein over nucleoplasm and cytoplasm is determined using SDS-PAGE. Similar experiments using native [20–22] or in vitro synthesized proteins [23] have established the karyophilic nature of a large number of proteins. It will also be possible to use the in vitro generated protein to determine a number of its possible characteristics, such as its DNA binding capacity or recombinase activity. Thus, based on these four criteria, it should be possible to select cDNA clones which are strong candidate regulatory genes and to predict in which developmental transition they are involved. The actual testing of these predictions will involve gene transfer in appropriate cell cultures or cell lines which represent early stages of B-cell development and which have retained their capacity to develop to mature sIg$^+$B cells. Several such systems have been described [24–27]. We are confident that some of these will be useful to study the function of B-lineage-specific cDNA clones in B-cell development.

One group of regulatory molecules we hope to isolate by the strategy outlined in this paper are those regulating the transcription of the Ig light chain and MHC class II genes. We predict that at least in part those regulatory genes are B-lineage-specific and are expressed in the B-cell stage but not in the pre-B stage. However, we unexpectedly found RNA transcripts related to the Ig lambda and kappa genes and the MHC class II genes in a large proportion of the AbLV-transformed pre-B-cell lines. This suggests that in most cell lines which are used as in vitro models for the pre-B-cell stage, much of the regulatory apparatus for Ig light chain and MHC class II genes is already functional. It is interesting that the majority of the pre-B lines tested express a lambda 1 or 4 but not a lambda 2 or 3 related transcript (see Table II). This might reflect the uneven use of lambda isotypes in the mouse (75% of the serum lambda light chains are lambda 1). It is also possible, however, that the pre-B lines represent a restricted subpopulation of pre-B cells. We are presently determining the expression of Ig and class II genes in both in vivo derived and freshly cultivated pre-B cells to determine whether our findings extend to normal, nontransformed cell populations.

ACKNOWLEDGMENTS

We thank Kathy Redman for preparation of the manuscript, Robert Perry for help with the cell surface staining, and George Tidmarsh for providing us with the AbLV-transformed cell lines.

This work was supported by grants to M.M.D. from the American Cancer Society and the PEW Memorial Trust Fund. Jan Jongstra is a recipient of a Senior Postdoctoral Fellowship from the American Cancer Society, California Division.

REFERENCES

 1. Kincade PW: Adv Immunol 31:177, 1981.
 2. Owen JJT, Wright DE, Habu S, Raff MC, Cooper MD: J Immunol 118:2067, 1977.
 3. Burrows P, Lejeune M, Kearney JF: Nature 280:838, 1979.
 4. Levitt D, Cooper MD: Cell 19:617, 1980.
 5. Landreth KS, Rosse C, Clagett J: J Immunol 127:2027, 1981.
 6. Alt F, Rosenberg N, Lewis S, Thomas E, Baltimore D: Cell 27:381, 1981.
 7. Lala PK, Johnson GR, Battye FL, Nossal GJV: J Immunol 122:334, 1979.
 8. Mond JJ, Kessler S, Finkelman FD, Paul WE, Scher I: J Immunol 124:1675, 1980.
 9. Kincade PW, Lee G, Watanabe T, Sun L, Scheid MP: J Immunol 127:2262, 1981.
10. Lanier LL, Warner NL, Ledbetter JA, Herzenberg LA: J Immunol 127:1691, 1981.
11. McKenzie IFC, Zola H: Immunol Today 4:10, 1983.
12. McKearn JP, Baum C, Davie JM: J Immunol 132:332, 1984.
13. Davis MM, Cohen DI, Nielsen EA, Defranco AL, Paul WE: In Vitteta E, Fox CF (eds): "B and T Cell Tumors." UCLA Symp 24:215, 1982.
14. Davis MM, Cohen DI, Nielsen EA, Steinmetz M, Paul WE, Hood L: Proc Natl Acad Sci USA 81:2194, 1984.
15. Mengle-Gaw L, McDevitt HO: Annu Rev Immunol 3:367, 1985.
16. Singer PA, Lauer W, Dembic Z, Mayer WE, Lipp J, Koch N, Hammerling G, Klein J, Dobberstein B: EMBO 3:873, 1984.
17. Hieter PA, Korsmeyer SJ, Waldmann TA, Leder P: Nature 290:368, 1981.
18. Coleclough C, Perry RP, Karjalainen K, Weigert M: Nature 290:372, 1981.
19. Krieg PA, Melton DA: Nucleic Acids Res 123:7057, 1984.
20. Gurdon JB: Proc Soc Lond [Biol] 176:303, 1970.
21. Bonner WM: J Cell Biol 64:431, 1975.
22. DeRobertis EM, Longthorne RF, Gurdon JB: Nature 272:254, 1978.
23. Dabauvalle M-C, Franke WW: Proc Natl Acad Sci USA 79:5302, 1982.
24. Whitlock CA, Witte ON: Proc Natl Acad Sci USA 79:3608, 1982.
25. Kurland JI, Ziegler SF, Witte ON: Proc Natl Acad Sci USA 81:7554, 1984.
26. Palacios R, Steinmetz M: Cell 41:727, 1985.
27. Spalding DM, Griffin JA: Cell 44:507, 1986.

28. Feinberg AP, Vogelstein B: Anal Biochem 132:6, 1983.

NOTE ADDED IN PROOF

Since the submission of this paper we have isolated a cDNA clone of the Ig lambda light chain related RNA transcript from the pre-B cell line 220.2. DNA sequence analysis of the cDNA clone shows that the transcript derives from a novel Ig lambda related gene which we call Lambda 5 (J. Jongstra et al, submitted).

Cellular and Molecular Biology of Tumors and Potential
Clinical Applications 269–274 (1988)

Virally Induced Hematopoietic Cell Transformation: Multistep Leukemogenesis and Growth-Factor-Independent Cell Proliferation

Allen Oliff and Steven Anderson

Merck Sharp and Dohme Research Laboratories, West Point, Pennsylvania 19486

Friend murine leukemia virus (F-MuLV) induces a rapidly fatal nonlymphocytic leukemia in mice. Although the disease caused by F-MuLV is highly virulent, leukemia cells obtained from diseased animals do not grow in vitro in the absence of exogenous growth factors. F-MuLV-infected leukemia cells also fail to transplant into syngeneic animals. However, if interleukin-3 or WEHI-3 cell conditioned media is added to cultures of F-MuLV-induced leukemia cells, immortal cell lines develop. These cell lines are absolutely dependent on exogenous growth factors for their survival, and they will not form tumors if injected into syngeneic mice. We superinfected these growth-factor-dependent cell lines with a variety of mammalian retroviruses. Both Abelson leukemia virus and a mammalian *src* containing retrovirus eliminate the cell lines' requirement for interleukin-3. Concomitant with the loss of growth factor dependence in vitro, the AbLV- and *src*-infected cell lines became tumorogenic in syngeneic mice. Harvey sarcoma virus, Kirsten sarcoma Virus, FBJ osteosaroma virus, Moloney murine sarcoma virus, feline sarcoma virus, and a mammalian *myc*-containing virus failed to alter the growth properties of the F-MuLV-infected cell lines.

Key words: friend leukemia virus, oncogenes, mitogenesis

Friend murine leukemia virus (F-MuLV) is a replication-competent, type C retrovirus [1]. Newborn NIH Swiss mice inoculated with F-MuLV rapidly develop acute nonlymphocytic leukemia characterized by circulating hematopoietic blasts, severe anemia, and hepatosplenomegaly [2,3]. NIH Swiss and NFS/n mice are particularly susceptible to F-MuLV-induced leukemias. One hundred percent of these mice die from their leukemias within 3 months following inoculation with F-MuLV. Despite the extreme virulence of F-MuLV-induced disease, leukemia cells taken from these animals do not exhibit all of the characteristics normally associated with malignant cells. Specifically, F-MuLV-infected leukemia cells will not grow in cell culture, and they will not transplant into syngeneic mice. It is possible to isolate rare

Received February 20, 1986.

($< 1/10^6$) leukemia cells from F-MuLV-infected animals that do grow in cell culture and form tumors in syngeneic animals. However, these cells are only found in diseased mice that are given supportive therapy in the form of packed red blood cell transfusions. Diseased mice that receive red blood cell transfusions survive 6–8 weeks longer than untreated mice. Fifty percent of the transfused animals develop transplantable leukemia cells [4]. We use these functional criteria—transplantability and explantability—to separate the disease caused by F-MuLV into two stages. Stage I disease and stage II disease are pathologically and histologically indistinguishable. However, stage I cells do not grow in syngeneic mice and do not grow in cell culture. Stage II cells are both transplantable and explantable.

To define the genetic events responsible for the different growth characteristics of stage I and stage II cells, we attempted to isolate large numbers of pure stage I and stage II cells for biochemical analysis of their nucleic acids. Pure stage II cells are easily obtained from cell culture. Stage I cells are more difficult to purify since they do not grow in vitro under standard cell culture conditions. However, it is possible to propagate stage I cells in vitro if the culture medium is supplemented with either conditioned media from WEHI-3 cells [5] or with purified interleukin-3 (IL-3) [6]. One hundred percent of F-MuLV-infected mice with stage I disease yield immortal cell lines when their hematopoietic tissues are explanted into IL-3-containing media [7]. While these cell lines are immortal, they nonetheless remain absolutely dependent on IL-3 for proliferation and survival. If stage I cells are removed from culture and plated in fresh media devoid of IL-3, they cease to divide and die within 24 hr. Stage I cell lines grown in the presence of IL-3 exhibit a cell doubling time of 18–20 hr. The cell population in these cultures consist primarily of myeloblasts, with only 1–5% of the cells spontaneously differentiating into more mature elements in the myeloid lineage. Most importantly, stage I cell lines do not cause leukemia or any other tumors if inoculated into syngeneic animals. In contrast to the stage I cell lines, stage II cells are immortal in vitro with or without IL-3, and stage II cells cause donor cell leukemias in syngeneic mice. Stage II cells also undergo rapid cell division with a doubling time of 18 hr. Stage II cells are entirely blastic in morphology with no evidence of spontaneous differentiation.

It is possible to propagate normal bone marrow cells in vitro using IL-3. These cultures are similar to the stage I cell lines in that they are absolutely dependent on IL-3 for proliferation, and they do not cause disease in syngeneic mice. However, normal bone marrow precursors will only proliferate in media containing IL-3 for 4–6 weeks under our culture conditions. Normal bone marrow cultures grow more slowly (cell doubling time = 48–72 hr) than either stage I or stage II cell cultures. These normal cell cultures contain predominantly differentiated elements from the myeloid series and 1–5% hematopoietic blasts. We call the cells obtained from normal bone marrow cultures stage 0 cells. Stage 0 cells appear to represent the normal hematopoietic counterpart of the F-MuLV-infected stage I and stage II cells. The growth characteristics of stage I, II, and 0 cells are summarized in Table I.

In an attempt to identify genes that are preferentially expressed in the normal (stage 0), abnormal (stage I), or malignant (stage II) cells in our culture system, we purified cytoplasmic RNAs from these cells. The poly-A$^+$ fraction [8] of each cell lines' RNA was analyzed by dot blots and filter hybridization [9] using the following radiolabeled oncogene and growth factor genes as probes: Harvey *ras*, Kirsten *ras*, N-*ras*, *mos*, *abl*, *fes*, *fms*, *raf*, *fos*, *sis*, *src*, *myc*, *myb*, *erb-a*, *erb-b*, *ski*, *myc*, B-*lym*, *p-53*, *transferrin*, *EGF*, and *IL-3*.

TABLE I. Growth Characteristics of Stage 0, Stage I, and Stage II Cells

	Stage 0	Stage I	Stage II
Tissue source	Normal BM[a]	Leukemic BM	Leukemic BM/transfused mice or Stage I cell lines
Transplantation in syngeneic mice	NED[b]	NED	Donor cell leukemia
Survival in culture + WEHI-3 CM	3–5 wk	Immortal	Immortal
− WEHI-3 CM	24 hr	24 hr	Immortal
Cell doubling time (hr)	48–72	18–24	18–20
Blast cell count (%)	1–2	95–99	100
Viruses	0	F-MuLV (Fr-MCF)	F-MuLV Fr-MCF

[a]Bone Marrow.
[b]NED = no evidence of disease.

No clear pattern of oncogene expression is evident from these studies. Approximately, half of these genes are expressed at higher levels in either stage I or stage II cells relative to stage 0 cells. The remaining genes are expressed either at the same levels in all three cell cultures or at higher levels in stage 0 cells than in stage I or stage II cells. For example, *myc* expression is higher in stage 0 cells than in stage II cells, while Ki-*ras* is expressed at higher levels in stage II cells than in either stage I or stage 0 cells. What is clear is that many genes rather than only one or a few genes are expressed at different levels in stage 0, stage I, and stage II cell cultures.

To analyze the contribution of individual genes to the growth properties of stage I and stage II cells, it is necessary to introduce these genes into cells one at a time. We used retroviruses to introduce viral oncogenes into either stage 0 or stage I cell lines. These genes are infected into the recipient cell lines using amphotropic [10] pseudotypes of mammalian retroviruses. Viral penetration and replication within the stage 0 and stage I cells is monitored by recovery of biologically active virus from the culture media of the infected cell lines (Table II). Once a productive infection is established, the infected cells are tested for the ability to grow in the absence of IL-3 and for their transplantability in syngeneic mice. The following viruses were infected into both stage 0 and stage I cell lines: Harvey sarcoma virus (HaSV), Kirsten sarcoma virus (KiSV), Abelson leukemia virus (AbLV), AS (a mammalian retrovirus carrying the Rous sarcoma virus *src* gene) [11], Moloney sarcoma virus (MoMSV), McDonough strain of feline sarcoma virus (FeSV, carrying the *Fms* oncogene), *myc*-containing mammalian virus, and FBJ murine osteosarcoma virus (carrying the *fos* oncogene).

Only the AbLV and AS retroviruses altered the growth properties of stage I cells [12,13]. Two independent stage I cell lines infected with either AbLV or AS virus lose their dependence on IL-3 for growth in culture. Concomitant with the loss of growth factor dependence in vitro, both cell lines become tumorogenic in syngeneic mice. The transplanted tumors in each case were analyzed by cytogenetic markers and found to be of donor cell origin. In other words, the AbLV- and AS-infected stage I cell lines now behave like stage II cells. The *abl* and *src* genes present in these viruses must be responsible for the abrogation of growth factor dependence since infection of the same stage I cells with non-oncogene-containing helper virus does not affect

TABLE II. Viral Titers of Infected Cell Lines

Cell line[a]	Viral titer[b]
IO-3	$< 10°$
OZ-3	$< 10°$
ST-0	$< 10°$
IO-3—Ampho	$< 10°$
OZ-3—Ampho	$< 10°$
ST-0—Ampho	$< 10°$
IO-3—AbLV/Ampho	10^1
OZ-3—AbLV/Ampho	10^1
ST-3—AbLV/Ampho	10^1
IO-3—AS/Ampho	10^1
OZ-3—AS/Ampho	10^1
ST-0—AS/Ampho	10^1
IO-3—HaSV/Ampho	10^2
OZ-3—HaSV/Ampho	10^2
ST-0—HasV/Ampho	10^1
IO-3—KiSV/Ampho	10^2
OZ-3—KiSV/Ampho	10^2
ST-0—KiSV/Ampho	10^2
IO-3—MoMSV/Ampho	10^2
OZ-3—MoMSV/Ampho	10^2
ST-0—MoMSV/Ampho	10^1
IO-3—FBJ/Ampho	10^2
OZ-3—FBJ/Ampho	10^2
ST-0—FBJ/Ampho	10^1
IO-3—FeSV/Ampho	$5 \times 10°$
OZ-3—FeSV/Ampho	NT[c]
ST-0—FeSV/Ampho	NT
IO-3—myc/Ampho	NT
OZ-3—myc/Ampho	NT
ST-0—myc/Ampho	10^{3d}

[a]Each cell line was infected with the indicated virus. IO-3 and OZ-3 are independent clonally derived stage I cell lines. ST-0 = stage 0 cells. Ampho = amphotropic murine leukemia virus.
[b]Viral titers were determined on NIH 3T3 cells by counting foci [14] of transformed cells 14–21 days postinfection with 1 ml of freshly harvested culture media.
[c]NT = not tested.
[d]myc/Ampho titers were determined by reverse transcriptase assay [15] on serially diluted samples of freshly harvested culture media. The values listed indicate the highest dilution of media that still contain detectable reverse transcriptase activity.

their growth properties. None of the other viruses used in our studies affect the growth properties of stage I cells. Interestingly, none of the viruses, including AbLV and AS affect the growth characteristics of the stage 0 cells. Retrovirus-infected stage 0 cells do not form tumors in mice and die out after 4–6 weeks in culture even in the presence of IL-3.

We conclude that the growth factor dependence of murine leukemia cells can be overcome by specific oncogenes (Fig. 1). In the case of F-MuLV-infected myeloid leukemia cells, both *src* and *abl* but not *myc*, *fos*, *fms*, *H-ras*, *Ki-ras*, or *mos* abrogate the IL-3 dependence of these cells. Presumably, a similar phenomena is at work during the spontaneous generation of growth-factor-independent leukemia cells in F-

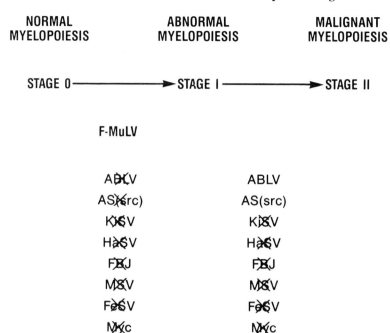

Fig. 1.   Schematic representation of leukemia cell progression from normal to malignant myelopoeisis. Only F-MuLV infection converts normal bone marrow cells to abnormal leukemia cells in vivo. Only AbLV or AS virus converts the abnormal cell population into fully malignant myeloblasts in vitro.

MuLV-diseased mice that receive transfusion therapy. The transfused mice survive longer, which allows more time for rare genetic events to occur in the leukemia cell population. One such event could be the activation of a cellular gene that behaves like *abl* or *src* and bypasses the need for growth factors that stimulate leukemia cell division. Unfortunately, our studies do not shed light on the nature of the genetic event(s) which convert normal bone marrow precursors into Stage I leukemia cells. It is possible to induce this change in mice by infection with F-MuLV. But none of the retroviruses tested in our model system altered the growth properties of the normal bone marrow cells in culture. We are currently examining the sites of integration of F-MuLV in multiple stage I cell lines looking for common cellular sequences that may be affected by the insertion of F-MuLV DNA into the host cell genome.

REFERENCES

1. Troxler DH, Scolnick EM: Virology 85:17–27, 1978.
2. MacDonald MR, Mak TW, Bernstein A: J Exp Med 151:1493–1503, 1980.
3. Oliff A, Hager GL, Chan EH, Scolnick EM, Chan HW, Lowy DR: J Virol 33:475–586, 1980.
4. Oliff A, Ruscetti S, Douglass EC, Scolnick EM: Blood 58:244–254, 1981.
5. Moore MAS: J Cell Physiol [suppl] 1:53–64, 1982.
6. Ihle JN, Keller J, Henderson L, Klein F, Palaszynski E: J Immunol 129:2431–2434, 1982.
7. Oliff A, Oliff I, Schmidt B, Famulari N: Proc Natl Acad Sci USA 81:5464–5467, 1984.
8. Aviv H, Leder P: Proc Natl Acad Sci USA 69:1408, 1972.
9. Alwine JC, Kemp DJ, Stark GR: Proc Natl Acad Sci USA 74:5350–5354, 1977.

10. Rasheed S, Gardner MB, Chan E: J Virol 19:13–18, 1976.
11. Anderson SM, Scolnick EM: J Virol 46:594–605, 1983.
12. Oliff A, Agranovsky O, McKinney MD, Murty VVVS, Bauchwitz R: Proc Natl Acad Sci USA 82:3306–3310, 1985.
13. Anderson SM, Agranovsky O, Oliff A: (submitted to press), 1987.
14. Bassin RH, Simons PJ, Chesterman FC, Harvey JJ: Int J Cancer 3(2):265–272, 1968.
15. Scolnick EM, Rands E, Aaronson SA, Todaro GJ: Proc Natl Acad Sci USA 67:1789–1796, 1970.

Workshop Summary: Growth Factors and Tumors

David Givol

Department of Chemical Immunology, The Weizmann Institute, Rehovot 76100, Israel

A central problem in tumor growth is its dependence on or independence of growth factors. In many systems the abrogation of growth-factor dependence is the critical step which leads to continuous growth in culture as well as to tumorigenicity. This elimination of the requirement for external growth factors for cell growth and division can be achieved by either an autocrine mechanism or by somehow making this growth factor superfluous for cell proliferation. Several aspects of this problem were discussed in this workshop.

A. Oliff (Merck Sharp & Dohme) analysed this question in the Friend virus-induced myeloid leukemia in NFS/n mice. The disease can be divided into two stages based on the growth properties of the leukemic cells. Stage I cells are unable to grow in culture and are not tumorigenic. Stage II cells will form a continuous line in culture and will transplant into syngeneic mice. Stage I cells will grow as an immortal cell line only if supplemented with interleukin 3 (IL-3), but will not form tumors in vivo. A. Oliff has shown that superinfection of stage I cells with Abelson murine leukemia virus (Ab-MuLV), but not with Harvey murine sarcoma virus (Ha-MuSV), will abrogate the IL-3 dependence and confer tumorigenicity on these cells. Analysis of the Ab-MuLV-infected lines did not show any altered IL-3 transcript or IL-3 gene rearrangement, and conditioned medium obtained from these lines did not support the growth of stage I cells. Hence, this study does not support the autocrine model and suggests a circumvention of the IL-3 requirement in Ab-MuLV-infected cells.

J. Schrader (Walter and Elisa Hall Institute, Australia), on the other hand, described myeloid cell lines which arose in vivo in mice exposed to mineral oil (WHEI-3B) or AB-MuLV (WHEI-274.14). These lines showed constitutive expression of IL-3, which was due to aberrant activation of the IL-3 gene. In WHEI-3B an intracisternal A-particle genome was inserted into the IL-3 gene. In WHEI-274.14, the IL-3 gene also showed gene rearrangement and a larger RNA transcript. Another series of leukemic lines were spontaneously derived in vitro from nonleukemogenic, IL-3-dependent mast cell lines. These variants synthesize IL-3 mRNA and secrete a growth factor, which appeared to be identical with IL-3. This study provides support

Received February 25, 1986.

for the autocrine model and suggests the possible use of antibodies to IL-3 as antileukemic agents. In this context it is worth mentioning that in another lecture of the symposium *F. Cuttita* (NIH) described the use of antibombesin antibodies as an antitumor agent. Bombesin (gastrin-releasing peptide) is a growth factor secreted by small cell lung carcinoma (SCLC). The injection of SCLC into nude mice will result in tumors. Antibodies to the C-terminal heptapeptide of bombesin inhibited tumor formation by SCLC in nude mice.

J. Pierce (NIH) described the construction of a recombinant murine retrovirus containing chicken v-erbB (MuLV/erbB). Transfection of NIH 3T3 with this construct induced at high frequency transformed foci which were tumorigenic in mice. MuLV/erbB retrovirus was generated by superinfection with MuLV and was used to infect several cell lines. J. Pierce found that erbB abrogates growth factor dependence; and this includes EGF, IL-2, and IL-3 in various cell lines. Young mice developed lymphoma 5–6 wk after injection of MuLV/erbB. Somehow the tissue specificity of MuLV/erbB in mice is different from that of Avian erythroblastosis virus (AEV) in chickens.

A mechanism to explain the elevated amount of IL-2 receptors in human T cell leukemia virus 1 (HTLV-1)-infected T cells (adult T cell leukemia) was described by *W. Green* (NIH). It turned out that the protein *tat*, the product of pX in HTLV-1, transactivates a hidden promoter in the IL-2 receptor gene. The gene for IL-2 receptor (located on chromosome 10) was characterised; and in normal activated T cells it is transcribed from two promoters, P1 and P2. W. Green constructed a retrovirus containing pX and demonstrated that upon infection of Jurkat (a T cell line) but not Raji (a B cell line), with this retrovirus IL-2 receptors are made. The transcription initiation site was at a new promoter, P3, which is upstream of P2. The protein *tat* also transactivates other genes (eg, DR), and it is possible that the effect of HTLV-1 on T cells occurred in two steps: (1) transactivation by *tat* of the IL-2 and the IL-2 receptor genes and (2) rendering the cells IL-2 independent.

M. Haas (University of California, San Diego) described a new lymphoma growth factor (LGF) produced by an x-ray-induced T-cell lymphoma. LGF differs from known interleukins or tumor growth factors (TGFs). His studies suggest that the initiation of the lymphoma state is due to activation of an autocrine loop in which the cells produced their own growth factor. Newly established human T cell acute lymphocytic leukemia (T-ALL) lines were also shown to secrete LGF. In addition to the main discussion about mechanisms that release tumor cells from growth-factor requirement, several speakers discussed properties of growth factors or their receptors.

J. Massague (University of Massachusetts Medical School) described the properties of TGFβ, a 25-kilodalton (kD) polypeptide found in normal and transformed cells and abundantly in blood platelets. TGFβ can induce untransformed cells to adopt a transformed phenotype, but this requires a concomitant stimulation by a mitogenic growth factor. TGFβ can also inhibit the growth of tumor cells and can block adipogenic cell differentiation without affecting cell growth, suggesting that the role of TGFβ may be to modulate cell development. One of the primary effects of TGFβ is to increase expression of fibronectin and collagen. This effect is rapid (4–6 hr) and not mimicked by other growth factors. Since cell growth in soft agar ("anchorage independence") depends on the extracellular matrix, he suggested that TGFβ exerts some of its transforming effect by increasing fibronectin synthesis. Indeed, the addition of fibronectin (100 μg/ml) to soft agar increases the number of colonies. A hexapeptide, Gly-Arg-Gly-Asp-Ser-Pro, which binds to fibronectin receptors, inhibits colony formation. He suggested that TGFβ action is based on the control of extracellular matrix in the target cells and facilitate the establishment of a local environment which allows cell proliferation.

A.M. Lebacq (NCI-Navy) analysed the gastrin-releasing peptide (GRP) in a small cell lung carcinoma (SCLC) cell line. GRP (bombesin) is synthesized in SCLC (0.8-kilobase [kb] mRNA). Although it is encoded by a single gene, at least three different cDNA clones were obtained from SCLC. The structure of pro GRP is as follows: a 23 amino acid signal peptide followed by 27 amino acids (GRP), a processing signal (GlyLysLys), and a 3′ region coding for 85–95 amino acids of the GRP-associated peptide. The three forms of pro GRP arise from a single primary transcript by alternative splicing in the region coding for the associated peptide. All three mRNA are present in SCLC line NCI-H209. The biological function of the associated peptides is not known. GRP acts as an autocrine growth factor in SCLC.

Two speakers described aberrant expression of growth factor receptors in tumors. *P. Steck* (M.D. Anderson Hospital, Texas) described an elevated amount of a p190 glycoprotein in cultured human glyoma. This protein is distinct from EGF-receptor and its tyrosine kinase activity was not stimulated by EGF. It was suggested that p190 may be the product of the *neu* oncogene.

F. Hendler (University of Texas, Dallas) found that EGF-receptor level is increased in squamous cell malignancy. The increase was observed in cultured lines and in most tumor biopsy specimens. Amplification of EGF-receptor gene was observed in 9/9 biopsy specimens. The receptor gene was rearranged in at least three cell lines with the synthesis of a 2.8-kb transcript. Many of the squamous cell lines with increased EGF receptors are EGF independent. These cell lines, however, synthesize TGFα, an EGF analogue with high affinity for EGF receptor. He suggested that the increase in EGF receptor is functional in epidermoid tumors where the elevated level of receptors and the production TGFα may be the mechanism by which autocrine regulation is achieved.

The material presented at the workshop as well as the discussion clearly indicated the importance of understanding mechanisms that release tumor cells from the requirement for external growth factors. It seems that different mechanisms may operate in different systems. These include a) aberrant expression of a growth factor which is not the natural product of this cell type. This generates an autocrine loop which continuously stimulates cell growth. b) Abrogation of growth-factor requirement without the stimulation of its endogenous production. This circumvents the need for the growth factor by some as yet unknown route. c) Aberrant or amplified expression of growth factor receptors which stimulate the cell in the absence of growth factor or respond to "wrong" stimuli. Since growth factors are extracellular, it is likely that a better understanding of the above mechanisms will also help applications in diagnosis and therapy.

Cellular and Molecular Biology of Tumors and Potential
Clinical Applications 279–285 (1988)

H-*ras* Expression and Metastasis Formation

**Sean E. Egan, Grant A. McClarty, Lenka Jarolim, Jim A. Wright, Ira Spiro,
Gordon Hager, and Arnold H. Greenberg**

*The Manitoba Institute of Cell Biology, University of Manitoba, Winnipeg, Manitoba,
Canada R3E 0V9 (S.E.E., G.A.M., L.J., J.A.W., A.H.G.); Division of Radiation Oncology,
George Washington University, Washington, DC 20037 (I.S.); Laboratory of Tumor Virus
Genetics, National Cancer Institute, Bethesda, Maryland 20205 (G.H.)*

Using three independent approaches, we have studied the effects of H-*ras* on
metastasis formation. Transformation of two nonsenescing murine fibroblasts
10T½ and NIH-3T3, by H-*ras* oncogenes consistently produced metastatic tumor
lines. Analysis of five in vitro *ras*-transfected 10T½ clones revealed a relationship
between metastatic potential and H-*ras* expression. Four metastatic variants derived from a poorly metastatic, low H-*ras*-expressing line all express high levels
of H-*ras* RNA. Activation of H-*ras* expression in the metastatic tumors had
occurred through amplification and rearrangement of H-*ras* sequences. In addition, preinduction of p21 synthesis in NIH-3T3 line 433, which contained v-H-*ras*
under the transcriptional control of the glucocorticoid-sensitive mouse mammary
tumor virus long terminal repeat (MMTV LTR), significantly increased metastatic
efficiency. This study demonstrates a correlation between metastatic potential and
H-*ras* expression, suggesting that progression to the metastatic phenotype may
occur through selection of variants with enhanced oncogene expression.

Key words: fibroblasts, oncogene expression

Metastasis is a complex process that results in tumor growth at sites distant to
the primary neoplasm. Much effort has been directed at understanding the metastatic
cascade, yet little is known about the mechanisms involved. On the other hand, the
critical events in cell immortalization and transformation have been partially elucidated and attributed to mutation or disregulation of a group of genes collectively
known as oncogenes. These genes are normally responsible for maintenance of
control over diverse cellular functions including proliferation, differentiation, morphology, communication, and motility [1–5]. Consequently, they are good candidates
for study of the metastatic process which also requires alterations of many of these
functions [6,7]. Recent studies have shown that NIH-3T3 cells transformed by
activated *ras* sequences can form metastases [8–10]. We report here that the level of
ras oncogene expression in H-*ras*-transfected 10T½ and NIH-3T3 cells is critical in
determining metastatic potential.

Received March 6, 1986.

MATERIALS AND METHODS
Gene Transfer, Plasmids, and In Vitro Derived Cell Lines

DNA-mediated gene transfer or transfection was carried out using the calcium phosphate method as previously described [11]. The plasmid pAL8A was constructed by introducing the 6.6-kilobase (kb) T24 H-*ras* insert into the BamH1 site of pSV2neo. Following transfection of pAL8A into 10T½, three morphologically transformed cell lines were established and cloned from foci observed at confluence. These cell lines, designated CIRAS-1, -2, and -3, were subsequently shown to be resistant to 400 μg/ml of G418 sulphate. Two other cell lines were isolated through selection in 400 μg/ml G418. These two lines, NR3 and NR4, were morphologically nontransformed. MDS.R cell lines are radiation-transformed 10T½ cells which were selected for anchorage-independent growth and tumorigenicity [12]. All 10T½-derived cell lines were grown in either αMEM or F12 media supplemented with 10% fetal calf serum (FCS). NIH-3T3 line 433, which contains v-H-*ras* under control of the glucocorticoid-sensitive MMTV LTR (plasmid pA9) [13], was grown in RPMI-1640 and 10% FCS with or without 2×10^{-6} M dexamethasone for 7 days prior to injection into Balb/c nu/nu mice. Growth with dexamethasone under these conditions results in a 20-fold increase in p21 synthesis [13]. Experimental metastases assay was performed as described below, using a 5×10^5 cell inoculum. All cells were kept in culture for a maximum of approximately 2 months before they were discarded and returned to frozen stocks to minimize drift from the original clones.

Experimental and Spontaneous Metastasis Assays

Metastatic potential was determined by the experimental metastasis assay using a 3×10^5 tumor cell inoculum injected in 0.2-ml volume into the tail vein of mice [14]. Cells were lightly trypsinized from subconfluent cultures, washed, and adjusted to the appropriate concentration in Hanks' balanced salt solution. Recipient animals were sacrificed by ether anesthesia 21 days later, and Bouin's solution was injected intratracheally. The stained lungs were then removed, and metastatic foci were counted under a dissecting microscope.

Spontaneous lung metastasis formation was assayed between 30 and 60 days after subcutaneous injection. Lung metastases were occasionally visible but normally detected as micrometastases by culturing lung cells in 400 μg/ml G418.

In Vivo Derived Cell Lines

In vivo derived lines were obtained by dissecting out the tumor, physically and enzymatically disaggregating it (800 μg/ml collagenase, 10 U/ml hyaluronidase, and 0.05% trypsin), followed by selection of plasmid-carrying cells in 400 μg/ml G418 sulphate for 3 days. NR3.1L lines were derived from 2 C3H/HeN mice with rare experimental lung metastases following intravenous injection of 10^6 NR3 cells. NR3.3 and NR3.4 were isolated from nonregressing tumors 40–45 days after subcutaneous injection of NR3 into C3H/HeN mice.

Northern and Southern Blot Analysis

Total RNA was prepared by the guanidinium/cesium chloride method previously described [15] and 20 μg electrophoresed on formaldehyde gels [16]. RNA was then transferred to nitrocellulose and hybridized at 68°C for 16 hr to a ^{32}P-labeled (3 $\times$

108 cpm/μg) nick-translated v-H-*ras* probe (Oncor Inc., Gaithersberg, MD). The filters were washed in 2 × SSC, .1% SDS (2 × 15 min at room temperature [RT]) followed by 0.1 × SSC, .1% SDS (1 × 30 min RT, 1 × 30 min 65°C). Autoradiography was carried out at −70°C using Kodak X-Omat AR film and Cronex lightning plus intensifying screens.

Twenty micrograms of genomic DNA were digested with BamH1 and electrophoresed on 0.6% agarose gels. DNA was then transferred to nitrocellulose and hybridized at 42°C (50% formamide/10% dextran sulfate) for 16 hr to a ^{32}P-labeled (Klenow extension) [17] (1 × 10^9 cpm/μg) v-H-*ras* probe. Following hybridization, filters were washed in 2 × SSC, 0.1% SDS (2 × 15 min RT) and 0.1 × SSC, 0.1% SDS (2 × 30 min 50°C, 1 × 30 min 65°C).

RESULTS

Survival and tumor latency data indicates that CIRAS-2 and -3 are the most tumorigenic of the five lines obtained through transfection of pAL8A into 10T½ (Table I). In contrast, morphologically nontransformed NR3 was poorly tumorigenic, and many of the tumors regressed. Subcutaneous injection of up to 10^7 cells of control 10T½ into either syngeneic C3H/HeN or immunodeficient BALB/c nu/nu mice did not result in tumor formation. Spontaneous metastasis were detected in all transfected lines except NR3. Using the more quantitative experimental metastasis assay, CIRAS-

TABLE I. Tumorigenicity and Metastatic Characteristics of H-*ras*-Transformed 10T½ in C3H/HeN Mice

Line[a]	Lung metastases[b]		Tumorigenicity[c]		
	Mean ± SE	Frequency	Latency (days ± SE)	Frequency	Survival (days ± SE)
10T½	0 ± 0	0/13	—	0/12	—
CIRAS-1	28 ± 11	6/12	10.0 ± 1.0	13/13	66.5 ± 7.0
CIRAS-2	117 ± 5	8/8	6.5 ± 0.7	11/11	58.2 ± 9.5
CIRAS-3	142 ± 26	14/14	6.5 ± 0.7	11/11	36.2 ± 4.2
NR4	5 ± 1	12/19	10.7 ± 1.4	10/10	58.5 ± 12.4
NR3	0 ± 0	0/13	49.6 ± 2.0	6/8	106 ± 7.0
MDS.R1	0	0/3	7.1 ± 0.9	5/5	NT
MDS.R5	0	0/6	8.1 ± 1.1	5/5	NT
MDS.R9	0	0/3	8.7 ± 1.3	5/5	NT
MDS.R25	0	0/4	4.0 ± 0	5/5	NT
NR3.1LA	49 ± 7	6/6	6.8 ± 0.5	5/5	NT
NR3.1LB	40 ± 18	6/6	9.8 ± 1.5	5/5	NT
NT3.1LC	30 ± 6	6/6	6.7 ± 0.7	5/5	NT
NR3.1LD	13 ± 7	6/6	5.8 ± 0.6	5/5	NT
NR3.3	16 ± 5	4/4	9.8 ± 0.5	5/5	NT
NR3.4	42 ± 19	4/4	13.8 ± 2.2	5/5	NT

[a]MDS lines are radiation-induced 10T½ transformants. R1 and R5 were negative for activated *ras* in the NIH-3T3 transfection assay. NR3.1L lines were derived from lung metastases, while NR3.3 and 3.4 were isolated from progressively growing subcutaneous tumors of the NR3 parent.
[b]10T½, *ras*-transfected 10T½, and all NR3-derived tumors were injected in a 3 × 10^5 cell inoculum intravenously. MDS lines were injected at a 10^6 cell inoculum I.V.
[c]All tumors were injected at a 3 × 10^5 cell inoculum. One-half of the NR3 tumors regressed. NR3 latency was calculated from the six mice with tumors. NT = not tested.

2 and -3 were the most metastatic; CIRAS-1 and NR4 were intermediate and low, respectively; and NR3 was virtually nonmetastatic with only 3 out of 43 mice injected producing lung tumors and only at the highest cell inoculum (10^6). Control 10T½ and 10T½-transfected with pSV2neo (not shown) produced only rare experimental metastasis. Radiation-transformed 10T½ cell lines (MDSR) were tumorigenic but not metastatic (Table I).

Southern blot analysis revealed the presence of novel H-*ras* sequences in all five lines (not shown); however, gene copy number did not correlate with in vivo behavior. A correlation between expression of H-*ras* and metastatic potential was detected on Northern blots. Highly metastatic lines CIRAS-2 and CIRAS-3 exhibited high levels of H-*ras* RNA, while the least metastatic line NR3 was very low, comparable to 10T½. The other two lines expressed intermediate levels (Fig. 1).

Four lung metastases and two subcutaneous tumor lines derived from NR3 were next examined. All six in vivo derived cell lines were highly tumorigenic and metastatic (Table I). These lines all expressed high levels of H-*ras* RNA as compared to the poorly expressing NR3 from which they were derived (Fig. 2a). Evidence that gene rearrangement and amplification had occurred in the lung metastasis was found on Southern blotting (Fig. 2b). In contrast, the subcutaneous tumors NR3.3 and NR3.4 were likely not activated by the same mechanism. Although DNA restriction patterns were different from NR3, no amplification of H-*ras* sequences was observed. All four lung metastasis (NR3.1L) lines showed complex and nearly identical restriction patterns with novel H-*ras* sequences indicating that they were of clonal origin. Both NR3.3 and NR3.4 also exhibited an identical restriction band suggesting a common origin.

The relationship between activated H-*ras* expression and metastatic potential was then confirmed in the NIH-3T3 system using line 433. Preinduction of v-H-*ras* prior to injection into BALB/c nu/nu by incubation in dexamethasone for 7 days resulted in a significant 2.5–3-fold increase in metastatic potential (Table II).

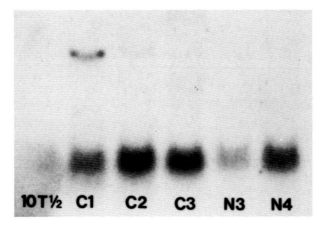

Fig. 1.   Northern blot analysis of T24 H-*ras*-transfected cell lines. Comparison of H-*ras* RNA levels from original transfectant lines with 10T½ control (C1, CIRAS-1; C2, CIRAS-2; C3, CIRAS-3; N3, NR3; N4, NR4).

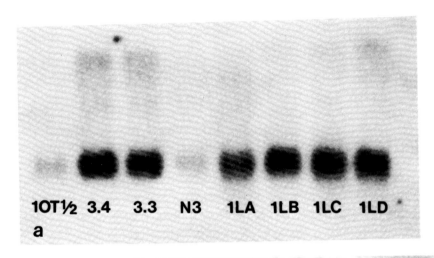

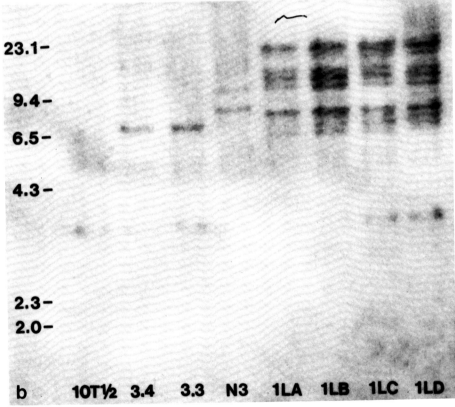

Fig. 2. **a:** Comparison of H-*ras* RNA levels from NR3-derived subcutaneous tumor lines (3.4, 3.3) and NR3-derived lung metastases lines (1LA, 1LB, 1LC, and 1LD) with NR3 (N3) and 10T½ controls. **b:** Southern blot analysis of BamH1 digested DNA from NR3 (N3) derived lung metastases (1LA–D) and subcutaneous tumor lines (3.3 and 3.4).

TABLE II. Lung Colony Formation Following v-H-*ras* Induction in Line 433

	Lung metastases[a]	
	No.	Mean $\pm$ SE
2×10^{-6} M dexamethasone	150, 152, 168, 175, 178, 227, 250	185 $\pm$ 14*
Nil	24, 33, 66, 76, 89, 98, 103	70 $\pm$ 12

[a]5×10^5 cells were injected intravenously into BALB/c nu/nu mice.
*P < .001.

DISCUSSION

We have studied the effects of activated H-*ras* on metastatic potential in both 10T½ and NIH-3T3 cells and report that metastatic efficiency is closely related to the level of H-*ras* expression. H-*ras* RNA levels correlated with both the tumorigenicity and metastatic potential of a series of T24 H-*ras*-transfected 10T½ cell lines. The correlation is not absolute since the nontransformed NR4 cells are less metastatic than the CIRAS-1, which expresses the same amount of H-*ras* RNA, and are only somewhat more metastatic than the non-H-*ras*-expressing NR3. This is partially due to natural killer (NK) cell regulation of lung metastasis formation, as we have found that in NK-deficient beige (C3H bg/bg) mice both CIRAS-1 and NR4 lines are now highly metastatic, while NR3 remains very weakly able to form lung tumors. The rank order of metastatic efficiency of these lines, however, was identical with that seen in the immunocompetent bg/+ host (Greenberg, unpublished results). In addition, one must consider possible post-translational suppression of activated *ras* which has been observed in flat revertants similar to the NR4 line and may contribute to its lower metastatic rate [18–20]. The six NR3-derived in vivo lines were all highly tumorigenic, metastatic, and expressed high levels of H-*ras* RNA, indicating that selection of metastatic cells also resulted in selection for high H-*ras* expressing cells. The existence of common restriction banding patterns on Southern blots (Fig. 2b) suggests that all four NR3.1L lines likely arose from the same cell, while the two subcutaneous tumor lines were derived from a different but common variant. Activation of H-*ras* expression may have occurred within the in vitro NR3 population, giving rise to preexisting high H-*ras*-expressing subpopulations that preferentially formed tumor on inoculation. Derivation of lung metastasis and subcutaneous lines were carried out using parental NR3 cells of different passage number; thus, selection of different high H-*ras*-expressing variant populations may have occurred from both subcutaneous tumors and lung metastases. The alternative explanation that transcriptional activation occurred during in vivo passage via unique mechanisms in each instance is also possible.

The relationship between *ras* expression and metastatic potential was also evident in the NIH-3T3 system using line 433 which contains v-H-*ras* under transcriptional control of the glucocorticoid-sensitive MMTV LTR. Induction of v-H-*ras* p21 synthesis prior to intravenous injection resulted in a significant increase in metastatic potential. Physiological glucocorticoids [13] presumably induced v-H-*ras* in vivo and are thus responsible for metastases from cells not incubated in dexamethasone prior to injection. Although both lines were expressing v-H-*ras* in vivo, in vitro induction provided a kinetic advantage that allowed more cells to survive and form lung tumors.

It has been shown that a single copy of activated H-*ras* can fully transform NIH-3T3 cells even when regulated by the normal cellular promotor [21]. Enhanced H-*ras* expression from strong promotors increases the tumorigenic potential of recipient cells [22]. Our studies indicate that the presence of activated *ras* sequences is not sufficient to confer a highly metastatic phenotype. Elevated expression appears to be necessary, since only cells containing high level of H-*ras* RNA were highly metastatic and this was proportional to the level of expression.

Other types of transformation of 10T½ (MDSR lines) or NIH-3T3 [8] are not sufficient for expression of the metastatic phenotype, suggesting that the H-*ras* oncogene is inducing some phenotypic alterations in the cells that are necessary for metastasis formation. Our findings also suggest that in vivo progression to the metastatic phenotype may occur by selection of variants with enhanced oncogene expression. It will be important to determine whether these findings are applicable to other cell types and/or any other oncogenes.

ACKNOWLEDGMENTS

We wish to thank Dr. Mike Mowat for his invaluable advice. This work was supported by the National Cancer Institute of Canada, the Manitoba Health Research Council, and the Winnipeg Children's Hospital Research Foundation. A.H.G. and J.A.W. are Terry Fox Cancer Research Scientists.

REFERENCES

1. Mulcahy LS, Smith MR, Stacey DW: Nature 313:241–243, 1985.
2. Weissman B, Aaronson SA: Mol Cell Biol 5:3386–3396, 1985.
3. Rohrschneider L, Reynolds S: Mol Cell Biol 5:3097–3107, 1985.
4. Chang C-C, Trosko JE, Kung H-J, Bombick D, Matsumura F: Proc Natl Acad Sci USA 82:5360–5364, 1985.
5. Martinet Y, Bitterman PB, Mornex J-F, Grotendorst GR, Martin GR, Crystal RG: Nature 319:158–160, 1986.
6. Roos E: Biochim Biophys Acta 738:263–284, 1984.
7. Poste G, Fidler IJ: Nature 283:139–145, 1980.
8. Thorgeirsson NP, Turpeenniema-Hujanen T, Williams JE, Westin EH, Heilman CA, Talmodge JE, Liotta LA: Mol Cell Biol 5:259–262, 1985.
9. Greig G, Koestler TP, Trainer DL, Corcuin SP, Miles L, Kline T, Sweet R, Yokoyama S, Poste G: Proc Natl Acad Sci USA 82:3698–3701, 1985.
10. Muschel RJ, Williams JE, Lowy DR, Liotta LA, Am J Pathol 121:1–8, 1985.
11. Wigler M, Silverstein S, Lee LS, Pellier A, Cheng Y, Axel R: Cell 11:223–232, 1977.
12. Raaphorst GP, Vadasz JA, Azzams E, Sargent MD, Borsa J, Einspenner M: Cancer Res 45:5452–5456, 1985.
13. Huang AL, Ostrowski MC, Berard D, Hager G: Cell 27:245–255, 1981.
14. Fidler JJ, Kripke ML: Science 197:893–895, 1977.
15. Chirguin JM, Przbyla AE, McDonald RJ, Rutter WJ: Biochemistry 18:5294–5299, 1979.
16. Lehrach H, Diamond D, Wozney JM, Boedtker H: Biochemistry 16:4743–4751, 1977.
17. Feinberg A, Vogelstein B: Anal. Biochem. 132:6–13, 1982.
18. Craig RW, Sager R: Proc Natl Acad Sci USA 82:2062–2066, 1985.
19. Noda M, Selinger Z, Scolnick EM, Bassin RH: Proc Natl Acad Sci USA 80:5602–5606, 1983.
20. Hsiao W-L.W., Gattoni-Celli S, Weinstein IB: Science 226:552–555, 1984.
21. Tabin, CJ, Weinberg RA: J Virol 53:260–265, 1985.
22. Spandidos DA, Wilkie NM: Nature 310:469–475, 1984.

Cellular and Molecular Biology of Tumors and Potential
Clinical Applications 287–296 (1988)

Multidrug Resistance in Human Cells: The Role of the *mdr*1 Gene

I.B. Roninson, D.-W. Shen, J.E. Chin, K. Choi, A. Fojo, R. Soffir, N. Richert, P. Gros, D.E. Housman, M.M. Gottesman, and I. Pastan

Center for Genetics, University of Illinois College of Medicine at Chicago, Chicago, Illinois 60612 (I.B.R., J.E.C., K.C., R.S.); Laboratory of Molecular Biology, National Cancer Institute, Bethesda, Maryland 20892 (D.-W. S., A.F., N.R., M.M.G., I.P.); Center for Cancer Research and Department of Biology, Massachusetts Institute of Technology, Cambridge, Massachusetts 02139 (P.G., D.E.H.)

The ability of tumor cells to develop simultaneous resistance to multiple cytotoxic drugs constitutes a major problem in cancer chemotherapy. The expression of the multidrug-resistant phenotype in Chinese hamster cell lines was found to correlate with amplification and increased expression of the gene designated *mdr*. Analysis of multidrug-resistant sublines of human KB carcinoma cells, selected with colchicine, adriamycin, or vinblastine, reveals amplification of two different DNA sequences homologous to the hamster *mdr* gene, designated *mdr*1 and *mdr*2. Cloned *mdr*1 but not *mdr*2 probes hybridize to a 4.5 kilobase (kb) mRNA, the expression of which correlates with the degree of cellular drug resistance. During selection for increased drug resistance, the increase in the *mdr*1 mRNA level precedes the amplification of *mdr*1 DNA. Acquisition of the multidrug-resistant phenotype in mouse NIH 3T3 cells transfected with DNA from multidrug-resistant human cells correlates with the transfer and amplification of the human *mdr*1 gene. Amplification and increased expression of the *mdr*1 gene were also observed in multidrug-resistant cell lines derived from a human leukemia cell line (CEM) and an ovarian carcinoma cell line, 2780. These results suggest that *mdr*1 gene is likely to be responsible for multidrug resistance in human tumor cells.

Key words: cancer chemotherapy, anthracyclines, vinca alkaloids, colchicine

The development of drug resistance by neoplastic cells is a major factor in limiting the efficiency of cancer chemotherapy. Among different types of drug resistance, multidrug resistance, also known as pleiotropic drug resistance, constitutes a particularly important clinical problem, since it involves cross-resistance to many drugs that are widely used as anticancer agents. This group of drugs includes anthracyclines, vinca alkaloids, epipodophyllotoxins, maytansine, actinomycin D, puromycin, and colchicine. Studies with multidrug-resistant sublines of mammalian

Received April 1, 1986.

cells indicate that multidrug resistance is due to decreased intracellular drug accumulation, apparently as a result of alterations in the plasma membrane [1–3]. The most common biochemical characteristics of multidrug-resistant cells is the increased expression of a 170 kilodalton (kd) membrane glycoprotein, or P-glycoprotein [1–6] and, in some cases, a 19–21-kd cytosolic protein [1,17]. Double minute chromosomes and homogeneously staining regions, cytogenetic markers of gene amplification, are found in some multidrug-resistant cell lines [1,7–10], indicating that multidrug resistance may result from amplification of some unknown genes.

We have used the technique of in-gel DNA renaturation, which allows one to detect, compare, and clone amplified genomic DNA sequences in the absence of cloned probes [11] to analyze the DNA of two independently derived multidrug-resistant Chinese hamster cell lines, selected with either adriamycin or colchicine [12]. Both cell lines were found to contain amplified DNA sequences, some of which were amplified in common in these cells. We have cloned a contiguous region of over 120 kb of the commonly amplified DNA and shown that it contains a transcription unit, which encodes an mRNA of approximately 5-kb size [13]. This mRNA is overexpressed in multidrug-resistant sublines of Chinese hamster cells. This transcription unit has been designated *mdr*.

To investigate the mechanism of multidrug resistance in human cells, we have isolated multidrug-resistant sublines of human KB carcinoma cells, selected with colchicine, vinblastine, or adriamycin. These cells are characterized by decreased accumulation of different drugs and by several biochemical changes [14–16] which include increased expression of P-glycoprotein [17] and of a protein which is capable of binding vinblastine and co-migrates with the P-glycoprotein [18]. Some of the multidrug-resistant KB sublines contain double minute chromosomes, and in-gel DNA renaturation analysis indicated the presence of amplified DNA sequences in the genomes of these cells [10]. In the present study we have analyzed the amplification and expression of DNA sequences homologous to the hamster *mdr* gene in multidrug-resistant KB cells, as well as in mouse NIH 3T3 cells transfected with genomic DNA from multidrug-resistant human cells. Our data indicate that the human homologue of the *mdr* gene, designated *mdr*1, is likely to be responsible for the multidrug-resistant phenotype in human tumor cells.

MATERIALS AND METHODS

Derivation and characterization of multidrug-resistant sublines of KB carcinoma, CEM leukemia, and 2780 ovarian carcinoma cells has been described previously [3,14–19]. The cloning and hybridization procedures used in this study have been presented elsewhere [20,21]. Mouse NIH 3T3 cells were cotransfected with genomic DNA and pSV$_2$neo using the calcium phosphate precipitation procedure [22]. Cells were initially selected for resistance to 0.8 mg/ml G418, and the resulting neo^R colonies were pooled and reselected in 30 ng/ml colchicine, with subsequent multistep selection for resistance up to 1 μg/ml colchicine. DNA from primary transfectants at the highest level of resistance was used to obtain secondary transfectants by the same protocol, except that the selection was done in 80 ng/ml colchicine.

RESULTS

To obtain an *mdr* probe hybridizing to human DNA, a cosmid clone cosDR3A, containing a 5′ portion of the hamster *mdr* gene [13] was mapped with several restriction enzymes and individual subfragments were isolated and used as probes for Southern [23] hybridization with human genomic DNA. Most probes, including some that contained transcriptionally active regions, produced no detectable hybridization signal, indicating a low degree of evolutionary conservation in this part of the *mdr* gene. However, a subclone containing a 4.7-kb XbaI fragment (pDR4.7; Fig. 1a), hybridized to discrete bands in restriction digests of human DNA under conditions of low hybridization stringency (4 × SSC; 0.5% SDS at 65°C in the last wash). The pDR4.7 clone was used as probe for hybridization with DNA from drug-sensitive KB carcinoma cells (line KB-3-1) and different multidrug-resistant sublines of these cells, as shown in Figure 1B. pDR4.7 hybridizes to two EcoRI fragments of 13.5 and 4.5 kb, both of which are amplified in colchicine-resistant sublines KB-8-5-11, KB-8-5-11-24, KB-C3, and KB-C4 (see Table I for characterization of the sublines), but not in the revertant subline KB-C1-R1. Only the 13.5-kb, but not the 4.5-kb fragment was amplified in vinblastine-resistant KB-V1 and adriamycin-resistant KB-A1 and KB-A2 cells. Analysis with other restriction enzymes (not shown) indicated that the two EcoRI bands correspond to two different related DNA sequences, possibly different members of a multigene family, rather than to two different parts of one contiguous hybridizing region. The sequence corresponding to the 13.5-kb and 4.5-kb fragments were designated *mdr*1 and *mdr*2, respectively.

Fragments of *mdr*1 and *mdr*2 loci were cloned by screening recombinant phage libraries, containing complete EcoRI or HindIII digests of KB-C3 DNA, with the hamster pDR4.7 probe. The resulting clones were further characterized with regard to the location of repeated sequences and of the evolutionary conserved sequences that hybridized to the hamster *mdr* DNA. Repeat-free fragments of both clones that hybridized to the pDR4.7 hamster probe were subcloned and designated pMDR1 and pMDR2. pMDR1 and pMDR2 were found to cross-hybridize with each other under conditions of low hybridization stringency, but not under high stringency (0.1 × SSC; 0.5% SDS at 65°C) conditions. These subclones were tested for the presence of transcriptionally active sequences by Northern hybridization [24] with poly (A)$^+$ RNA from multidrug-resistant KB cells. pMDR1 hybridized to a 4.5–kb mRNA, which was expressed in multidrug-resistant cells, but could not be detected in the parental drug-sensitive cells (Fig.. 2).

No expression of *mdr*2-specific RNA has been detected in any of the cell lines analyzed, when either the pMDR2 clone or DNA sequences immediately adjacent to pMDR2 sequences in the genome were used as probes. If *mdr*2 is indeed unexpressed in our cell lines, amplification of *mdr*2 DNA in some of these lines could be explained as co-amplification with the functional *mdr* 1 gene, provided that *mdr*1 and *mdr*2 are linked within the same amplified unit. We have analyzed the linkage between *mdr*1 and *mdr*2 by Southern hybridization with DNA from KB-C3 cells in which both of these sequences are amplified. DNA was digested with infrequently cutting restriction enzymes and separated by pulse field gradient gel electrophoresis [25]. By this assay, both pMDR1 and pMDR2 were found to be linked within less than 350 kb of DNA (data not shown). This result suggests that *mdr*2 may indeed be a "passenger gene" which is amplified coincidentally owing to its linkage to *mdr*1. It is also interesting to note that in two cell lines, KB-A1 and KB-V1, one of the alleles of the *mdr*2 locus has undergone a rearrangement, which appears to be identical or nearly identical in these independently derived cell lines (data not shown). However, while the rearranged *mdr*2 remains at single copy level in KB-V1, it has been amplified in KB-A1

A.

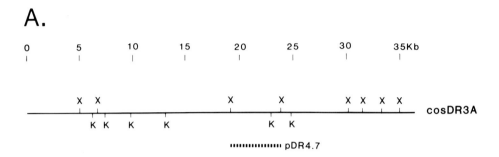

B.   pDR4.7 probe, EcoRI digest

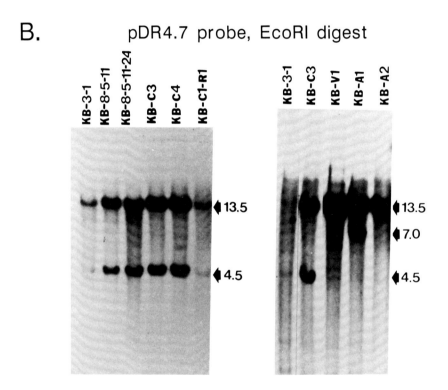

Fig. 1. **A:** Restriction map of the cosmid clone cos DR3a, containing a 5' portion of the Chinese hamster *mdr* gene [13]. Position of the 4.7-kb XbaI fragment (pDR4.7), containing DNA sequences hybridizing to human DNA, is indicated. Restriction sites: X-XbaI; K-KpnI. **B:** Southern hybridization of pDR4.7 with EcoRI-digested DNA from multidrug-resistant KB cells. See Table I for characterization of the sublines. Each lane contains 5 μg of DNA. The filter was hybridized with the gel-purified insert of pDR4.7 hamster *mdr* clone under conditions of low hybridization stringency (4 × SSC, 0.5% SDS at 65°C in the last wash). Fragment sizes (in kb) are indicated. The 13.5-kb band corresponds to the *mdr*1 gene, and the 4.5-kb band represents a cross-hybridizing *mdr*2 sequence. The 7.0–kb band in the KB-A2 digest corresponds to the rearranged and amplified allele of *mdr*2 (see text for details). (This figure is reproduced from Roninson et al [20].

TABLE I. Characterization of Multidrug-Resistant Cell Lines*

	Relative resistance to —			*mdr*1 Gene copy No.	*mdr*1 mRNA expression
Cell line	Colchicine	Adriamycin	Vinblastine		
KB-3-1 (parental)	1	1	1	1	<0.1
KB-8	2.1	1.1	1.2	1	1
KB-8-5	3.8	3.2	6.3	1	3
KB-8-5-11	40	23	51	7–8	80
KB-8-5-11-24	128	26	20	9	n/d
KB-C1	263	162	96	10	270
KB-C1.5	324	n/d	142	15	340
KB-C3	487	141	206	20	n/d
KB-C4	1750	254	159	30	n/d
KB-C6	2100	320	370	80	820
KB-C1-R1	6	3	4	1	1
KB-V1	171	422	213	100	320
KB-A1	19	97	43	70	270
KB-A2	n/d	140	n/d	80	n/d
CEM (parental)	1	1	1	1	<0.1
CEM-V1b 100	45	124	420	5–10	250
2780 (parental)	1	1	1	1	<0.1
2780-Ad	n/d	167	15	10–15	260

*Derivation and characterization of multidrug-resistant sublines of KB carcinoma, CEM lymphoblastoid leukemia, and 2780 ovarian carcinoma cell lines has been described before [3,14–18]. Relative resistance was determined by measuring the concentration of drug that reduced the cloning efficiency of the cells to 10% of the value in the absence of drug (LD_{10}) and dividing the LD_{10} of the resistant cells by the LD_{10} of the parental cells [14]. The copy number of the *mdr*1 gene was determined by comparing the intensity of the signal obtained upon Southern or slot blot hybridization of pMDR1 or pDR4.7 probes with serially diluted DNA from the resistant sublines and from the parental drug-sensitive cells. The levels of *mdr*1 mRNA expression were determined by slot blot hybridization of total or $poly(A)^+$ RNA from different cell lines with pMDR1 probe. The signal intensity was determined by densitometry. Since no expression of *mdr*1 mRNA could be detected in any of the parental cell lines, the mRNA levels are expressed relative to KB-8 cell line, corresponding to the first step of colchicine selection, which was arbitrarily assigned a value of 1. n/d = not done.

cells. The significance of this specific rearrangement and its possible relationship to the amplification of the *mdr*1/*mdr*2 locus remain to be elucidated.

The copy number of the *mdr*1 gene and the degree of *mdr*1 mRNA expression have been estimated in different independently selected sublines of KB cells, as well as in a vinblastine-resistant subline of human lymphoblastoid leukemia, CEM-VLB$_{100}$ [3], and an adriamycin-resistant subline of human ovarian carcinoma, 2780-Ad [19]. The results are summarized in Table I. The expression of *mdr*1 mRNA appears to parallel closely the degree of relative drug resistance in all the cell lines. On the other hand, there is no precise correlation between the degree of *mdr*1 gene amplification and the level of mRNA expression. For example, a similar (320–340-fold) level of *mdr*1 mRNA expression corresponds to 100-fold level of gene amplification in KB-V1 cells, but only to 15-fold amplification in KB-C1.5 cells. Most interestingly, no amplification of the *mdr*1 gene was observed in the cells at a low (2–6-fold) level of drug resistance: KB-8, KB–8-5, and KB-C1-R1. It appears that in KB-8 and KB-8-5 cell lines, corresponding to the first two steps of colchicine selection, transcriptional

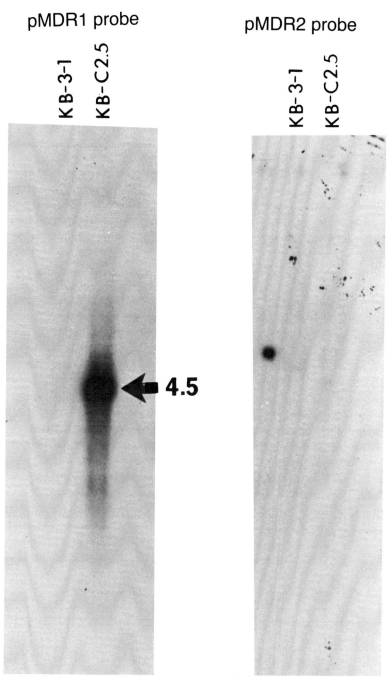

Fig. 2.   Analysis of *mdr*1 and *mdr*2 RNA expression. Poly(A)$^+$ RNA was extracted from the parental drug-sensitive KB-3-1 cells and from the colchicine-resistant KB-C2.5 subline. One microgram of each RNA preparation was electrophoresed in a 1.5% glyoxal agarose gel. The filters were hybridized with gel-purified inserts of pMDR1 and pMDR2 clones under conditions of high hybridization stringency (0.1 × SSC, 0.5% SDS at 65°C in the last wash). The size of the *mdr*1-specific RNA band was determined from its mobility relative to the positions of 28S and 18S ribosomal RNA. No *mdr*2-hybridizing RNA has been detected. (This figure is reproduced from Roninson et al [20]).

activation of the *mdr*1 gene has occurred in the absence of gene amplification. The *mdr*1 gene becomes amplified only at the later stages of selection, resulting in the further increase in mRNA expression. The revertant cell line KB-C1-R1 has lost all the extra copies of the *mdr*1 gene, but it has nevertheless retained detectable expression of this gene and a corresponding low level of multidrug resistance. These observations may be especially relevant for tumor cells that have acquired drug resistance in the course of chemotherapy. Such cells are expected to have acquired a low level of drug resistance, similar to KB-8 and KB-8-5 cells, since even a 2–4-fold level of resistance would still be sufficient to give clinically refractory tumors. Analysis of the role of *mdr*l in clinical drug resistance should therefore involve quantitation of its expression at the RNA or protein level rather than assaying for amplification of the *mdr*1 gene.

In an independent series of experiments, we have tried to identify the essential gene responsible for multidrug resistance by DNA transfection assays. In these experiments, multidrug-resistant human KB-C1.5 cells were used as the DNA donor, and mouse NIH 3T3 cells served as the recipients. In order to increase the efficiency of selection and to decrease the background of spontaneous drug-resistant variants of NIH 3T3 cells, we have used a two-step selection protocol. In this protocol, genomic DNA from drug-sensitive or drug-resistant cells was cotransfected with the plasmid pSV$_2$neo, carrying a dominant selectable marker encoding resistance to the antibiotic G418. A population of approximately 10,000 G418-resistant cells was pooled and selected for resistance to 30 ng/ml colchicine. In these experiments, only those cells that were transfected with DNA from drug-resistant, but not from drug-sensitive human cells, gave rise to colchicine-resistant colonies. The primary transfectants were then selected in multiple steps for increased levels of colchicine reistance (up to 1 μg/ml), with an expectation that this protocol would result in amplification of the transfected gene. The highly resistant primary transfectants were then used as DNA donors for the second round of transfection, using the same protocol for selection, and secondary transfectants were isolated. Both primary and secondary colchicine-resistant transfectants were tested for cross-resistance to other drugs and found to express the multidrug-resistant phenotype, the pattern of which was similar to the donor cell line (data not shown).

DNA from primary and secondary transfectants at different steps of colchicine selection was analyzed by Southern hybridization with pMDR1 probe. A typical experiment is shown in Figure 3. All the DNA preparations in this experiment were digested with HindIII. Human cell lines, as well as primary and secondary transfectants, but not the parental NIH 3T3 cells and the control cells selected with G418 alone, show a 4.4-kb band characteristic of the human *mdr*1 gene. This band is amplified during the selection of transfectants for increased colchicine resistance. Analysis with different restriction enzymes indicated that this band corresponds to the human but not the mouse *mdr* gene, judging not only by the size of the bands, but also by their hybridization to pMDR1 under high stringency conditions, when no cross-hybridization with the mouse gene could be detected (data not shown). Only *mdr*l but not the linked *mdr*2 gene was found in the transfectants. Hybridization with the human *Alu* repetitive sequence (not shown) indicated that the total size of human DNA present in secondary transfectants is approximately 100–200 kb, which is close to our current estimate for the size of human *mdr*1 gene. Analysis of the RNA from primary and secondary transfectants indicated that the human *mdr*1 gene, but not its

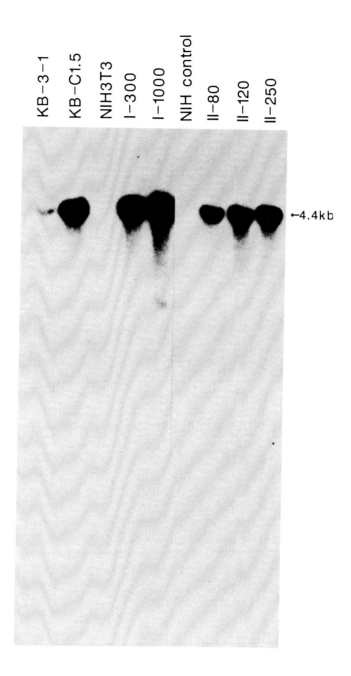

Fig. 3.   DNA-mediated gene transfer of the multidrug-resistant phenotype correlates with the transfer of the *mdr*1 gene. A Southern blot of 2 μg of DNA from parental (KB-3-1), drug-resistant DNA donor (KB-C1.5), recipient (NIH 3T3) and transformant cells. NIH controls is a mixed population of G418-resistant mouse cells obtained after transfection. I-300, I-1000 are primary NIH 3T3 transformants selected in 300 ng/ml and 1,000 ng/ml colchicine, respectively. II-80, II-120, and II-250 are secondary transformants selected in 80 ng/ml, 120 ng/ml, and 250 ng/ml colchicine, respectively. The filter was hybridized with the ^{32}P-labeled insert of pMDR1 clone.

mouse homolog, is overexpressed in these cells, and the level of *mdr*1 expression correlates with the degree of cellular drug resistance.

DISCUSSION

The experiments described above demonstrate that *mdr*1 DNA sequences are intimately associated with the multidrug-resistant phenotype in human tumor cells. These sequences are characterized by increased mRNA expression in multidrug-resistant cell lines of different origins selected with colchicine, adriamycin, or vinblastine. The *mdr*1 gene is amplified in the genomes of the cell line with a 20–40-fold or higher level of relative drug resistance. The transfer of the transcriptionally active human *mdr*1 gene, but not of the linked *mdr*2 DNA sequences, correlates with the acquisition of multidrug resistance in mouse NIH 3T3 cells transfected with DNA from multidrug-resistant human cells. Taken together, these results indicate that *mdr*1 gene is likely to be responsible for multidrug resistance in human cells, though a formal possibility that this phenotype may be encoded by another gene which is tightly linked to *mdr*1 cannot yet be excluded. The role of the *mdr*1 gene will be analyzed directly once a full length cDNA clone of *mdr*1 is isolated and tested for the ability to confer multidrug resistance using an eukaryotic expression vector. We have recently constructed cDNA libraries from the multidrug-resistant KB-C3 and KB-V1 cells and isolated a number of partial *mdr*1 DNA clones. The isolation of a functional full-length cDNA clone of *mdr*1 is anticipated in the near future.

The results with the human *mdr*1 gene parallel our findings in the Chinese hamster and mouse systems, where increased expression and amplification of *mdr* DNA sequences correlate with multidrug resistance in several independently selected cell lines [12,13 and unpublished data]. Furthermore, we have found that the multi-drug-resistant phenotype can be transferred from multidrug-resistant Chinese hamster to drug-sensitive mouse cells by the metaphase chromosome transfer procedure, and the resulting mouse transfectants carry multiple copies of the hamster *mdr* gene (Gros and Housman, unpublished data). One difference between the human KB carcinoma and Chinese hamster systems is that amplification of the *mdr* gene accompanies a low level of relative drug resistance in hamster cells, both at the early stages of selection and in the revertants obtained upon prolonged growth in the absence of the drug, but in human KB cells the corresponding low levels of resistance correlate with increased expression of *mdr*1 mRNA without *mdr*1 gene amplification. It is interesting to note in this regard that *mdr* mRNA expression occurs at a low but detectable level in parental drug-sensitive hamster cell lines [13], but expression of *mdr* 1 mRNA is below the limits of detection with nick-translated pMDR1 probe in the unselected KB carcinoma and several other human tumor-derived cell lines. The absence or very low level of *mdr*1 expression in at least some drug-sensitive human tumor cells is highly encouraging with regard to the possible diagnostic use of *mdr*1-specific probes.

The nature of the protein encoded by the *mdr* gene(s) is still unknown. Several indirect arguments suggest that *mdr* may be identical with or related to the gene for the membrane P-glycoprotein, a cDNA clone of which was recently isolated from multidrug-resistant hamster cells [6]. Both genes were found to be amplified in two independently derived sets of multidrug-resistant Chinese hamster cells [12,26] and in multidrug-resistant human leukemia cell line [26]. The sublines of KB carcinoma cells used in our studies were analyzed with an anti-P-glycoprotein monoclonal antibody [27] and found to have an increased amount of P-glycoprotein in their membranes [17]. Both *mdr*1 and P-glycoprotein encode a mRNA of approximately 4.5–5-kb size. It was recently reported [28] that the P-glycoprotein gene maps to human chromosome 7. We have found that both *mdr*1 and *mdr*2 genes are also localized in chromosome 7 [29]. If the *mdr* gene product is indeed an integral component of the cell membrane, it could be used as a target for an immunotherapy, which might selectively destroy multidrug-resistant tumor cells.

ACKNOWLEDGMENTS

We would like to thank Carol Cardarelli for help with the development and maintenance of the multidrug-resistant KB cells. This work was supported in part by grant CA40333 from the National Cancer Institute.

REFERENCES

1. Biedler JL, Chang T, Meyers MB, Peterson RHF, Spengler BA: Cancer Treat Rep 67:859–868, 1983.
2. Ling V, Kartner N, Sudo T, Siminovitch L, Riordan JR: Cancer Treat Rep 67:869–875, 1983.
3. Beck WT, Muellen TJ, Tanzer LR: Cancer Res 39:2070–2076, 1979.
4. Kartner N, Riordan JR, Ling V: Science 221:1285–1289, 1983.
5. Debenham PG, Kartner N, Siminovitch L, Riordan JR, Ling V: Mol Cell Biol 2:881–889, 1982.
6. Robertson SM, Ling V, Stanners CP: Mol Cel Biol 4:500–506, 1984.
7. Baskin F, Rosenberg RN, Dev V: Proc Natl Acad Sci USA 78:3654–3658, 1981.
8. Kopnin BP: Cytogenet Cell Genet 30:11–14, 1981.
9. Grund SH, Patil SR, Shah HO, Pauw PG, Stadler JK: Mol Cell Biol 3:1634–1647, 1983.
10. Fojo AT, Whang-Peng J, Gottesman MM, Pastan I: Proc Natl Acad Sci USA 82:7661–7665, 1985.
11. Roninson IB: Nucleic Acids Res 11:5413–5431, 1983.
12. Roninson IB, Abelson HT, Housman DE, Howell N, Varshavsky A: Nature 309:626–628.
13. Gros P, Croop JM, Roninson IB, Varshavsky A, Housman DE: Proc Natl Acad Sci USA 83:337–341, 1986.
14. Akiyama S-I, Fojo A, Hanover JA, Pastan I, Gottesman, MM: Somatic Cell Mol Genet 11:117–126, 1985.
15. Fojo A, Akiyama S-I, Gottesman MM, Pastan I: Cancer Res 45:3002–3007, 1985.
16. Richert N, Akiyama S-I, Shen D-W, Gottesman MM, Pastan I: Proc Natl Acad Sci USA 82:2330–2334, 1985.
17. Shen D-W, Cardarelli C, Hwang J, Richert N, Ishii S, Pastan I, Gottesman MM: J Biol Chem 261:7762–7770, 1986.
18. Cornwell M, Safa A, Felsted R, Gottesman MM, Pastan I: Proc Natl Acad Sci USA, 83:3847–3850, 1986.
19. Rogan AM, Young RC, Klecker RW, Ozols RF: Science 224:994–996, 1984.
20. Roninson IB, Chin JE, Choi K, Gros P, Housman DE, Fojo A, Shen D, Gottesman M, Pastan I: Proc Natl Acad Sci USA 83:4538–4542, 1986.
21. Shen D, Fojo A, Chin JE, Roninson IB, Richert N, Pastan I, Gottesman MM: Science 232:643–645, 1986.
22. Wigler M, Sweet R, Sim GK, Wold B, Pellicer A, Lacey E, Maniatis T, Silverstein S, Axel R: Cell 16:777–785, 1979.
23. Southern EM: J Mol Biol 98:503–517, 1975.
24. Thomas PS, Proc Natl Acad Sci USA 80: 1194–1198, 1980.
25. Schwartz DC, Cantor CR: Cell 37:67–75, 1984.
26. Riordan JR, Deuchars K, Kartner N, Alon N, Trent J, Ling V: Nature 316:817–819, 1985.
27. Kartner N, Evernden-Porelle D, Bradley G, Ling V: Nature 316:820–823, 1985.
28. Trent J, Bell D, Willard H, Ling V: Human Gene Mapping 8 40:761, 1985.
29. Fojo A, Lebo R, Shimizu N, Chin JE, Roninson IB, Merlino GT, Gottesman MM, Pastan I: Somatic Cell Mol Genet 12:415–420, 1986.

Cellular and Molecular Biology of Tumors and Potential
Clinical Applications 297–299 (1988)

Tumor Progression and Resistance to Drug Therapy

Adi F. Gazdar

*NCI-Navy Medical Oncology Branch, National Cancer Institute and Naval Hospital,
Bethesda, Maryland 20814*

Tumors are dynamic processes, constantly undergoing alterations, both in vivo and in vitro. Tumor progression events include changes in morphology, growth rate, cytogenetic abnormalities, oncogene amplification/expression, metastatic ability, and the development of drug resistance. Several aspects of these events were addressed during the workshop.

Adi Gazdar (National Cancer Institute) presented an overview of tumor progression, using small cell lung carcinoma (SCLC) as an example. For some years it has been noted that SCLC frequently undergoes morphological alterations, especially to large cell undifferentiated carcinoma. Variant tumors have rampant growth, decreased survival time, and poor response to therapy. Their corresponding cell lines are characterized by poor cell-to-cell adhesion, alterations in cell surface protein phenotype, short doubling times, high cloning efficiencies, selective loss of neuroendocrine properties and relative radioresistance. There is a high frequency of amplification and expression of the c-myc gene, with cytogenetic evidence of gene amplification (double minute chromosomes or homogeneously staining regions). In addition to the changes associated with variant morphology, there is a high incidence of amplification/ expression of other myc family genes (N-myc, L-myc) in SCLC cell lines from previously treated patients. At the present time it is not known whether cytotoxic therapy helps induce these changes directly or whether it enables the patients to live long enough for tumor progression events to occur spontaneously.

Julia Ibson (Ludwig Institute for Cancer Research, Cambridge) characterized twelve SCLC lines derived in Cambridge and compared them to the NCI lines. The English lines all were of the classic or biochemical variant phenotype (no morphological variants were identified). Several lines had N-myc amplification, but there was no correlation with phenotype (findings similar to those of the NCI group). Of great interest, all lines of the classic phenotype had a 3p deletion, and they located the breakpoint more precisely than other investigators to 3p 23-24.

Received April 22, 1986.

The latter report sparked a lively debate on whether a specific cytogenetic abnormality was associated with SCLC. Jackie Whang-Peng, in her earlier analysis of the NCI cell lines, reported a 100% incidence of 3p deletion irrespective of phenotype. This finding has been confirmed, but in widely varying incidences, in SCLC tumors and cell lines by other centers, both in the United States, and worldwide including Japan, the United Kingdom, Germany, and Sweden. However, the Dartmouth group found an incidence of only 14%, and June Beidler, in her reexamination of a few of the NCI lines, could not confirm Whang-Peng's findings. All of the investigators conceded that cytogenetic analyses of SCLC cells were complex and difficult, and subject to differing interpretations. Some unpublished work was cited from Susan Naylor (Houston) and York Miller (Denver) using restriction enzyme fragment polymorphism and amino acylase-1 expression. Both of these studies suggested that deletions of 3p are frequently present in SCLC tumors and cell lines.

Sean Egan (University of Manitoba, Winnipeg) reported on the role of H-ras activation and metastasis formation. C3H 10T½ mouse cells were transfected with T24 H-ras and colonies were selected having both refractile and flat morphologies. The morphologically transformed colonies gave rise to highly tumorigenic and metastatic lines, whereas the phenotypically flat NR3 line was poorly tumorigenic and rarely metastatic. However, four sublines of NR3 were highly tumorigenic and metastatic. While the parent 10T½ and the NR3 lines have very low expression of H-ras mRNA, all metastatic sublines have high transcription. These results indicate that transcription of activated H-ras can result in tumorigenic transformation and a metastatic phenotype. As other (radiation induced) transformants do not have activated H-ras transcripts, expression of H-ras may be necessary, but not sufficient, for the development of the metastatic phenotype.

The remaining papers dealt with multidrug resistance. Adi Gazdar (NCI, Bethesda) introduced the topic, once again citing SCLC as a model. SCLC tumors are usually highly responsive to cytotoxic therapy initially, but develop clinical resistance at time of relapse or tumor progression. In general, cell lines from untreated patients are sensitive in vitro to two or more drugs, while lines from previously treated patients usually are resistant. In addition, a subgroup of lines from untreated patients are highly resistant initially. All four such patients failed to respond to initial therapy. Thus, in vitro testing can identify a resistant subgroup of untreated patients having a poor prognosis. In addition, cell lines reflect the clinical responses of the patients from whom they were derived.

Peter Twentyman (MRC Unit, Cambridge) reported on the development of multidrug-resistant (MDR) variants of three human lung carcinoma sublines (one small cell, one adenocarcinoma, one large cell). The variants were isolated by exposure to increasing concentrations of adriamycin. In addition, the lines were resistant to vincristine and colchicine, and were deficient in adriamycin uptake. Resistance could be partly overcome by the use of the calcium transport blocker verapamil. In both human and rodent MDR lines multiple changes in cellular protein composition were observed.

Several reports described gene amplification associated with MDR. June Beidler (Memorial Sloan Kettering, New York) reported studies on the chromosomal location of one such gene, pVCR5L-18, cloned from vincristine-resistant cells. Chinese hamster ovary (CHO) hamster cells were probed with cloned cDNA to determine the location of single copy and amplified pVCR5L-18 genes. The native gene was localized to 1q. In MDR lines the amplified genes were localized to regions of homogeneously staining or abnormally banded regions. In contrast to results obtained with dihydrofolate reductase gene amplification, pVCR5L-18 gene amplification occurred in loco in at least two lines. Alexander Van der Bliek (Netherlands Cancer Institute, Amsterdam) presented data indicating that MDR is complex and consists of several components. A cDNA library was prepared from a colchicine-resistant CHO subline. Clones representing overexpressed mRNAs were isolated by differential screening with cDNA probes from parental and resistant lines. RNA blot hybridizations indicated that five overexpressed genes were involved, amplified 10–30-fold. One of the genes appears to code for the 170-kilodalton (kD) p-glycoprotein described previously. The genes appear to be linked in one large ($>$ 600 kilobase [kb]) domain of which a segment has been triplicated prior to amplification of the whole domain. Finally, Douglas Clark (NCI, Bethesda) reported on the isolation of cDNA clones for *mdr1*, the multidrug resistance gene from human KB cells. A number of sublines selected independently for resistance to colchicine, adriamycin, and vinblastine show cross-resistance to the selecting drugs as well as actinomycin-D and vincristine. Each line has amplified sequences, some of which have been cloned. One clone recognizes a gene, *mdr1*, expressed at high levels in several MDR human lines. The probe was used to screen a cDNA library from a MDR line. Several large cDNA inserts were isolated and are currently being analyzed.

From these presentations it is apparent that cloning the gene(s) for MDR from human and rodent cells has shown considerable progress, and these studies have greatly aided our understanding of this fascinating phenomenon, which has considerable clinical and biological interest.

Cellular and Molecular Biology of Tumors and Potential
Clinical Applications 301–305 (1988)

Patterns of Proto-Oncogene Expression: A Tool to Subtype Histopathologically Similar Solid Tumors

Carol J. Thiele, Catherine McKeon, Lee Helman, and Mark A. Israel

Molecular Genetics Section, Pediatric Branch COP, National Cancer Institute, National Institutes of Health, Bethesda, Maryland 20892

Monoclonal antibodies and other biochemical markers have revolutionized the manner in which we view the normal development of the hematopoetic system. The delineation of these developmental pathways has enabled researchers to suggest that various lymphoid and other hematopoetic malignancies correspond to clones of cells arrested at discrete points during differentiation. It is possible that specific genetic alterations are closely associated with the patterns of differentiation which have been observed. For example, tumors such as Burkitt's lymphoma, which corresponds to a pre-B cell [1], and chronic myelogenous leukemia, which corresponds to an early hematopeotic stem cell [2], each contain a unique cytogenetic alteration which is similar among most examples of these tumors. The fact that proto-oncogenes are located at or near the sites of these chromosomal alterations is particularly interesting [3].

Analysis of solid tumors has been less fruitful. This is due, in part, to the paucity of developmental markers which phenotypically define the transitions from stem cell to a highly specialized, fully differentiated cell of nonhematopoetic origin. Since the expression of many proto-oncogenes is developmentally regulated [4,5], we explored the possibility that solid tumors also correspond to different stages of maturation and, therefore, might have characteristic profiles of proto-oncogene expression. Analysis of proto-oncogene expression may enable us to determine developmental subtypes among the solid tumors of any given tissue when analyzed in conjunction with defined biochemical and immunocytochemical markers.

Towards this end, we have been studying cell lines of tumors derived from embryonic neural crest, neuroblastoma(NB) and neuroepithelioma(NE), and pheochromocytoma(PC) tumor tissue. In addition, we have examined cell lines from Ewing's sarcoma(ES), a tumor whose origin is unknown. NB, NE, and ES belong to a class of tumors known as "small-, round-, blue-cell tumors," whose differential diagnosis at both the clinical and histopathological level is often difficult.

Received April 1, 1986.

Neuroblastoma (NB) is a tumor of the sympathetic nervous system which generally occurs in children less than 5 yr of age. It is most commonly detected in the adrenal medulla, extra-adrenal retroperitoneal abdominal areas, the thorax, and cervical ganglia. Abdominal NB is often associated with high levels of urinary catecholamines. Advanced stage NB presents as widely metastatic disease involving the bone marrow, lymph nodes, skeleton and less frequently, other organs. NB has been termed a "dysontogenic" neoplasm since it is characterized by tissue with varying degrees of morphological differentiation ranging from homogeneous patterns of primitive, small, round cells to well-differentiated ganglion cell formations containing extensive neuritic processes and Schwann cells. Several neural crest derivatives such as melanocytes, Schwann-like cells, and neurons have been cultured in vitro from NB cell lines suggesting that this may even be a tumor of a pluripotent stem cell [6,7].

Neuroepithelioma (NE) is histopathologically indistinguishable from NB. NE has often been called adult neuroblastoma, since it occurs clinically in somewhat older children and adults. Typically it presents with metastatic disease, although involvement of the adrenal gland or other known sites of sympathetic tissue is not seen. Whang-Peng et al [8] have described a rcp(11;22) in NE which cytogenetically differentiates it from NB. This rcp(11;22) is also cytogenetically indistinguishable from the translocation found in Ewing's sarcoma, a tumor of unknown histogenesis.

Ewing's sarcoma (ES) is the second-most-common bone tumor of children and young adults. It frequently occurs in the midshaft of the long bones or in the trunk. While ES can be immunocytochemically differentiated from NE, both tumors contain a cytogenetically indistinguishable chromosomal translocation. This is particularly intriguing since the tissue of origin of ES is an unknown [9,10].

Pheochromocytoma (PC) is a rare tumor which occurs in the sympathetic nervous system. It presents most commonly during adulthood, typically in the adrenal medulla. This tumor is rarely invasive or metastatic and is most strikingly characterized by excessive production of catecholamines. These two clinical features, as well as its chromaffinlike histologic appearance, suggest that PC corresponds to a more mature neural crest derivative than NB.

Recently, it has been shown that the proto-oncogene N-myc is amplified and expressed at high levels in virtually all NB cell lines [11–13] and in a subset of NB tumors [14]. Our study showing that NB cell lines induced to differentiate had reduced levels of N-myc expression [15] suggested that N-myc may be developmentally regulated. This was supported by the finding that N-myc is expressed early during embryogenesis [16] and at high levels in fetal kidney, brain, intestine, heart, and adrenal but not in their adult counterparts [7]. We studied NB, NE, and ES cell lines and PC tumor tissue RNA by Northern blot analysis to determine the relative levels of N-myc expression. The results are shown in Figure 1. As expected, NB cell lines (containing amplified N-myc sequences) expressed high levels of N-myc RNA compared to NE, ES, and PC. The levels of N-myc expression in NE and ES (which contain single-copy N-myc DNA) are somewhat elevated compared to other tissues containing a single copy of the N-myc proto-oncogene (data not shown). We could not detect N-myc expression in PC under these assay conditions.

The proto-oncogene c-myc is both structurally and functionally related to N-myc [18], yet its expression during development is quite distinct [17]. For example, expression of N-myc decreases during development of the adrenal gland while expression of c-myc increases [7]. In contrast to the pattern of N-myc expression in

A   B   C

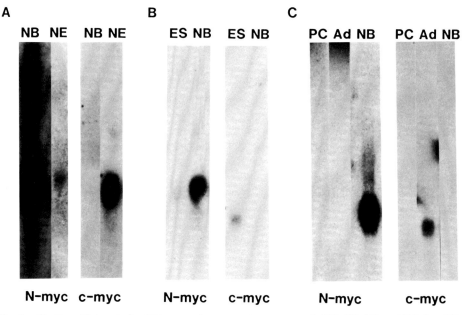

Fig. 1. Northern blot analysis of N-myc and c-myc proto-oncogenes in NB, NE, ES, and PC. 2 µg NB and 15 µg NE poly(A) + (**A**); 2 µg ES poly(A) +, and 5 µg NB total RNA(**B**); and 30 µg PC total RNA, 30 µg adrenal(Ad) total RNA, and 5 µg NB total RNA(**C**) were electrophoresed on 1% formaldehyde-agarose gels, blotted onto nitrocellulose paper, hybridized to ^{32}P-labeled pNB-1(N-myc)[11] and pMC41-3RC(c-myc)[1] plasmid DNA, washed at 0.1× standard saline citrate, 0.1% sodium-dodecyl-sulfate, and exposed to Kodak XAR film and a lightening plus intensifying screen.

NE and ES cell lines, the levels of c-myc expression in these cell lines was quite high relative to NB cell lines. PC tumor tissue did not express detectable levels of c-myc RNA (Fig. 1C).

We have also studied the expression of the c-sis and c-myb proto-oncogenes. Since the c-sis proto-oncogene is located distal to the breakpoint in NE and ES, we examined these cell lines as well as NB cell lines for c-sis expression. We were unable to detect c-sis in any of the cell lines examined [20]. High levels of c-myb expression have been detected primarily in immature cells of the myeloid lineage, and these levels decline upon differentiation [21]. We have been able to detect c-myb expression in NB, NE, and ES at approximately equivalent levels.

In Table I we have summarized the profiles of relative proto-oncogene expression as well as several other known morphological and immunocytochemical properties of these cell lines and tumor tissue. Analysis of this table reveals several striking differences and similarities among these tumor cell lines. The most striking differences were between the histopathologically similar tumor cell lines, NB and NE. While both appear as small, round tumor cells with neuronal features and contain detectable neuron specific enolase, NB cell lines express high levels of N-myc mRNA yet do not express easily detected c-myc mRNA: NE cell lines express low levels of N-myc and relatively high levels of c-myc mRNA. Further contrast between these tumors can be noted by the expression of class I histocompatability antigens (HLA) [22] on NE cell lines while these antigens are only weakly detected on NB cell lines [23]. The low levels of N-myc mRNA and expression of HLA in NE suggest that it is a more mature neural crest derivative than NB. Thus, although NB and NE are

TABLE I. Characterization of Selected Solid Tumor Tissues*

	Neuroblastoma	Neuroepithelioma	Ewing's sarcoma	Pheochromocytoma
Morphology				
Light microscopy	Small, round cells neural features	Small round cells	Small round cells	Chromaffin cells
Electron microscopy	Neural features	Neural features	Undifferentiated	Chromaffin features
Immunocytochemistry				
Neuron-specific enolase	+	+	–	+
HLA-class I	–	+	+	NT[a]
Cytogenetics				
Rearrangements	1p–	rcp(11;22)(q24;q12)	rcp(11;22)(q24;q12)	–
Frequency HSRs/DMs[b]	High	Low	Low	–
Proto-oncogene expression				
N-myc[c]	++++	+	+	–
c-myc	–	++	++	–
c-myb	+	+	+	–
c-sis	–	–	–	NT

*NB, NE, ES are pediatric solid tumors, while PC is an adult tumor which is used in this analysis to represent a neural tumor derived from mature adrenal medullary tissue. PC cell lines are not available and these results are for tumor tissue.
[a]Not tested. [b]HSRs, homogeneously staining regions; DMs, double minute bodies.
[c]+, indicates amount detected in SK-N-SH, a cell line with a single copy of the N-myc gene [12]; –, indicates not detected.

histopathologically indistinguishable, their proto-oncogene expression profiles and expression of HLA clearly differentiate them.

The other striking pattern that emerges from this analysis is the similarities betwen NE and ES. The similarities in proto-oncogene expression profiles, expression of HLA antigens, and their common cytogenetic alteration strongly suggests that NE and ES may be tumors of closely related or identical cell types. A neuronal origin for ES is supported by the recent report that ES expresses receptors for nerve growth factor and neural cellular adhesion molecules [24].

With this type of analysis, we have started to develop a proto-oncogenetic phenotype for ontogenetically related and histopathologically similar solid tumors. As more becomes known about developmental expression of proto-oncogenes in normal tissue, it may be possible to expand this approach and further delineate developmentally related tumors. Molecular genetic analysis of this type is important since current clinical and histopathological descriptions of certain tumors do not reflect many aspects of tumor cell heterogeneity which may be of diagnostic and prognostic importance.

REFERENCES

1. Dalla Favera R, Bregni M, Erikson J, et al: Proc Natl Acad Sci USA 79:7824, 1982.
2. deKlein A, vanKessel AG, Grosveld G, et al: Nature (Lond) 300:765, 1982.
3. Yunis JJ, Soreng AL: Science 226:1199, 1984.
4. Muller R, Slamon D, Trembly J, et al: Nature (Lond) 299:640, 1982.
5. Slamon D, Cline MJ: Proc Natl Acad Sci USA 81:7141, 1984.
6. Ross RA, Biedler JL: In Evans AE, D'Angio G, Seeger RC (eds): "Advances in Neuroblastoma Research."New York: Alan R. Liss, Inc., 1985, pp 13–37.
7. Reynolds CP, Maples J: In Evans AE, D'Angio G, Seeger RC (eds): "Advances in Neuroblastoma Research." New York: Alan R. Liss, Inc., 1985, pp 13–37.
8. Whang-Peng J, Triche TJ, Knutsen T, et al: N Engl J Med 311:584, 1984.
9. Aurias A, Rimbaut C, Buffe A, et al: N Engl J Med 309:496, 1983.
10. Turc-Carel C, Philip I, Berger MP, et al: N Engl J Med 309:497, 1983.
11. Schwab M, et al: Nature (Lond) 305:245, 1983.
12. Kohl NE, et al: Cell 35:359, 1983.
13. Kohl NE, Gee C, Alt FW: Science 226:1335, 1984.
14. Broedeur GM, Seeger RC, Schwab M, et al: Science 224:1121, 1984.
15. Thiele CJ, Reynolds CP, Israel M: Nature (Lond) 313:404, 1985.
16. Jakobovits A, Schwab M, Bishop JM, Martin G: Nature (Lond) 318:188, 1985.
17. Zimmerman KA, Yancopoulos GD, Collum DG, et al: Nature (Lond) 319:780, 1986.
18. Kohl NE, Legouy E, DePinho R, et al: Nature (Lond) 319:73, 1986.
19. Yancopoulos GD, Nisen PD, Tesfaye A, et al: Proc Natl Acad Sci USA 82:5455, 1985.
20. Thiele CJ, Whang-Peng J, Kao-Shan C, et al: Cancer Genet Cytogenet 24:119, 1987.
21. Westin E. Gallo RC, Arya SK, et al: Proc Natl Acad Sci USA 79:2194, 1982.
22. Natali PG, Bigotti A, Nicotra MR, et al: Cancer Res 44:4679, 1984.
23. Donner L, Triche TJ, Israel MA, et al: In Evans AE, D'Angio G, Seeger RC (eds): "Advances in Neuroblastoma Research." New York: Alan R. Liss, Inc., 1985, pp 347–366.
24. Lipinski M, Braham K, Philip I, et al: J Cell Biochem [Suppl] 10A:39, 1986.

Cellular and Molecular Biology of Tumors and Potential
Clinical Applications 307–312 (1988)

Monoclonal Antibodies Against the Receptor for Epidermal Growth Factor as Potential Anticancer Agents

J. Mendelsohn, H. Masui, H. Sunada, and C. MacLeod

Memorial Sloan Kettering Cancer Center, New York, New York 10021 (J.M., H.M., H.S.); Cornell University Medical College, New York, New York 10021 (J.M.); University of California at San Diego Cancer Center, La Jolla, California 92093 (C.M.)

Epidermal growth factor (EGF) stimulates the proliferation of fibroblasts and most epithelial cell types, whereas it profoundly inhibits the growth of A431 epidermoid carcinoma cells. The growth of 8 EGF receptor-bearing human tumor cell lines was measured following the addition of EGF or monoclonal anti-EGF receptor antibody 528 IgG2a (which blocks EGF binding). Epidermoid carcinoma cell lines from lung (T222), skin (T423), and vulva (A431) were growth-inhibited by both EGF and 528 IgG. Proliferation of the other five human tumor cell lines tested was not blocked by either EGF or 528 IgG. Xenografts of the three cell lines inhibited by EGF and 528 IgG in culture were inhibited by 528 IgG treatment in vivo, whereas the other five tumors were unaffected. Differences in the number of EGF receptors expressed on the cell surface did not account for the inhibition of selected receptor-bearing tumor cells. Monoclonal antibody 225 IgG1 also prevented proliferation of A431 cells in culture and xenografts. Screening for complement-mediated and cellular mechanisms of cytotoxicity demonstrated cytolytic effects of macrophages upon A431 cells in the presence of 528 IgG2a, but we could find no immune mechanism to explain the antitumor effect on 225 IgG1. Thus, the antiproliferative activity may be related to direct effects upon the receptor. In summary, immunotherapy of xenografts with anti-EGF receptor antibody is effective against a subset of receptor-bearing cells, which are also, in all cases, inhibited in vitro.

Key words: antireceptor antibody, tyrosine kinase, EGF, xenografts, antibody therapy, nude mouse xenograft, A431 carcinoma, immunotherapy, EGF receptor

RATIONALE

We have produced a panel of monoclonal antibodies (mAbs) against the epidermal growth factor (EGF) receptor, which have the capacity to inhibit EGF-related

Received March 19, 1986.

biochemical processes and proliferation of cells bearing receptors for this ligand. The research project was stimulated by the observations of Sato and others that the requirement of cell lines for serum in the culture medium could be obviated, in many cases, by addition of a mixture of 5–7 growth factors, hormones, and transport proteins [1,2]. This body of research clearly demonstrated that access to essential growth-promoting agents is essential for the proliferation of malignant cells in vitro. Furthermore, different cell types appear to require differing, individually tailored "cocktails" of growth factors. From these observations it is clear that cell surface membranes have receptors for different growth factors and hormones each of which are, in fact, surface membrane antigens. We reasoned that monoclonal antibodies which could bind to surface membrane receptors for essential growth-promoting agents might block access to the natural ligand and thereby interfere with cell function.

This hypothesis was supported by data in the experimental literature, and, most importantly, by the existence of three disease states in which antireceptor antibodies produce abnormal physiology in man. These include 1) myasthenia gravis, in which autoantibodies against the receptor for acetyl choline result in abnormal nerve signal transmission; 2) hyperthyroidism or hypothyroidism resulting from the action of autoantibody against the receptor for thyroid-stimulating hormone (LATS); and 3) a rare form of diabetes in which autoantibodies against the insulin receptor cause insulin resistance [3–6].

A second line of evidence which stimulated this research was the observation of Todaro and collaborators that a number of cultured tumor cells have the capacity to produce autostimulatory growth-promoting factors with the apparent capacity to bind to receptors on the cells synthesizing the factors, resulting in "autocrine" growth stimulation [7]. One of the first of these factors was transforming growth factor alpha, which is closely related to EGF.

The discovery of oncogenes provided additional evidence for the potential utility of antibodies against growth factor receptors. At the present time three oncogenes are known to code for receptors or for growth factors: erb-B (EGF receptor), fms (colony-stimulating factor-1 receptor), and sis (platelet-derived growth factor). In addition a number of oncogenes code for protein kinases which appear to act in a manner similar to kinases linked to the receptors for insulin, the somatomedins, and platelet-derived growth factor [8].

Finally, research from a number of laboratories has demonstrated the presence of increased numbers of receptors for EGF on human tumor cells obtained from non-small-cell lung cancers [9] as well as a number of other malignancies. In some cases the increase in receptors is at a level of two logs above the normal values. This increase in the amount of specific antigen to which an antireceptor antibody could react supplies the potential for substantial selectivity in antibody activity.

OBSERVATIONS
Production of Monoclonal Antibodies Against the EGF Receptor

We have produced four mAbs against the human EGF receptor (Table I)[10, 11]. These antibodies were raised against affinity-purified receptors obtained from A431 cells, an epidermoid carcinoma cell line which contains 2 million EGF receptors per cell. The first three antibodies in the table bind to the receptor with high affinity

TABLE I. Monoclonal Antibody Characteristics

Ligand	A431 binding		% inhibition of binding of ligand	
	$(K_D \times 10^9 M)$	Sites $(\times 10^{-6}/\text{cell})$	^{125}I-EGF	[125]I-528
528 IgG2A	2.0	1.6	100	100
225 IgG1	0.9	1.5	100	100
579 IgG2A	1.5	1.2	100	100
455 IgG1	20	1.8	0	0
EGF	2.5	1.5–2.0	100	95

and compete effectively for the binding of labeled EGF or labeled antibody. They appear to react with the polypeptide backbone chain of the receptor [12], at a site near but not identical with the binding site for EGF. The latter is presumed to be the case because the antibodies (unlike EGF) show species specificity. The fourth antibody in the table reacts with a carbohydrate residue on the receptor [12], binds with a weaker affinity, and does not compete for the binding of EGF or the other antibodies. Each of the antibodies precipitates a cell membrane protein with molecular weight 170,000 which has the capacity to autophosphorylate itself on tyrosine residues [11].

Antibody Effects Upon Receptor Tyrosine Kinase Activity

Whereas EGF stimulation results in autophosphorylation of the receptor on tyrosine residues, none of the antibodies stimulates this enzymatic activity in intact cells [14]. However, each of the three blocking antibodies has the capacity to prevent EGF-induced activation of tyrosine kinase [13].

Antibody Effects Upon EGF Receptor Expression

When EGF binds to its receptors on the cell surface membrane, the great majority of receptor-ligand complexes are internalized by endocytosis into organelles known as endosomes. This results in decreased expression of receptor on the cell surface, a process known as "down-regulation." When A431 cells (2×10^6 receptors per cell) or KB cells (5×10^4 receptors per cell) are exposed to antireceptor antibody, down-regulation occurs with kinetics comparable to that observed with the natural ligand [14]. Between 80% and 95% of EGF binding capacity is removed within an hour. Analysis of cell lysates following incubation with labeled EGF or labeled mAb demonstrates that each of these ligands sediments in the location of endosomes on Percoll gradients. This is an important characteristic of the antigen-antibody system under study, because binding of mAbs to some surface antigens has been observed to result in shedding into the culture medium rather than internalization.

Monoclonal Antibody Effects Upon Cell Proliferation in Culture

Cultures of human foreskin fibroblasts grow poorly under serum-free conditions but can divide every 24 hr in the presence of insulin, transferrin, and EGF. Addition of any of the three antireceptor antibodies which block EGF binding can completely inhibit the EGF-induced proliferation of these fibroblasts [11]. In contrast, the antibodies have no intrinsic inhibitory effect upon the slow fibroblast proliferation observed in the absence of EGF. The inhibition is cytostatic rather than cytosidal and excess EGF can reverse the inhibitory effects of anti-EGF receptor mAb. Comparable effects are observed with cultured human tumor cells which exhibit stimulation in response to EGF.

A431 cells are unusual in that they express 2 million receptors for EGF [15], and they have another unusual property: exposure to physiologic (1 nM) concentrations of EGF results in inhibition of cell proliferation in culture [16]. Concentrations of anti-receptor mAbs which block EGF binding to A431 cell can prevent the EGF-induced inhibition of cell proliferation. Moreover, the three blocking antireceptor antibodies exhibit a direct inhibitory effect upon the proliferation of A431 cells when added to the cells in the absence of EGF [10,11]. Thus the antibodies mimic the antiproliferative effect of EGF upon A431 cells. We believe that this effect is through a different mechanism than the inhibition produced by the natural ligand, because the antibodies (at intermediate concentrations) can reverse the inhibition produced by EGF [10,11, 17] and because the antibodies, unlike EGF, do not stimulate receptor tyrosine kinase activity. At first we believed that this inhibitory effect could be related to the high number of receptors on A431 cells. However, two other tumor cell lines— T222 (carcinoma of the lung) and T423 (carcinoma from the inner ear)—have a normal number of EGF receptors, but are inhibited by EGF and the three blocking antireceptor antibodies (Table II). In summary, the blocking mAbs have the capacity to prevent EGF-induced effects upon cell proliferation; in addition, for those tumor

TABLE II.   Studies of Human Tumor Cells in Culture and in Xenografts[*]

Cells[a]	Effects of ligands on proliferation in culture		Receptor No. on cultured cells[d]	Effect of treating xenografts with 528 IgG[e]
	EGF[b]	528 IgG[c]		
HFF	S	N	Lo	—
Epidermoid carcinoma				
A431	I	I	Hi	I
T222	I	I	Lo	I
T423	I	I	Lo	I
HeLa	S	N	Lo	N
T323	S	N	Lo	N
Other malignant				
Li-7	N	N	Lo	N
T84	N	N	Lo	N
T24	S	N	Lo	N

[*]I = inhibition; N = no effect; S = stimulation; Lo = low or typical number ($3-5 \times 10^4$); Hi = high number ($0.5-2 \times 10^6$).
[a]The cell types are as follows: HFF = human foreskin fibroblasts; A431 = vulvar epidermoid carcinoma; T222 = lung epidermoid carcinoma; T423 = epidermoid carcinoma (ear); HeLa = cervical adenocarcinoma; T323 = epidermoid carcinoma (larnyx); Li-7 = hepatoma; T84 = colon carcinoma; T24 = astrocytoma.
[b]Cells were cultured in serum-free medium, or in 0.5% serum, containing approximately 5 pM EGF, which is ordinarily not stimulatory. Proliferation was assayed in the presence or absence of 2 and 20 nM EGF.
[c]Cells were cultured in the presence or absence of 10 and 100 nM 528 IgG.
[d]Receptor number was determined by Scatchard analysis after incubation with ^{125}I-EGF at varying concentrations.
[e]Mice bearing xenografts were treated intraperitoneally twice weekly with 2 mg of 528 IgG, for 3–6 wk.

cells which are inhibited by EGF, the antibodies demonstrate an intrinsic inhibitory capacity.

Antibody Effects Upon the Growth of Human Tumor Xenografts

Studies were carried out to examine the antitumor activity of antireceptor mAbs against human tumor xenografts placed subcutaneously in athymic mice. Intraperitoneal injection of antireceptor antibody at a concentration of 2 mg, three times weekly, produces a marked inhibition of tumor growth, compared with control animals treated with an irrelevant antibody [18]. When therapy is delayed until 4 wk after subcutaneous implantation, antibody treatment results in a plateauing of tumor growth, which resumes when therapy is discontinued. Further studies demonstrated that antibody therapy effectively prevents the proliferation of tumor xenografts in those situations where the antibody (and EGF) produces inhibition of tumor cell growth in culture. In contrast, antixenograft activity is not observed in situations where the antibody does not display intrinsic inhibitory effects upon cultures of the tumor cells (Table II).

Mechanism of Antitumor Activity Against the Xenografts

In order to explore the mechanism of antitumor activity, we compared the results of a number of in vitro assays utilizing 528 IgG2A and 225 IgG1 as antiproliferative agents. The two antibodies are comparable in binding affinity, in the number of receptors detected, in precipitation characteristics, in down-regulation and internalization patterns, in antiproliferative effects on cultured cells, and in antiproliferative activity against tumor xenografts. They differ only in their isotype and therefore provide an interesting model system for comparing the mechanism of antitumor activity in IgG1 and IgG2A monoclonal antibodies. While 528 IgG2A demonstrates some cytotoxic activity against A431 cells in the presence of activated macrophages or compliment, these effects cannot be demonstrated with 225 IgG1 [19]. These observations, plus the finding that activity against the tumor xenografts is demonstrable only for a particular subpopulation of EGF receptor-bearing cells, suggest that the antiproliferative activity in vivo might be related to specific effects upon the physiologic function of the EGF receptor, rather than to nonspecific immune processes activated by the Fc fragments of bound antibodies. Clearly, immune-related mechanisms might account for some of the activity of the 528 IgG2A, supporting the observations of previous investigators.

FUTURE DIRECTIONS

We are examining the EGF receptors on various types of tumor cells, to determine whether there is genomic rearrangement, abnormal messenger RNA synthesis, or abnormal receptor kinetics in the susceptible subpopulation of EGF receptor-bearing cells. Combination immunotherapy against xenografts with antireceptor mAbs to the EGF and transferrin receptors is planned. It should be stressed that the in vivo test system utilized in these experiments is artificial, in the sense that the antireceptor mAbs employed do not react with murine EGF receptors. EGF receptors are present on a variety of normal human tissues, including liver, gastrointestinal epithelium, and lung. Prior to contemplating the use of antireceptor antibodies in a therapeutic setting, it will be necessary to test for toxic effects on normal tissues. In the meantime, antibodies to the EGF receptor provide a unique analytical tool for examining the biochemical and physiologic function of the EGF receptor on normal cells, and in tumor cells which often bear increased receptor numbers and may have atypical growth responses to EGF.

ACKNOWLEDGMENTS

This research was supported by NIH grants CA 37641 and CA 42060. C.M. is a Clayton Foundation investigator; the research was conducted in part by the Clayton Foundation for Research, California division.

REFERENCES

1. Barnes D, Sato G: Cell 22:649–655, 1980.
2. Sato G, Pardee AB, Sirbasku D: "Growth of Cells in Hormonally Defined Media." Cold Spring Harbor Conferences on Cell Proliferation, Vol. 9. New York: Cold Spring Harbor Laboratory, 1982.
3. Appel SH, Anwyl R, McAdams MW, Elias SB: Proc Natl Acad Sci USA 74:2130, 1977.
4. Volpe R: Clin Endocrinol Metab 7:3, 1978.
5. Dexhage HA, Bottazzo GF, Bitensky L, Chayen J, Doniach D: Nature 289:594, 1981.
6. Flier JS, Kahn CR, Jarrett DB, Roth J: J Clin Invest 58: 1442–1449, 1976.
7. Sporn MB, Todaro GJ: N Engl J Med 303:878, 1980.
8. Sefton MB, Hunter T: In Greengard P, Robinson GA (ed): Adv Cyclic Nucleotide Protein Phosphorylation Res 18:195, 1984.
9. Hendler FS, Ozanne BW: J Clin Invest 74:647–651, 1984.
10. Kawamoto T, Sato JD, Le A, Polikoff J, Sato GH, Mendelsohn J: Proc Natl Acad Sci USA 80:1337–1341, 1983.
11. Sato JD, Kawamoto T, Le AD, Mendelsohn J, Polikoff J, Sato GH: Mol Biol Med 1:511–529, 1983.
12. Gooi HC, Hounsell EF, Lax I, Kris R, Liebermann TA, Schlessinger J, Sato JD, Kawamoto T, Mendelsohn J, Feizi T: Biosci Rep 5:83–94, 1985.
13. Gill GN, Kawamoto T, Cochet C, Le A, Sato JD, Masui H, MacLeod C, Mendelsohn J: J Biol Chem 259:7755–7760, 1984.
14. Sunada H, Magun BE, Mendelsohn J, MacLeod CL: Proc Natl Acad Sci USA 83:3825–3829, 1986.
15. Fabricant RN, De Larco JE, Todaro GJ: Proc Natl Acad Sci USA 74:565–569, 1977.
16. Barnes DW: J Cell Biol 93:1–4, 1982.
17. Kawamoto T, Mendelsohn J, Le A, Sato GH, Lazar CS, Gill GN: J Biol Chem 259:7761–7766, 1984.
18. Masui H, Kawamoto T, Sato JD, Wolf B, Sato G, Mendelsohn J: Cancer Res 44:1002–1007, 1984.
19. Masui H, Takamasa M, Mendelsohn J: Cancer Res 46:5592–5598, 1986.

Cellular and Molecular Biology of Tumors and Potential
Clinical Applications 313–315 (1988)

Workshop: Antibodies and Other Biological Response Modifiers as Preventive, Diagnostic, and Therapeutic Agents

John Mendelsohn

Memorial Sloan Kettering Cancer Center, New York, New York 10021

Biological reagents with potential utility for the diagnosis and treatment of human malignant disease were discussed in this workshop. For the most part attention continues to focus on monoclonal antibodies. However, it is clear that recombinant DNA technology is providing biochemical tools which can clarify cancer pathogenesis and enable production of specific antitumor cytokines. The ten presentations at this workshop demonstrate these developments.

Stephen Smith of the Division of Surgery and Biology, City of Hope, Duarte, California, presented data suggesting that stable alterations in the methylation of repeated DNA sequences may provide a clonal marker in neoplastic cells. With the aid of cloned repetitive DNA sequences as probes, altered methylation patterns were found in Southern blots of restriction digests of a number of tumor DNA's. Patterns for squamous carcinoma and adenocarcinoma of the lung differed, as did patterns obtained from pulmonary metastases of colon carcinoma. These preliminary data suggest that differences in methylation patterns may be characteristic of particular tumor types.

Two presentations were concerned with the use of monoclonal antibodies and recombinant DNA probes to classify human tumors. Carol Thiele and her colleagues in the laboratory of Mark Israel, from the National Cancer Institute Bethesda, Maryland reviewed data differentiating neuroepithelioma from neuroblastoma. Neuroblastoma cell lines and primary tumors express increased mRNA for N-myc, have amplified N-myc gene sequences, and contain enzymes characteristic of cholinergic (parasympathetic) neurons. In contrast, neuroepitheliomas express increased mRNA for C-myc, have amplified C-myc genes, contain enzymes characteristic of adrenergic (sympathetic) neurons and have a different karyotypic abnormality involving a t (11;22). These two tumors, which affect different age groups but are similar under the light microscope, can now be distinguished on the basis of biochemical parame-

Received March 11, 1986.

ters. Marc Lipinski and colleagues of the Institute Gustave Roussy, Villejuif, France, reported evidence linking Ewing's sarcoma to the neuroectodermal malignancies. Ewing cell lines contain ganglioside GD_2, a marker of neuroectodermal tumors, and are stained by HNK-one and other monoclonal antibodies that detect carbohydrate epitopes present on several glycoconjugates of the nervous system, including the N-CAM adhesion molecule. These cells also are characterized by a t (ll;22) translocation similar to that observed in neuroepitheliomas. At a plenary session, Mark Israel reported encouraging preliminary results when patients with neuroepitheliomas were treated with chemotherapy regimens that are successful in Ewing's sarcoma.

Two presentations explored the use of monoclonal antibodies to diagnose malignancy. Brian Liu in the laboratory of John Fahey of the UCLA School of Medicine, Los Angeles, California, reported on E7, an IgM murine monoclonal antibody generated against human bladder cancer. The antibody reacts with some, but not all, bladder cancer cell lines and cross-reacts with other malignancies, but does not react with blood group antigens or normal tissues. The antigen has a molecular weight of 200,000 by Western blot. Preliminary data show that a trypsinized, reduced fragment of the IgM can detect tumor antigen in the urine of patients with metastatic transitional cell (bladder) carcinoma, and a clinical trial is ongoing to test its specificity and sensitivity.

Thomas Tursz reported new data derived with his monoclonal antibody 38.13 against a phospholipid on 50% of Burkitt's lymphoma cells. There was no cross-reactivity with Epstein-Barr virus (EBV)-transformed cells, including viral-trans-formed B cells from patients with Burkitt's lymphoma. The antigen is a glycolipid, globotriaosylceramide, which is the blood group antigen Pk. A careful screen of normal tissues detected cells reactive with 38.13 in human tonsils, but not blood, bone marrow, lymph nodes, or spleen. The tonsilar B cell is IgM^+, IgD^-, and $CALLA^+$. It was hypothesized that the glycolipid antigen on the cell surface might promote homing of normal and malignant B cells.

Monoclonal antibodies active against oncogene products and growth factors were the subject of three presentations at the workshop. Monoclonal antibody, 45-2D9, generated by Robert S. Ames of the National Cancer Institute, Bethesda, Maryland, and collaborators reacts with NIH-3T3 cells transformed by c-Ha-ras transfection. The antibody detects a glycophosphoprotein with molecular weight 74,000, which is not the ras gene product and does not bind GTP. It binds to a variety of adenocarcinomas, with some cross-reactivity with normal cells. Preliminary studies demonstrated cytotoxicity with ricin A chain conjugates and xenograft localization by ^{125}I-labeled antibody. Production of monoclonal antibodies against oncogene trans-formed cells may provide a useful approach to developing reagents for immu-notherapy.

John Mendelsohn's laboratory group at Memorial Sloan-Kettering Cancer Center, New York, has produced monoclonal antibodies against the EGF receptors on human A431 cervical carcinoma cells, which block EGF binding to its receptor and inhibit both EGF-induced tyrosine kinase activity and EGF-depedent alterations in cell proliferation. A subpopulation of EGF receptor-bearing cells, which are inhibited by EGF in culture, are also inhibited from proliferation by the antireceptor antibodies, both in vitro and as xenografts in athymic mice. While immune mechanisms may contribute to the antitumor activity of 528 IgG2a, they do not account for the comparable activity of 225 IgG1. These antibodies may act by blocking the physio-logic function of the EGF receptor.

Bombesin is a growth factor for many small cell carcinoma cells. John Minna's group of the National Cancer Institute, Navy Medical Oncology Branch, Naval Hospital, Bethesda, Maryland, has provided evidence, reviewed in a plenary session, that it may stimulate proliferation through an autocrine mechanism. May-Kin Ho and colleagues at E.I. Dupont DeNemours, Inc., No. Billerica, Massachusetts, have produced human monoclonal antibodies against bombesin by immunizing cultured human splenic B cells and fusing them to mouse myeloma cells. The in vitro immunization system has been refined, and it is anticipated that human monoclonal antibodies against a variety of antigens will be available in the near future for clinical trials.

A novel form of antitumor therapy involves stimulation of malignant clonogenic cells to differentiate to the point where proliferative capacity is lost. Barbara Zimmerman of the University of Colorado Health Sciences Center, Denver, Colorado, and her collaborators have found that ouabain induces maturation of a murine embryonal carcinoma cell line PCC4-ayal. Other agents which alter NA^+, K^+ ATPase activity did not produce this effect. It was postulated that maturation may have resulted from a change in the energy charge (relative high-energy phosphate content) of the cells.

Therapy with cytokines was the subject of work by Arthur Bollum of Wadley Institutes of Molecular Medicine, Dallas, Texas, who has isolated and expressed the gene for tumor necrosis factor (TNF) from human peripheral blood leukocyte DNA. The material is produced as a 17,700-dalton monomer, which dimerizes to the active form. Recombinant TNF shows direct cytotoxic activity against some cell lines in preliminary studies. Antitumor activity is potentiated by alpha- or gamma-interferon, and by sodium butyrate, but not by chemotherapeutic agents. Animal studies have established an LD50 of 6×10^7 U/kg, and human phase I clinical trials have been initiated.

The investigators who participated in this workshop presented explorations into new methods of diagnosing and treating cancer, taking advantage of recent technical and conceptual advances in molecular genetics and immunology. *The theme in each case was specificity.* It is apparent that during the next five years we will be performing highly individualized phenotypic characterizations of tumor cells, based on alterations in DNA structure, content, and arrangement; differences in messenger RNA production and size; changes in synthesis and activation of specific proteins in the plasma membrane and in the enzymatic apparatus of the cell; altered proliferative characteristics in the presence and absence of growth factors; and more. This is truly a remarkable change from the picture five years ago, when there was still argument about whether significant biochemical differences existed between normal and malignant cells. The differences are clear, both qualitatively and quantitatively. How to exploit them in the future diagnosis and treatment of cancer was the subject of the workshop as well as the entire meeting.

Index

317